INTERNATIONAL REVIEW OF CHILD NEUROLOGY SERIES

Neonatal Seizures

Managing Director: Ann-Marie Halligan
Editor/Production Manager: Udoka Ohuonu
Project Management: Lumina Datamatics

First published in this edition 2016

British Library Cataloguing-in-Publication data

A catalogue record for this book is available from the British Library

ISBN: 978-1-909962-67-5

Printed by Heny Ling Ltd. Dorset Press, Dorchester, UK

INTERNATIONAL REVIEW OF CHILD NEUROLOGY SERIES

Neonatal Seizures

Edited by Lakshmi Nagarajan

Princess Margaret Hospital for Children,
Perth, Australia

2016
Mac Keith Press

CONTENTS

AUTHORS' APPOINTMENTS

Geraldine B. Boylan   Director and Professor of Neonatal Physiology, Irish Centre for Fetal and Neonatal Translational Research, Department of Paediatrics & Child Health, University College Cork, Ireland

Maria Roberta Cilio   Professor of Neurology and Pediatrics, School of Medicine, University of California, San Francisco, USA
Director of Research in Pediatric Epilepsy, UCSF Epilepsy Center, University of California, San Francisco, USA

Linda S. de Vries   Professor in Neonatal Neurology, Department of Neonatology, Wilhelmina Children's Hospital, University Medical Center Utrecht, The Netherlands

Jarred Garfinkle   Resident in Pediatrics, Montreal Children's Hospital, McGill University Health Center, Canada

Soumya Ghosh   Clinical Professor, Centre for Neuromuscular and Neurological Disorders, University of Western Australia, Australia
Consultant Neurologist, Western Australian Neuroscience Research Institute, Princess Margaret Hospital for Children, Sir Charles Gairdner Hospital and Fiona Stanley Hospital, Australia
Medical Director, Centre for Restorative Neurology, Western Australian Neuroscience Research Institute, QEII Medical Centre, Australia

Ellen Grant   Professor of Radiology, Harvard Medical School, USA
Director, Fetal-Neonatal Neuroimaging and Developmental Science Center, Boston Children's Hospital, USA

Lena Hellström-Westas Professor, Department of Women's and Children's Health, Uppsala University, Sweden

Thierry Huisman Professor of Radiology, Pediatrics, Neurology and Neurosurgery, Johns Hopkins University School of Medicine, USA
Chairman, Department of Imaging and Imaging Science, Johns Hopkins Bayview Medical Center, USA
Director, Division of Pediatric Radiology and Pediatric Neuroradiology, Johns Hopkins Hospital, USA
Co-Director, Neurosciences Intensive Care Nursery, Johns Hopkins Hospital, USA

Camilo Jaimes Radiologist, Department of Radiology, Massachusetts General Hospital, USA

Michael Johnston Chief Medical Officer and Director, Developmental Neuroscience Laboratory, Kennedy Krieger Institute, USA
Professor of Neurology, Pediatrics and Physical Medicine and Rehabilitation, Johns Hopkins University School of Medicine, USA

Shilpa Kadam Research Scientist, Developmental Neuroscience Laboratory, Kennedy Krieger Institute, USA
Assistant Professor of Neurology, Johns Hopkins University School of Medicine, USA

Barry Lewis Head, Department of Clinical Biochemistry, PathWest Laboratory Medicine WA, Princess Margaret Hospital for Children, Australia

Lakshmi Nagarajan Clinical Professor, School of Paediatrics and Child Health, University of Western Australia, Australia
Paediatric Neurologist and Epileptologist, Head of the Department of Neurology, Princess Margaret Hospital for Children, Australia

Linda Palumbo Neurophysiology Technologist, Department of Neurology, Princess Margaret Hospital for Children, Australia

Christos Papadelis Instructor in Pediatrics, Harvard Medical School, USA
Associate Scientific Researcher, Fetal-Neonatal Neuroimaging and Developmental Science Center, Boston Children's Hospital, USA

Andrea Poretti Assistant Professor, Russell H Morgan Department of Radiology and Radiological Science, Johns Hopkins University School of Medicine, USA

Shripada Rao Clinical Associate Professor, Neonatal Intensive Care Units, Princess Margaret Hospital for Children and King Edward Memorial Hospital for Women, Australia
Clinical Associate Professor, Centre for Neonatal Research and Education, University of Western Australia, Australia

Ingmar Rosén Professor Emeritus, Department of Clinical Neurophysiology, Lund University, Sweden

Michael Shevell Chairman, Department of Pediatrics and Professor (with Tenure), Departments of Pediatrics and Neurology/Neurosurgery, McGill University, Canada
Harvey Guyda Chair in Pediatrics and Pediatrician-in-Chief, Montreal Children's Hospital, McGill University Health Center, Canada

Nathan J. Stevenson Postdoctoral Researcher, Irish Centre for Fetal and Neonatal Translational Research, Department of Paediatrics & Child Health, University College Cork, Ireland

Xiaohe Yu Visiting Scholar, Developmental Neuroscience Laboratory, Kennedy Krieger Institute and Department of Neonatology, Johns Hopkins University School of Medicine, USA
Associate Professor of Neonatology, Department of Pediatrics, Xiang Ya Hospital, Central South University, China

FOREWORD

The highest risk of seizures across the lifespan is during the first few days after birth. Compared with seizures at older ages, neonatal seizures differ in etiology, semiology, electroencephalographic signature, response to antiepileptic drugs and outcome. Although neonatal seizures have been recognized for over a century, it is only during the last decade that we have begun to understand the developmental, molecular and physiological mechanisms that underpin neonatal seizures. An increased appreciation of the high incidence and poor outcome of neonatal seizures coupled with the development of animal models and identification of genetic mutations resulting in neonatal epilepsy has energized clinicians and scientists, resulting in remarkable advances in understanding the pathophysiological basis of neonatal seizures.

A comprehensive text which provides a critical review of new information on neonatal seizures is long overdue. Professor Lakshmi Nagarajan and her colleagues have beautifully filled this gap, with a highly authoritative review of neonatal seizures. Using a strong foundation in developmental neuroanatomy and neurophysiology, there are excellent chapters dealing with clinical assessment and diagnostic tools including continuous EEG and video monitoring, amplitude-integrated EEG, automated EEG seizure detection and neuroimaging. Whether it is a medical student assigned to the neonatal unit or a seasoned neonatologist, the state of the art information conveyed in this section of the book will be very helpful.

While many neonatal seizures are transient and resolve after a few days, there are a group of newborn infants that develop chronic epilepsy and epileptic encephalopathies. While these children represent only a small proportion of infants presenting with neonatal seizures, the mutations provide information on the mechanism causing the seizure and serve as an opportunity to develop novel therapeutics. The chapter on neonatal epilepsy and encephalopathies provides a current review of the genetic neonatal epilepsies and dovetails nicely with discussion of the mechanisms of neonatal seizures. Identifying mutated targets also adds new ideas that could lead to genetically determined individualized therapy.

There are two major gaps in our knowledge-base regarding neonatal seizures. The first is whether neonatal seizures are simply a reflection of the brain injury causing the seizures or whether the seizures contribute to the brain injury. In other words, are seizures an epiphenomenon of brain injury that can be ignored or should they be vigorously treated? The question is important since there are indications from animal models that antiepileptic drugs can have adverse effects on the developing brain. The second question is if antiepileptic drug therapy is initiated, which drug should be used. These controversial areas are intertwined and both are addressed by the authors in a balanced and impartial manner.

While developing strategies for neuroprotection following brain insults is important at any age, the stakes are much higher when looking at newborn infants who have their full life ahead of them. In addition, the approach to neuroprotection is much different in newborns when one is dealing with developing neural circuits with robust plasticity than in the adult brain where the neural circuitry is relatively fixed and less plastic. The authors provide compelling data on neuroprotective strategies in the neonatal brain, pointing to the likelihood that during the next decade our approach to brain injury will change dramatically.

Professor Lakshmi Nagarajan deserves great praise for bringing this book to fruition. It is a remarkable reminder of how far we have progressed in the last decade in the neonatal intensive care unit in understanding the biology of neonatal seizures. While the book shows our progress, which has been substantial, it also lays out challenges for the next generation of clinicians and scientists.

Gregory L. Holmes, MD
Professor and Chair, Department of Neurological Sciences
University of Vermont College of Medicine
Vermont, USA

PREFACE

Neonatal seizures are an important manifestation of neuronal dysfunction. They contribute to and worsen brain injury from other insults, leading to significant neurodevelopmental sequelae. Seizures occur more frequently in the neonatal period than at any other time in life. Neonatal seizures are difficult to recognize clinically and this may result in both — underestimation and overdiagnosis. To complicate the issue further, a large proportion of neonatal seizures are electrographic only, with no clinical correlates. The Electroencephalogram (EEG) is an essential tool in accurately identifying neonatal seizures, estimating the seizure burden and evaluating response to therapy. Treatment of neonatal seizures is complicated: what to treat, what not to treat and what to treat with, is still being explored.

There have been major advances in the art and science of fetal and neonatal neurology. The brain of a neonate is in a state of rapid growth, development and organisation, driven by genetic, epigenetic and environmental influences. Rapid advances in our understanding of developmental neuroplasticity and neonatal seizure genesis, evolving diagnostic tools and prognostic markers, exciting neuroprotective strategies and promising new therapeutic options inspired me to undertake this book.

It has been a pleasure and privilege to work with the renowned and talented authors who have contributed to this book, aimed at being both practical and scholarly. The chapters are focused on the many unique aspects of neonatal seizures: brain maturation, aetiology, semiology, electrographic features, diagnostic dilemmas, neuroimaging, genetics, response to antiepileptic drugs and interventions such as therapeutic hypothermia, prognostic indicators and neurodevelopmental outcomes. The book highlights new horizons in this dynamic field. It emphasizes the importance of the EEG (challenging to interpret, but essential), recent advances in the diagnosis and approach to a neonate with seizures, novel options in treatment and neuroprotection. The book illustrates current concepts, provides clinical guidelines and outlines the gamut of challenges for the future.

This book has incorporated and integrated basic neuroscience with the clinical profile and management of neonates with seizures. It should be useful at the cot side of a neonate with seizures, but also valuable as a reference that enhances knowledge and provokes development of new and more effective strategies in this arena. The book has been designed to cater to a wide audience in neonatal neurology: scientists and clinicians, the novice and the expert. We hope it is effective, interesting and stimulating.

ACKNOWLEDGEMENTS

I wish to thank Robert Ouvrier for instigating this book, Charles Newton for his guidance and Annie Bye for her encouragement and comments. I would like to thank the co-authors for their excellent contributions. I want to express my gratitude to the staff of Mac Keith press, especially Udoka Ohuonu, without whose efficiency and professionalism this book would not have been possible.

Thank you to the newborn infants and their families — you are the reason for this book. To my many mentors across the world, especially BNS Walia, Annie Bye, Chris Burke, Abe Chutorian, Sasson Gubbay, John Dunne and Peter Walsh — a big thank you. I wish to acknowledge the support of all my colleagues in the Department of Neurology at PMH in this endeavour, especially Sarala Kumari and Patricia Cannell. I would like to acknowledge the helpful library staff as well as my collaborators in Neonatology and other departments in PMH. I am sure Linda Palumbo and Soumya Ghosh have enjoyed the camaraderie, our arguments and discussions as much as I have. Special thanks to my friends, for being there.

My heartfelt thanks to my wonderful family: my husband, Soumya and our sons Varun and Gaurav for providing a haven that not only cocoons, buffers and supports, but also inspires and challenges. With pride I acknowledge my parents and extended family in India.

LN

Chapter 4

Lena Hellström-Westas, Ingmar Rosén and Linda S de Vries acknowledge the financial support of Uppsala University and the Linnéa and Josef Carlsson Foundation.

Chapter 5

Nathan Stevenson and Geraldine Boylan acknowledge the support of the Science Foundation Ireland (10/IN.1/B3036 and 12/RC/2272) and of the Wellcome Trust UK (098983).

1
DEVELOPMENT OF THE NEONATAL CEREBRAL CORTEX

Soumya Ghosh

The neonatal period is a unique time of brain development. The cortical neuron undergoes major changes in the first few weeks after birth. It is a period of rapid growth, formation of new connections and progressive maturation of electrical and synaptic activity that translates into the formation of functional modules and networks in the brain. It is also a period when genetically programmed activity patterns are influenced by early environmental influences that result in the development of cortical maps. The neonatal brain is known to be vulnerable to injury and seizures, which are likely to disrupt normal development. There is a greater potential for neuroplasticity and modification of the developing networks in response to injury. The interaction of drugs with developing neurotransmitter and neuromodulatory systems may also influence normal maturation of the cortex. Therefore, a better understanding of the maturation of neural activity and the development of cortical connections and networks in the neonatal cortex is an important prerequisite for our ability to evaluate the cause and effect of neonatal seizures and their treatment.

Embryonic development

The embryonic development of the human cerebral cortex involves a complex sequence of events that starts at the rostral end of the neural tube around embryonic day 30, at the outer surface of the embryonic cerebral vesicle (Rakic 2006, Fox et al. 2010). These events include the proliferation of neuroepithelial cells in the regions near the cerebral ventricle (ventricular zone) and the formation of early developmental layers (subventricular zone, intermediate zone, subplate, cortical plate and marginal zone) through proliferation and migration (Bystron et al. 2008, Tiberi et al. 2012). Radial migration of neurons from the dorsal pallium accumulates in the cortical plate in an inside-out sequence to create a laminar structure and generate the projection neurons (pyramidal neurons) of the neocortex (Rakic 2006). Most GABAergic interneurons originate in and migrate tangentially from a different region of the forebrain, the subpallium or basal telencephalon. Migration is nearly complete by the beginning of the third trimester, and is followed by areal, laminar and cytological differentiation. Neurogenesis in the cerebral neocortex is seen till about gestational age of 28 weeks, when all cortical neurons have arrived in the cortical plate and are densely crowded together (Huttenlocher 1990). Spontaneous electrical activity begins in the late embryonic period (Luhman et al. 2003, Picken Bahrey and Moody 2003). Sensory signals (resulting from spontaneous fetal movements) start to influence cortical activity at this time (Milh et al. 2007).

Morphological changes in cortical neurons in the neonatal and infant brain

There is rapid expansion of cerebral cortical volume during the first four weeks after birth, which then continues at a slower pace for the next few years (Huttenlocher 1990, Levitt 2003). This increase in volume is because of growth of axons, dendrites and glia (Figs. 1.1 and 1.2), as well as myelination of axons (Huttenlocher and Dhabolkar 1997, Levitt 2003,

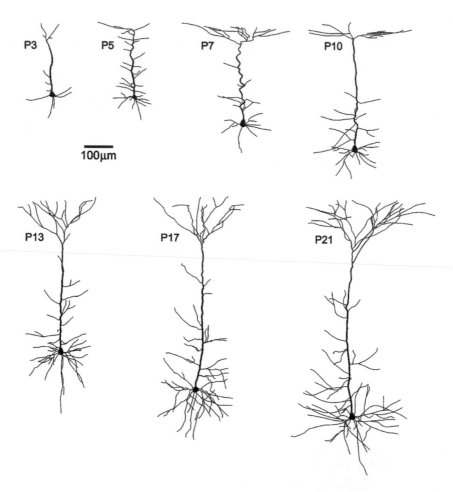

Figure 1.1. Morphology of layer V pyramidal neurons in the prefrontal cortex of the rat at various postnatal ages. Neurons were labelled with neurobiotin and reconstructed using the Neurolucida system. All neurons shown here were regular spiking cells. (Reproduced from *J Neurophysiol* Zhong-wei Z. Maturation of Layer V Pyramidal Neurons in the Rat Prefrontal Cortex: Intrinsic Properties and Synaptic Function 91: (3). © 2004, with kind permission of the American Physiological Society.)

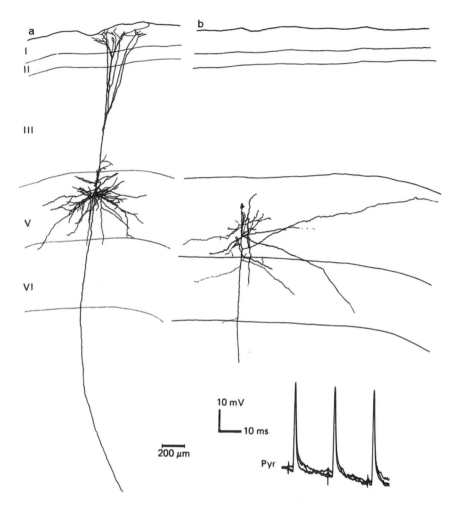

Figure 1.2. Camera-lucida reconstruction of a pyramidal neuron located in the motor cortex of the adult monkey. (a) Soma, dendrites and axon and (b) soma, axon and axon collaterals. The antidromic response to pyramidal tract (Pyr) stimulation is shown alongside. (Reproduced from *J Physiol* Ghosh S, Porter R. Morphology of Pyramidal Neurones in Monkey Motor Cortex and the Synaptic Actions of Their Intracortical Axon Collaterals. 400: 593–615. © 1988, with kind permission of John Wiley and Sons.)

Zhang 2004). Elongation of dendrites is associated with increased number and density of dendritic spines (Becker et al. 1984, Michel and Garey 1984). There is earlier growth and more elaborate branching of the dendritic tree in the deeper cortical layers. Growth of dendrites and dendritic spines occurs earlier and completes sooner in the occipital and auditory than the frontal cortex (Becker et al. 1984, Huttenlocher and Dhabolkar 1997). There is no evidence for overall regression of dendritic development; there is no reduction of the density of dentrites or dendritic spines (Becker et al. 1984). However, there is likely selective pruning and remodelling of dendrites, spines and synapses. Synaptic density (calculated as average number of synapses per neuron or per unit length of dendrite) increases greatly during late fetal life and early infancy to reach a maximum in the first year; it then declines to reach adult values by about 10–15 years. Synaptic density increases and declines later in the frontal than in the occipital and auditory cortices (Huttenlocher 1979, Huttenlocher et al. 1982, 1987, Huttenlocher and Dhabolkar 1997, Fox et al. 2010). Based on calculations of neuronal, dendritic and synaptic density and estimates of cortical volume, it appears likely that there is a loss of synapses after the first year (Huttenlocher 1990). Comparative studies in animals suggest that elimination of synapses is a more prominent developmental event as the complexity of the brain increases (Aghajanian and Bloom 1967, Changeux and Danchin 1976, Rakic et al. 1989). The large increase in the formation of synapses seen in the neonatal and infant brain and their later elimination during childhood is associated with greater plasticity in the brain. However, the activity in the exuberant synapses and their associated metabolic demands likely make the developing brain more vulnerable to metabolic and hypoxic insults, as well as to seizures (Holmes 2009).

Synaptic plasticity in the developing cortex

Development of the cortex is dependant on the synaptic plasticity driven by patterned physiological activity resulting from early experience (Fox et al. 2010). For example, refinement and maintenance of detailed sensory maps are dependant on early and continuing sensory experience (Khazipov et al. 2004, Milh et al. 2007, Fox et al. 2010). Nearly all activity-driven developmental events that involve gene expression are triggered initially by Ca++ influx into cells, and the effects are determined by the amplitude, frequency and spatial location of this influx (Greer and Greenberg 2008). This in turn is influenced by the excitability of neurons and the action of neurotransmitters and neuromodulators.

Excitability of cortical neurons

Experimental studies in animals suggest that many factors are developmentally regulated during the neonatal period to increase the excitability of neurons and neural networks. These include voltage-gated ion channels, neurotransmitter receptors and neuromodulators. This excitatory drive regulates spontaneous activity of neurons, dendritic growth and the formation and refinement of synaptic connections. These activity-dependant changes also result in transition to the mature physiological state.

Spontaneous electrical activity is required for the maturation of neuronal excitability and synaptic connectivity. For this reason configuration of ion channels and receptors in the neonatal cortex are optimized to mediate spontaneous activity, synchronize it among cells and allow Ca++ influx that transduces activity into development programs (Moody and Bosma 2005). During this time there is an increase in density of Na+ currents, increase in Ca++ activated K+ channels and the appearance of hyperpolarization-dependant cation channels (Picken Bahry and Moody 2003). There is an increase in the resting membrane potential and a reduction in input resistance and membrane time constant (Zhang 2004). As a result of these changes action potentials become larger in amplitude and shorter in duration (Fig. 1.3), and neurons gain the ability to fire repetitive action potentials

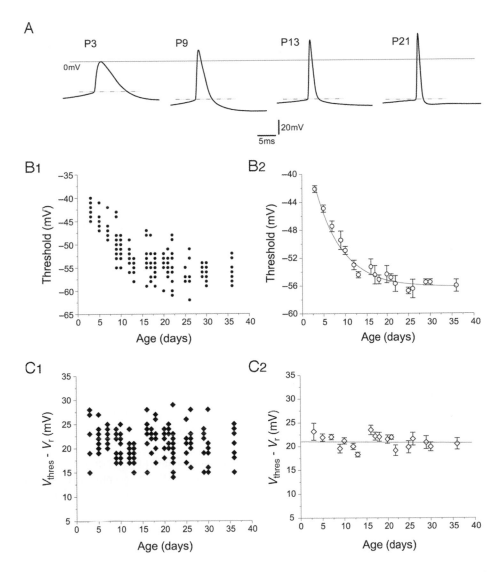

Figure 1.3. Developmental changes in action potential of pyramidal neurons in the rat prefrontal cortex. (A) Examples of action potential recorded at P3, P9, P13 and P21. Thin line indicates 0mV level, and spike threshold is shown by dashed lines; filtered at 2kHz and digitized at 8kHz. Please note increase in spike amplitude and reduction in spike duration during development; (B1) scatter plot of spike threshold at various ages; (B2) mean ± SE from cells recorded at a given age. Data can be fit to a single exponential function with a time constant of 6.2 d ($R2 \pm 0.98$); (C1) difference between spike threshold (V_{thres}) and resting potential (V_r), measured at various ages; (C2) mean ± SE. A linear fit gives a slope of ±0.006 mV/d, suggesting that the difference between V_{thres} and V_r remains stable during the first 5 weeks after birth. (Reproduced from *J Neurophysiol* Zhong-wei Z. Maturation of Layer V Pyramidal Neurons in the Rat Prefrontal Cortex: Intrinsic Properties and Synaptic Function 91: (3). © 2004, with kind permission of the American Physiological Society.)

spontaneously and to depolarizing stimuli (McCormick and Prince 1987, Picken Bahry and Moody 2003, Zhang 2004).

Neurotransmitters in the neonatal cortex

Gap junctions between dendrites appear early and transiently in the neonatal cortex, and increase synchronized activity between adjacent neurons to create local ensembles (Peinado et al. 1993, Dupont et al. 2006). This is followed by progressive increase in synaptic activity involving N-methyl D-aspartate (NMDA) and other glutaminergic receptors (Dupont et al. 2006).

Glutamate is the major excitatory neurotransmitter in the brain, and there are many types of glutamate receptors. Depending on their mechanisms of action, they are grouped into ionotropic and metabotropic receptors; the former include the α-amino-3-hydroxy-5-methyl-4-isoxazolepropionic acid (AMPA), kynurenic acid and NMDA receptors (Blanke and Van Dongen 2009). The metabotropic glutamate receptors are members of the G-protein receptor coupled superfamily (Niswender and Conn 2010). Because of their slow kinetics, voltage dependence and high permeability to Ca++ ions, NMDA receptors play a dominant role in activity-dependant synaptic plasticity and are critical for the development of the brain and the processes underlying learning and neuroplasticity. Studies in rats show that the density of NMDA receptors in the neocortex peaks in the first postnatal week (Haberny et al. 2002). The molecular subunit composition of the NMDA and other glutamate receptors also contributes to increased excitability in the neonatal period (Johnston 2005, Rakhade and Jensen 2009). AMPA receptors in the neonate are more permeable to Ca++ and may contribute to activity-dependant Ca++ influx into neurons (Rakhade and Jensen 2009). Enhanced excitability and activity of cortical neurons is important for development; experimental studies in rats show that blocking NMDA receptors, even transiently, in the early postnatal period is associated with apoptotic neurodegeneration and abnormal axonal arborization (Fox et al. 1996, Haberny et al. 2002).

GABA (gamma-Aminobutyric acid) is the predominant inhibitory neurotransmitter in the cortex. However, unlike in the adult brain, activation of GABA-A receptors during early postnatal development produces membrane depolarization (which may reach spike threshold), activation of voltage-gated Ca++ channels and removal of the voltage-dependant Mg++ block of NMDA channels, leading to Ca++ influx (Gaiarsa et al. 1995, Ben Ari et al. 2012). The developmental expression of cation-chloride importer NKCC1 and exporter KCC2 determines the depolarizing action of GABA in immature neurons; increased functional expression of NKCC1 and reduced expression of KCC2 result in a higher intracellular concentration of chloride and GABA-A receptor mediated depolarization. The excitatory action of GABA and its subsequent shift to inhibitory action are important for the maturation of neuronal morphology and cortical networks (Cancedda et al. 2007). In contrast, GABA-B mediated presynaptic inhibition is well developed at birth (Gaiarsa et al. 1995). Animal studies suggest that the density and molecular composition of GABA-A and GABA-B receptors vary during the early postnatal period, resulting in changes in receptor kinetics and function as well as their response to drugs such as benzodiazepines (Laurie et al. 1992, Gaiarsa et al. 1995).

Neurotrophic factors and peptides play an important role in neural activity and survival (Moody and Bosma 2005). These include brain-derived neurotrophic factor, parathyroid hormone-related peptide and pituitary adenylate cyclase activating polypeptide. Increased excitability of cortical neurons in the neonatal period may make them more vulnerable to stress and the influence of stress-related excitatory neuropeptides (e.g. corticotrophin-releasing hormone; Baram and Hatalski 1998).

Neonatal cortical development and seizures
It is most likely that the increased susceptibility of the neonate to seizures is caused by the intrinsic properties of cortical neurons and networks that are associated with increased excitability and their propensity to generate spontaneous and synchronized activity. The majority of neonatal seizures arise in the neocortex (Mizrahi 1999). Depending on their severity, neonatal seizures may disrupt normal activity-driven developmental processes and result in varying degrees of long-term neurological impairment (Glass et al. 2009, Nagarajan et al. 2010). Neonatal seizures are often symptomatic and associated with developmental or perinatal injury to the brain. However, seizures worsen outcomes, independent of the underlying injury (Glass et al. 2009, Payne et al. 2014).

Because of differences in neural and network properties, it is likely that consequences of seizures will be different in the neonatal period. Experimental studies in animals have found that prolonged seizures cause less neuronal loss and synaptic rearrangements in neonates than in adults (Sperber et al. 1991, Cataltepe et al. 1995, Haas et al. 2001). However, there is abnormal neurogenesis and axonal sprouting in neonatal animals subjected to seizures, and resultant impairment in memory and learning (Holmes and Ben-Ari, 1998, McCabe et al. 2001, Sayin et al. 2004). Recurrent neonatal seizures result in long-term increases in neocortical excitability and likelihood of seizures (Isaeva et al. 2010). Other studies have shown that hypoxic injury to the neonatal brain lowers seizure threshold and makes it more susceptible to recurrent seizures (Jensen 1999).

Neonatal seizures are hard to diagnose, may have variable or no motor features and are often refractory to pharmacotherapy (Misrahi 1999, Scher et al. 2003, Nagarajan et al. 2011, 2012). There is limited evidence regarding the best pharmacological treatment of neonatal seizures (Slaughter et al. 2013, Glass 2014, Thoresen and Sabir 2015). Since GABA is an excitatory neurotransmitter in the neonatal brain, effects of GABA-A receptor modulators are likely to be different than in adults (Dzhala et al. 2005, Rakhade and Jensen 2009, Glass 2014). In addition, GABA plays an important role in the development of patterns of activity, synaptogenesis and formation of functional circuits (Ben Ari 2006). Animal studies have shown that commonly used antiepileptic drugs (AEDs) that block voltage-gated sodium channels, enhance GABAergic inhibition or block glutamate mediated excitation cause apoptosis of neurons in the developing forebrain (Bittigau et al. 2002). NMDAr antagonists can impair motor and cognitive functions (Mares and Mikulecka 2009). There is less data from the clinic about the adverse effects of AEDs on brain development (Silverstein and Ferriero 2008). Phenobarbitone and other AEDs have been shown to depress cognitive performance in children (Farwell et al. 1990, Loring and Meador 2004, Loring et al. 2007). Thus, seizures as well as their treatment can impair normal brain development in the neonate, and there is a need for basic and clinical studies to assess the effects of seizures and pharmacotherapy on developmental outcomes.

Neonatal seizures and the associated aetiopathology (e.g. hypoxic-ischaemic encephalopathy) increase the risk of subsequent epilepsy (Rakhade and Jensen 2009, Nagarajan et al. 2010, Chapman et al. 2012). A better understanding of underlying mechanisms should aid in the development of AEDs.

The molecular, cellular and network changes underlying epileptogenesis are not completely understood and less so in the developing brain. Most animal studies of epileptogenesis, in both neonatal and adult brains, have focused on the hippocampus because of the region's well-characterized network architecture and cellular interactions. Such studies suggest that seizures (and associated Ca++ influx) activate and upregulate immediate early genes, alter ion channel and neurotransmitter function and activate inflammatory cascades. In neonatal animal models of epilepsy, observed changes include internalization of Kv2.1 channels, decreased expression of KCC2 cotransporters, GABA-A receptor endocytosis, modification of AMPA receptors, increase in neurotrophic factor expression, activation of inflammatory medicators and microglia and aberrant sprouting and network connectivity (Sanchez et al. 2005, Epzstein et al. 2008, Rakhade and Jensen 2009). These changes cause impaired inhibition, increased permeability of excitatory channels and increased network excitability and are thought to contribute to epileptogenesis. Based on these studies, inhibitors of cation-chloride cotransporters (e.g. bumetanide), AMPA receptor antagonists, antioxidants such as erythropoetin, and microglial inactivators have been explored as treatment to prevent seizures and epileptogenesis in such models (Koh et al. 2004, Rakhade and Jensen 2009, Chapman et al. 2012, Pressler and Mangum 2013).

Conclusion

The neonatal period is a unique time of brain development where there is rapid growth and maturation of cortical neurons, and formation of exuberant synapses and connections. It is a period when genetic programmes for development are influenced by early experiences. As a result, the brain reacts differently to injury and the consequences of injury include the interruption or modification of the proper sequence of development. Research studies in animals continue to provide important insights into cortical development and the dynamic changes in cellular and molecular processes that occur in the neonatal period. Animal and clinical studies have revealed significant immediate and long-term effects of injury to the brain during this vulnerable period. However, minimizing injury and its consequences continues to remain a challenge, and is an important focus for future research.

REFERENCES

Aghajanian GK, Bloom FE (1967) The formation of synaptic junctions in developing rat brain: A quantitative electron microscopic study. *Brain Res* 6: 716–727. doi: http://dx.doi.org/10.1016/0006-8993(67)90128-X.
Baram TZ, Hatalski CG (1998) Neuropeptide-mediated excitability: A key triggering mechanism for seizure generation in the developing brain. *Trends Neurosci* 21: 471–476. doi: http://dx.doi.org/10.1016/S0166-2236(98)01275-2.

Becker LE, Armstrong DL, Chan F, Wood MM (1984) Dendritic development in human occipital cortical neurons. *Devel Brain Res* 13: 117–124. doi: http://dx.doi.org/10.1016/0165-3806(84)90083-X.

Ben-Ari Y (2006) Basic developmental rules and their implications for epilepsy in the immature brain. *Epileptic Disord* 8 (2): 91–102.

Ben-Ari Y, Woodin MA, Sernagor E, et al. (2012) Refuting the challenges of the developmental shift of polarity of GABA actions: GABA more exciting than ever! *Front Cell Neurosci* 6: article 35. doi: http://dx.doi.org/10.3389/fncel.2012.00035.

Bittigau P, Sifringer M, Genz K, et al. (2002) Antiepileptic drugs and apoptotic neurodegeneration in the developing brain. *PNAS* 99 (23): 15089–15094. doi: http://dx.doi.org/10.1073/pnas.222550499.

Blanke ML, VanDongen, AMJ (2009) Activation Mechanisms of the NMDA Receptor. In: Van Dongen AM, editor. Biology of the NMDA Receptor. Boca Raton (FL): CRC Press/Taylor & Francis; 2009. Chapter 13. Available from: http://www.ncbi.nlm.nih.gov/books/NBK5274/

Bystron I, Blakemore C, Rakic P (2008) Development of the human cerebral cortex: Boulder committee revisited. *Nature Reviews Neuroscience* 9: 110–122. doi: http://dx.doi.org/10.1038/nrn2252.

Cancedda L, Fiumelli H, Chen K, Poo M (2007) Excitatory GABA action is essential for morphological maturation of cortical neurons in vivo. *J Neurosci* 27 (19): 5224–5235. doi: http://dx.doi.org/10.1523/JNEUROSCI.5169-06.2007.

Cataltepe O, Vannucci RC, Heitjan DF, Towfighi J (1995) Effect of status epilepticus on hypoxic brain damage in the immature rat. *Pediatr Res* 38 (2): 251–257. doi: http://dx.doi.org/10.1203/00006450-199508000-00019.

Changeux J-P, Danchin A (1976) Selective stabilization of developing synapses as a mechanism for the specification of neuronal networks. *Nature* 264: 705–712. doi: http://dx.doi.org/10.1038/264705a0.

Chapman KE, Raol YH, Amy Brooks-Kayal A (2012) Neonatal seizures: Controversies and challenges in translating new therapies from the lab to the isolette. *Eur J Neurosci* 35 (12): 1857–1865. doi: http://dx.doi.org/10.1111/j.1460-9568.2012.08140.x.

Dupont E, Hanganu IL, Kilb W, Hirsch S, Luhmann HL (2006) Rapid developmental switch in the mechanisms driving early cortical columnar networks. *Nature* 439 (5): 79–83. doi: http://dx.doi.org/10.1038/nature04264.

Dzhala VI, Talos DM, Sdrulla DA, et al. (2005) NKCC1 transporter facilitates seizures in the developing brain. *Nat Med* 11: 1205–1213. doi: http://dx.doi.org/10.1038/nm1301.

Epsztein J, Ben-Ari Y, Represa A, Crepel V (2008) Late-onset epileptogenesis and seizure genesis: Lessons from models of cerebral ischemia. *Neuroscientist* 14: 78–90. doi: http://dx.doi.org/10.1177/1073858407301681.

Farwell JR, Lee YJ, Hirtz DG, Sulzbacher SI, Ellenberg JH, Nelson KB (1990) Phenobarbitone for febrile seizures – effects on intelligence and on seizure recurrance. *NEJM* 322: 364–369. doi: http://dx.doi.org/10.1056/NEJM199002083220604.

Fox SE, Levitt P, Nelson CA (2010) How the timing and quality of early experience influence the development of brain architecture. *Child Dev* 81 (1): 28–40. doi: http://dx.doi.org/10.1111/j.1467-8624.2009.01380.x.

Fox K, Schlaggar BL, Glazewski S, O'Leary DDM (1996) Glutamate receptor blockade at cortical synapses disrupts development of thalamocortical and columnar organization in somatosensory cortex. *Proc Natl Acad Sci USA* 93: 5584–5589. doi: http://dx.doi.org/10.1073/pnas.93.11.5584.

Gaiarsa J-L, Mclean H, Congar P, et al. (1995) Postnatal maturation of gamma-aminobutyric acid $_A$ and $_B$-mediated inhibition in the CA3 hippocampal region in the rat. *J Neurobiol* 26: 339–349. doi: http://dx.doi.org/10.1002/neu.480260306.

Ghosh S, Porter R (1988) Morphology of pyramidal neurones in the monkey motor cortex and the synaptic actions of their intracortical axon collaterals. *J Physiol (Lond)* 400: 593–615. doi: http://dx.doi.org/10.1113/jphysiol.1988.sp017138.

Glass HC (2014) Neonatal seizures: Advances in mechanisms and management. *Clin Perinatol* 41 (1): 177–190. doi: http://dx.doi.org/10.1016/j.clp.2013.10.004.

Glass HC, Glidden D, Jeremy RJ, Barkovich AJ, Ferriero DM, Miller SP (2009) Clinical neonatal seizures are independently associated with outcome in infants at risk for hypoxic-ischemic brain injury. *J Pediatr* 155 (3): 318–323. doi: http://dx.doi.org/10.1016/j.jpeds.2009.03.040.

Greer PL, Greenberg ME (2008) From synapse to nucleus: Calcium-dependent gene transcription in the control of synapse development and function. *Neuron* 59: 847–860. doi: http://dx.doi.org/10.1016/j.neuron.2008.09.002.

Haas KZ, Sperber EF, Opanashuk LA, Stanton PK, Moshe SL (2001) Resistance of immature hippocampus to morphological and physiological alterations following status epilepticus or kindling. *Hippocampus* 11: 615–625. doi: http://dx.doi.org/10.1002/hipo.1076.

Haberny KA, Paule MG, Scallet AC, et al. (2002) Ontogeny of the N-Methyl-D-Aspartate (NMDA) receptor system and susceptibility to neurotoxicity. *Toxicol Sci* 68: 9–17. doi: http://dx.doi.org/10.1093/toxsci/68.1.9.

Holmes GL (2009) The long term effects of neonatal seizures. *Clin Perinatol* 36: 901–914. doi: http://dx.doi.org/10.1016/j.clp.2009.07.012.

Holmes GL, Ben-Ari Y (1998) Seizures in the developing brain: Perhaps not so benign after all. *Neuron* 21: 1231–1234. doi: http://dx.doi.org/10.1016/S0896-6273(00)80642-X.

Huttenlocher PR (1979) Synaptic density in human frontal cortex. Developmental changes and effects of aging. *Brain Res* 163: 195–205. doi: http://dx.doi.org/10.1016/0006-8993(79)90349-4.

Huttenlocher PR (1990) Morphometric study of human cerebral cortex development. *Neuropsychologia* 28: 517–527. doi: http://dx.doi.org/10.1016/0028-3932(90)90031-I.

Huttenlocher PR, De Coukten C, Garey LG, Van Der Loos H (1982) Synaptogenesis in human visual cortex – evidence for synapse elimination during normal development. *Neurosci Lett* 33: 247–252. doi: http://dx.doi.org/10.1016/0304-3940(82)90379-2.

Huttenlocher PR, Dhabolkar AS (1997) Regional differences in synaptogenesis in human cerebral cortex. *J Comp Neurol* 387: 167–178. doi: http://dx.doi.org/10.1002/(SICI)1096-9861(19971020)387:2<167::AID-CNE1>3.0.CO;2-Z.

Isaeva E, Savrasova A, Khazipov R, Holmes GL (2010) Recurrent neonatal seizures result in long-term increase of neuronal network excitability in the rat neocortex. *The Eur J Neurosci* 31 (8): 1446–1455. doi: http://dx.doi.org/10.1111/j.1460-9568.2010.07179.x.

Jensen FE (1999) Acute and chronic effects of seizures in the developing brain: Experimental models. *Epilepsia* 40 (Suppl. I): S51–S58.

Johnston MV (2005) Excitotoxicity in perinatal brain injury. *Brain Pathol* 15: 234–240.

Khazipov R, Sirota A, Leinekugel X, Holmes GL, Ben-Ari Y, Buzsaki G (2004) Early motor activity drives spindle bursts in the developing somatosensory cortex. *Nature* 432: 758–761.

Koh S, Tibayan FD, Simpson JN, Jensen FE (2004) NBQX or topiramate treatment following perinatal hypoxia-induced seizures prevents later increases in seizure-induced neuronal injury. *Epilepsia* 45: 569–575. doi: http://dx.doi.org/10.1111/j.0013-9580.2004.69103.x.

Laurie DJ, Wisden W, Seeburg PH (1992) The distribution of thirteen GABA$_A$ receptor subunit mRNAs in the rat brain. III. Embryonic and postnatal development. *J Neurosci* 12: 4151–4172.

Levitt P (2003) Structural and functional maturation of the developing primate brain. *J Ped* 143: S35–S45. doi: http://dx.doi.org/10.1067/S0022-3476(03)00400-1.

Loring DW, Marino S, Meador KJ (2007) Neuropsychological and behavioral effects of antiepilepsy drugs. *Neuropsychol Rev* 17: 413–425. doi: http://dx.doi.org/10.1007/s11065-007-9043-9.

Loring DW, Meador KJ (2004) Cognitive side effects of antiepileptic drugs in children. *Neurology* 62: 872–877. doi: http://dx.doi.org/10.1212/01.WNL.0000115653.82763.07.

Luhmann HJ, Hanganu I, Kilb W (2003) Cellular physiology of the neonatal rat cerebral cortex. *Brain Research Bulletin* 60: 345–353. doi: http://dx.doi.org/10.1016/S0361-9230(03)00059-5.

Mares P, Mikulecka A (2009) Different effects of two N-methyl-D-aspartate receptor antagonists on seizures, spontaneous behavior, and motor performance in immature rats. *Epilepsy Behav* 14: 32–9. doi: http://dx.doi.org/10.1016/j.yebeh.2008.08.013.

Mccabe BK, Silveira DC, Cilio MR, et al. (2001) Reduced neurogenesis after neonatal seizures. *J Neurosci* 21: 2094–2103.

Mccormick DA, Prince DA (1987) Post-natal development of electrophysiological properties of rat cerebral cortical pyramidal neurones. *J Physiol* 393: 743–762. doi: http://dx.doi.org/10.1113/jphysiol.1987.sp016851.

Milh M, Kaminska A, Huon C, Lapillonne A, Ben-Ari Y, Khazipov R. Rapid cortical oscillations and early motor activity in premature human neonate. (2007) *Cerebral Cortex* 17: 1582–1594.

Mizrahi EM (1999) Acute and chronic effects of seizures in the developing brain: Lessons from clinical experience. *Epilepsia* 40 (Suppl. 1): S42–S50. doi: http://dx.doi.org/10.1111/j.1528-1157.1999.tb00878.x.

Moody WJ, Bosma MM (2005) Ion channel development, spontaneous activity, and activity-dependent development in nerve and muscle cells. *Physiol Rev* 85: 883–941. doi: http://dx.doi.org/10.1152/physrev.00017.2004.

Nagarajan L, Palumbo L, Ghosh S (2010) Neurodevelopmental outcomes in neonates with seizures: A numerical score of background EEG to help prognosticate. *J Child Neurol* 25: 961–968. doi: http://dx.doi.org/10.1177/0883073809355825.

Nagarajan L, Palumbo L, Ghosh S (2011) Brief Electroencephalography Rhythmic Discharges (BERDs) in the neonate with seizures: Their significance and prognostic implications. *J Child Neurol* 26 (12): 1529–1533. doi: http://dx.doi.org/10.1177/0883073811409750.

Nagarajan L, Palumbo L, Ghosh S (2012) Classification of clinical semiology in epileptic seizures in neonates. *Eur J Paediatr Neurol* 16 (2): 118–125. doi: http://dx.doi.org/10.1016/j.ejpn.2011.11.005.

Niswender CM, Conn PJ (2010) Metabotropic glutamate receptors: Physiology, pharmacology and disease. *Ann Rev Pharmacol Toxicol* 50: 295–322. doi: http://dx.doi.org/10.1146/annurev.pharmtox.011008.145533.

Payne ET, Zhao XY, Frndova H, et al. (2014) Seizure burden is independently associated with short term outcome in critically ill children. *Brain* 137: 1429–1438. doi: http://dx.doi.org/10.1093/brain/awu042.

Peinado A, Yuste R, Katz LC (1993) Extensive dye coupling between rat neocortical neurons during the period of circuit formation. *Neuron* 10 (1): 103–114. doi: http://dx.doi.org/10.1016/0896-6273(93)90246-N.

Picken Bahrey HL, Moody WJ (2003) Early development of voltage-gated ion currents and firing properties in neurons of the mouse cerebral cortex. *J Neurophysiol* 89: 1761–1773. doi: http://dx.doi.org/10.1152/jn.00972.2002.

Pressler RN, Mangum B (2013) Newly emerging therapies for neonatal seizures. *Semin Fetal Neonatal Med* 18: 216–223. doi: http://dx.doi.org/10.1016/j.siny.2013.04.005.

Rakhade SN, Jensen FE (2009) Epileptogenesis in the immature brain: emerging mechanisms. *Nat Rev Neurol* 5 (7): 380–391. doi: http://dx.doi.org/10.1038/nrneurol.2009.80.

Rakic P (2006) A century of progress in corticoneurogenesis: From silver impregnation to genetic engineering. *Cerebral Cortex* 16 (Suppl.): 1–17. doi: http://dx.doi.org/10.1093/cercor/bhk036.

Rakic P, Bourgeois JP, Eckenhoff MF, et al. (1989) Concurrent overproduction of synapses in diverse regions of primate cortex. *Science* 232: 232–235. doi: http://dx.doi.org/10.1126/science.3952506.

Sayin U, Sutula TP, Stafstrom CE (2004) Seizures in the developing brain cause adverse long-term effects on spatial learning and anxiety. *Epilepsia* 45 (12): 1539–1548. doi: http://dx.doi.org/10.1111/j.0013-9580.2004.54903.x.

Scher MS, Alvin J, Gaus L, Minnigh B, Painter MJ (2003) Uncoupling of EEG-clinical neonatal seizures after antiepileptic drug use. *Paediatr Neurol* 28 (4): 277–280. doi: http://dx.doi.org/10.1016/S0887-8994(02)00621-5.

Silverstein FS, Ferriero DM (2008) Off-label use of antiepileptic drugs for the treatment of neonatal seizures. *Pediatr Neurol* 39 (2): 77–79. doi: http://dx.doi.org/10.1016/j.pediatrneurol.2008.04.008.

Slaughter LA, Patel AD, Slaughter JL (2013) Pharmacological treatment of neonatal seizures: A systematic review. *J Child Neurol* 28 (3): 351–364. doi: http://dx.doi.org/10.1177/0883073812470734.

Sperber EF, Haas KZ, Stanton PK, Moshe SL (1991) Resistance of the immature hippocampus to seizure-induced synaptic reorganization. *Dev Brain Res* 20: 88–93. doi: http://dx.doi.org/10.1016/0165-3806(91)90158-F.

Thoresen M, Sabir H (2015) Neonatal seizures still lack safe and effective treatment. *Nature Rev Neurol* 11: 311–312. doi: http://dx.doi.org/10.1038/nrneurol.2015.74.

Tiberi L, Vanderhaeghen P, Van Den Ameele J (2012) Cortical neurogenesis and morphogens: diversity of cues, sources and functions. *Curr Opin Cell Biol* 24: 269–276. doi: http://dx.doi.org/10.1016/j.ceb.2012.01.010.

Zhang Z-W (2004) Maturation of layer V pyramidal neurons in the rat prefrontal cortex: Intrinsic properties and synaptic function. *J Neurophysiol* 91: 1171–1182. doi: http://dx.doi.org/10.1152/jn.00855.2003.

2
THE ROLE OF THE VIDEO EEG IN NEONATES WITH SEIZURES

Lakshmi Nagarajan and Soumya Ghosh

Neonatal seizures are an important sign of neurological dysfunction in an infant. Neonatal seizures may be due to a variety of aetiologies with hypoxic ischaemic encephalopathy being the most common cause. Neonatal seizures are associated with long-term developmental sequelae – both morbidity and mortality (Volpe 2008, Uria-Avellanal et al. 2013). There is an increased incidence (15–75%) of neuromotor, neurosensory, neurocognitive and neurobehavioural impairment, and growth deficits on long-term follow-up, with the spectrum ranging from subtle to severe. The prevalence of post-neonatal epilepsy is increased in infants with neonatal seizures with estimates of 10–40% (Legido et al. 1991, McBride et al. 2000, Volpe 2008, Glass and Sullivan 2009, Nagarajan et al. 2010, 2011a, 2012, Garfinkle and Shevell 2011). Neonatal seizures are thought to contribute to and worsen adverse outcomes in infants with encephalopathy.

Seizures occur more frequently in the neonatal period than at any other time in life. The estimated incidence or prevalence of neonatal seizures varies from 1 to 65 per 1000 live births (Volpe 2008, Uria-Avellanal et al. 2013). This variance is partly due to the different baseline populations and methods of ascertainment (e.g. term vs. preterm, community vs. hospital based, clinical vs. electroencepahalography [EEG] confirmed). Accurate estimates of occurrence are difficult because neonatal seizures are a challenge to diagnose and manage.

Both under-recognition and over-reporting are known to occur with neonatal seizures (Volpe 1989, Wical 1994, Murray et al. 2008, Malone et al. 2009). Clinically diagnosed seizures include many paroxysmal phenomena that do not have surface EEG correlates. Some of these may be innocuous while others may reflect subcortical epileptiform activity or severe neurological impairment with brain stem release phenomenon (Scher 2002, Volpe 2008). Electrographic seizures without any clinical correlates occur frequently in the newborn infant (Mizrahi and Kellaway 1987, Bye et al. 1997, Nagarajan et al. 2010, Bragatti 2011, Nagarajan et al. 2011a). To treat or not to treat, what kind of seizures to treat, with what to treat and for how long to treat neonatal seizures are issues that are still debated (Sankar and Painter 2005, Wirrell 2005, Pressler and Mangum 2013, Shetty 2015). There is however universal consensus that correct identification of neonatal seizures and estimation of the epileptic burden are very important to better understand neonatal seizures, tailor effective therapeutic interventions and improve outcomes for infants with neonatal seizures.

The current gold standard for neonatal seizure detection is the conventional multichannel EEG with synchronised video recording (v-EEG) with visual interpretation by a neurologist with expertise in this area (Boylan et al. 2010, Boylan 2011, Shellhaas et al. 2011, Wusthoff 2013). This chapter outlines the role of v-EEG monitoring in the detection of neonatal seizures, estimation of seizure burden and assessing response to therapeutic interventions and its use in prognostication.

Clinically diagnosed neonatal seizures and clinical features of electroclinical seizures
Neonatal seizures may be difficult to recognise as non-epileptiform events can mimic seizures. Myoclonus, clonus and jitteriness are some of the paroxysmal movements that can mislead even the most experienced neonatal staff. This is well shown in a study (Malone et al. 2009) where 137 staff from several neonatal intensive care units were shown 20 video clips of infants with epileptiform and non-epileptiform events. Only about half were correctly identified, accurate responses were not necessarily dependant on the experience of the staff, and inter-observer agreements were poor. Mizrahi and Kellaway (1987) had previously shown that clinical events on video, diagnosed as clinical seizures based on Volpe's description (Volpe 1981) and classification, did not consistently have a time-synchronised EEG correlate: EEG correlates were only seen in 119 of the 415 events identified as clinical seizures. Focal clonic and focal tonic events were the most frequent phenomena associated with definite EEG correlates. Mizrahi and Kellaway felt that clinical manifestations thought to be clinical seizures are not all epileptiform events and that immediate EEG/polygraphic/video monitoring would provide information regarding the association of clinical behavioural events (called clinical seizures) to paroxysmal EEG events.

A diagnosis of neonatal seizures based on clinical features only is fraught with problems. A v-EEG is essential to confirm neonatal seizures in infants with clinical features suggestive of neonatal seizures, and continuous monitoring to quantify neonatal seizures.

In our study of 61 electroclinical seizures captured on v-EEG (Nagarajan et al. 2012), the majority had multiple clinical features. We found orolingual phenomenon (chewing, sucking, dry retching or grimacing/crying) to be the most common clinical feature associated with seizure onset (30%), whereas ocular phenomenon occurred most often during the seizure (70%). Seizure onsets with clonic, tonic and hypomotor features occurred in 20%, 8% and 18%, respectively; tonic and clonic features occurred at some stage during an electrographic seizure in 23% and 25% of the seizures. Focal clonic movements were the most frequent clinical feature in 13 infants with electroclinical seizures in another study (O'Meara et al. 1995). Specific EEG features such as ictal fast activity (Nagarajan et al. 2011b) have been shown to be correlated to the occurrence of clinical features during an electrographic seizure. Advances in neurophysiology may help further identify why and how some seizures are electroclinical whereas others are not, and promote better understanding of seizure genesis and epileptogenesis in the newborn infants.

The International League against Epilepsy has struggled with the characterisation and classification of neonatal seizures (Mastrangelo et al. 2005, Engel 2006, Berg et al. 2010) and had previously (Berg et al. 2010) proposed that neonatal seizures are no longer regarded as a separate entity. However in view of the complexity of neonatal seizures, a new task force on neonatal seizures was established in 2014, with the assignment to develop ways in which neonatal seizures and epilepsies can be integrated into the new classification of the epilepsies (ILAE Epigraph 2015). It is critical that we recognise the importance of the EEG in diagnosis, understand the electrographic as well as electroclinical features, incorporate aetiology, prognosis and specific treatments to develop a practical, universally accepted classification of neonatal seizures.

EEG seizures in neonates

An electrographic seizure in a neonate is conventionally defined as one in which a rhythmic EEG discharge lasts 10 seconds or longer, has an identifiable start and finish and could have variable morphology, frequency and field (Lombroso and Holmes 1993, Scher et al. 1993, Volpe 2008, Nagarajan et al. 2010, 2011a, McCoy and Hahn 2013). Examples of neonatal seizures are shown in Figures 2.1, 2.2 and 2.3. Clinicians need to beware of rhythmic

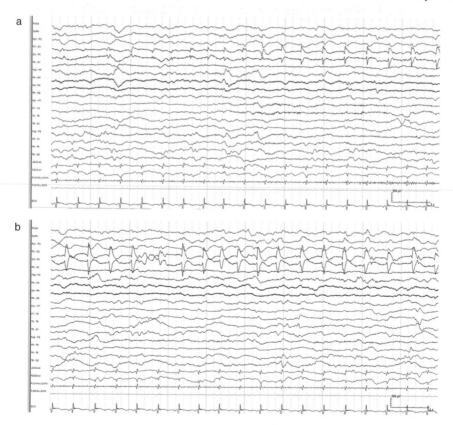

Figure 2.1. EEG epochs illustrate a focal seizure starting from the left hemisphere (C3), at onset (panel a) and 20 seconds later (panel b). Note increase in amplitude of the seizure discharge as it evolves. High frequency filter 70 Hz, low frequency filter 0.5 Hz. Calibration bars 100 uV and 1 s. Midline channels are in black, left sided channels in blue and right sided channels in red.

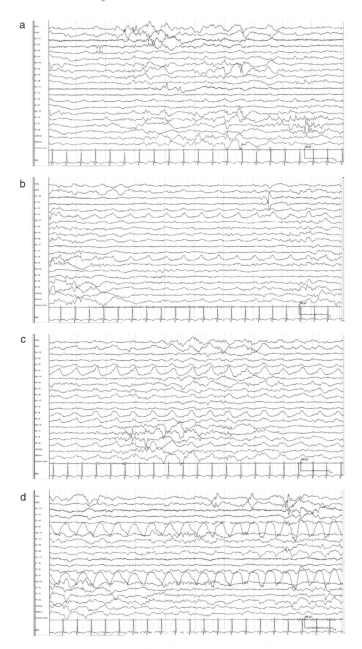

Figure 2.2. EEG epochs illustrate a focal seizure that evolves. (a) At the onset small amplitude rhythmic discharges from the left temporal leads are seen. Evolving seizure is seen (b) 40 seconds later (c) 80 seconds later and (d) 300 seconds later. The seizure discharge increases in amplitude and frequency, involves more regions in the left hemisphere and spreads to the right hemisphere. Note the morphology and field of the seizure discharge change during the seizure. Note the background asymmetry.

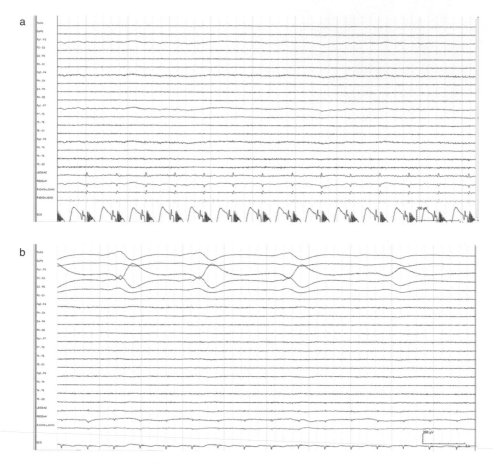

Figure 2.3. EEG epochs illustrate abnormal background with very low amplitude (panel a) in a neonate with severe hypoxic-ischaemic encephalopathy. Panel b shows a seizure discharge in the left parasagittal and midline leads. Please note amplitude calibration is different in each panel.

artefacts that can mimic electrographic seizures both on v-EEG and on amplitude integrated EEG (a-EEG). In Figure 2.4, panel a illustrates a patting artefact in one infant, whereas panel b shows an electroretinogram in response to photic stimulation in another infant with a severely abnormal background.

Neonatal seizures are invariably of focal origin – see Figures 2.1, 2.2, 2.5 and 2.6. Neonatal seizures can be complex in their discharge patterns (Nagarajan et al. 2011a). The ictal discharge may remain confined to a single electrode, spread to many electrodes, migrate to the other hemisphere, flip-flop between hemispheres, become bilateral or be complex with different seizure patterns in each hemisphere. Figures 2.1–2.3, 2.5 and 2.6 illustrate some of these characteristics. A neonatal seizure may have variable morphology, and a change in seizure pattern during the seizure occurs in the majority. The amplitude may be low and so

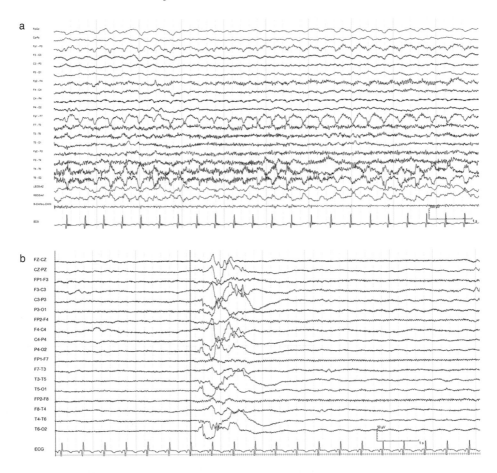

Figure 2.4. Beware of rhythmic artefacts. Panel a shows patting artefact that resembles a rhythmic seizure discharge. Panel b shows rhythmic electroretinogram waves in the frontal leads during photic stimulation at 20 Hz.

may be the frequency of the discharge (Nagarajan et al. 2011a). A sharp or slow-sharp discharge is reported to be the most frequent EEG seizure discharge (see Figs. 2.1, 2.2, 2.3 and 2.5). A spike and wave pattern is seen in less than 10% of neonatal seizures.

Electrographic seizures appear to occur more frequently in sleep: in one study (Nagarajan et al. 2011a) of 160 seizures, 40% occurred during sleep, 31% during wakefulness and the state was undetermined in 20%. Schmutzler et al. (2005) reported epileptiform activity most frequently in the unrecognised sleep state; when seen in sleep they found it occurred more frequently in active compared to quiet sleep. This is probably related to the sleep patterns in neonates and the shared mechanisms in the generation of sleep and epileptic discharges.

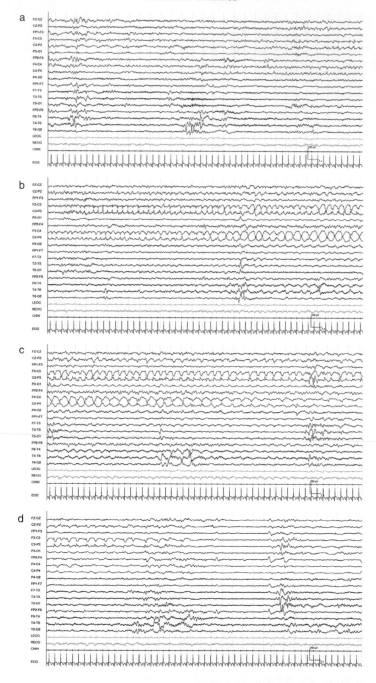

Figure 2.5. EEG epochs showing evolution of a complex seizure discharge. Seizure starts in panel a (initially right sided), and evolves to involve both hemispheres in panels b and c, and ends earlier in the right hemisphere (panel d). The seizure discharge has a different morphology and frequency in the two hemispheres.

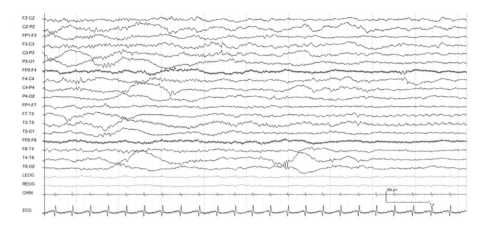

Figure 2.6. EEG shows seizure discharge from the left temporal area starting at β frequency and becoming slower.

Advances in neurophysiology have resulted in the development of newer analytical techniques such as density spectral array displays, envelope trend displays, neonatal automated seizure detection and background grading algorithms.

Electroclinical dissociation

Neonates with seizures have frequent electrographic seizures with no clinical correlates and these may constitute up to 90% of all neonatal seizures (Murray et al. 2008, Volpe 2008, Nagarajan et al. 2010, 2011a). This is referred to as electroclinical dissociation (ECD). Therefore a v-EEG is an important investigation to accurately identify, quantify and classify epileptiform activity in a neonate.

Infants with ECD may also have some seizures that have clinical correlates, and ECD is increased in preterms (Clancy et al. 1988, Bye and Flanagan 1995, McBride et al. 2000, Volpe 2008, Nagarajan et al. 2010, 2011a).

ECD is thought to arise from an impaired brain, with dissociation between neurons that are involved in EEG seizure generation and the neuronal circuitry and neuromuscular activity required to manifest clinical features (Zangaladze et al. 2008, Dichter 2009). ECD is reported in infants who have neuromuscular paralysis, those with diffuse encephalopathy, and those who have neonatal seizures after administration of antiepileptic drugs (AEDs) (Clancy et al. 1988, Tharp 2002, Volpe 2008). ECD can occur in infants who have not received AEDs (Scher 2003, Nagarajan et al. 2011a). The majority of seizures in infants undergoing therapeutic hypothermia do not have clinical correlates. Though seizure rates are similar in infants who undergo therapeutic hypothermia and those who have not, it has been shown that ECD is higher and the overall seizure burden is probably lower in the former (Boylan et al. 2015).

The high incidence of ECD in neonatal seizures may be because of the developmental profile and rostrocaudal pattern of maturation of the chloride cotransporters NKCC1 and

KCC2 (Sanchez and Jensen 2001, Dzhala et al. 2005). The mismatch between excitatory and inhibitory mechanisms in the neonatal brain may also contribute to ECD.

In keeping with the idea that ECD implies more severe brain impairment, electrographic-only seizures have been shown to have a lower maximum amplitude and frequency and tend to be more contained (less spread) than electroclinical seizures (Nagarajan et al. 2011a). They are less likely to show ictal fast frequency activity (Nagarajan et al. 2011b; see Fig. 2.7).

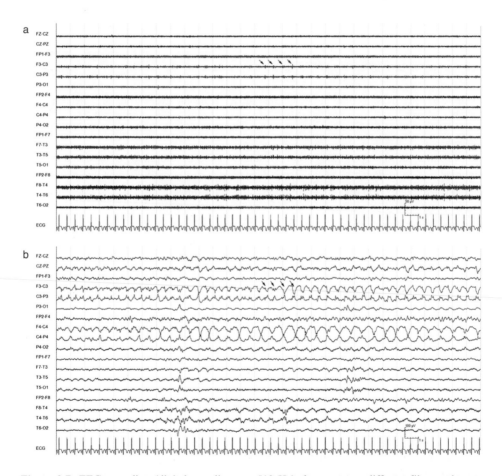

Figure 2.7. EEG recording (digital sampling rate 512 Hz) shown at two different filter settings to reveal fast frequency activity (FFA) during ictal discharge. In panel a, a high-pass finite impulse response filter at 30 Hz was used and shows FFA in the left hemisphere (arrowheads point to some FFA discharges). In panel b the same epoch with traditional filters (high-pass filter at 0.3 Hz and low-pass filter at 70 Hz) shows ictal discharges from both hemispheres (arrow heads point to the same ictal discharges as in panel a).

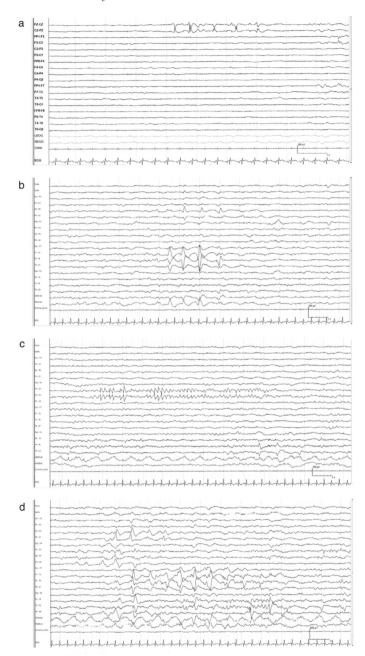

Figure 2.8. EEG epochs illustrate runs of sharps (panels a and b) and BERDs (panels c and d). Panel a illustrates runs of midline sharps on an abnormal background. Panels b, c and d show sharps, runs of sharps (1–5 s) and BERDs (5–9 s) from the same neonate. Panel b shows sharps with maximal amplitude over the left temporal region. Panels c and d illustrate BERDs (over the right hemisphere in panel c and over the left in panel d). Both neonates also had conventional electrographic seizures.

21

EEG for estimation of seizure burden

The fraction of the EEG with electrographic seizures as a percentage of the total duration of the recording is called the ictal fraction. Status epilepticus is defined as a seizure with a duration of more than 30 minutes or an ictal fraction greater than 50%. These measures are commonly used as an estimate of the seizure burden in neonatal seizures. Most studies have shown that higher ictal fractions and more frequent seizures and status epilepticus are associated with poorer outcomes (Legido et al. 1991, Bye et al. 1997, Pisani et al. 2007, Nagarajan et al. 2011a). The seizure/epileptic burden has been shown to correlate with neurodevelopmental outcomes and with post-neonatal epilepsy (Pisani et al. 2008, Volpe 2008, Nagarajan et al. 2011c, Uria-Avellanal et al. 2013).

It is difficult to quantify how much of the brain is involved during a neonatal seizure. Does the number of electrodes involved in an electrographic seizure on EEG reflect the percentage of the brain involved in seizure activity? Does the spread of ictal activity to the contralateral hemisphere or multiple foci of seizure activity correlate to outcome? The results are conflicting; in some studies (Bye et al. 1997, Pisani et al. 2008) it did, whereas in another it did not (Nagarajan et al. 2011a).

An electrographic seizure is conventionally defined as being at least 10 seconds in duration (Volpe 2008). However, brief rhythmic discharges (see Fig. 2.8) may share many of the features of a conventional seizure but last less than 10 seconds (Shewmon 1990, Nagarajan et al. 2010, 2011c). Nagarajan et al. (2011c) explored the significance and prognostic implications of 5–10 second discharges referred to as BERDs (brief EEG rhythmic discharges) in infants with neonatal seizures and concluded that they should be considered miniseizures. The prognostic implication of these brief discharges is probably the same as true seizures (Oliveira et al. 2000, Nagarajan et al. 2011c).

EEG for assessment of response to therapeutic interventions

Not only can the v-EEG identify and quantify seizures (Shellhaas et al. 2011) but EEG is also the best way to assess response to interventional therapy (e.g. AEDs, neuroprotective strategies), especially in infants with ECD. Changes in number, profile and type of neonatal seizures as well as changes in background can be monitored by v-EEG, either by repeated studies or by continuous monitoring.

EEG for clues to underlying aetiology

Specific features on an EEG may give clues to the aetiology of the neonatal seizures. A burst suppression pattern with short periods of activity and short interburst intervals in an infant with tonic seizures and other seizure types, with no convincing history of hypoxic-ischaemic encephalopathy (HIE), is suggestive of Ohtahara syndrome (Beal et al. 2012). Figure 2.9 shows a burst suppression pattern in an infant with Ohtahara syndrome due to an asymmetric brain malformation disorder in panel a and panel b (Fig. 2.9) demonstrates a burst suppression pattern in an infant with a metabolic disorder. Pyridoxine-dependant seizures (Volpe 2008) are thought to show a characteristic EEG pattern. Unilateral amplitude suppression and focal clonic electroclinical seizures in a neonate raise the possibility

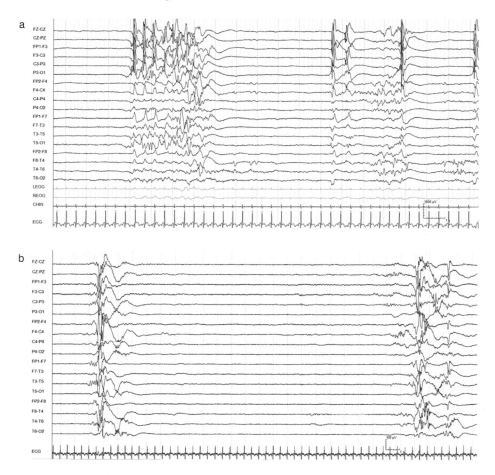

Figure 2.9. Panel a shows a burst suppression pattern in an infant with early infantile epileptic encephalopathy. Bursts are of higher amplitude over the left hemisphere, in keeping with a brain malformation disorder more severe on the left. Note the short bursts and interburst intervals. Panel b shows a burst suppression pattern in an infant with a metabolic disorder (non-ketotic hyperglycinemia).

of a stroke. Figure 2.2 shows a left hemispheric seizure onset and asymmetry of amplitude of the background in an infant with a left-sided neonatal stroke.

EEG for prognosis

The background on the EEG has been shown to be an excellent predictor of neurodevelopmental outcomes (Volpe 2008, Uria-Avellanal et al. 2013). Early EEGs demonstrate the extent and severity of initial brain impairment. Continuous monitoring or sequential EEGs provide information on persistence, worsening or improvement of the background and help assess response to any interventions. Conventional v-EEG with sampling of a large area of the brain is preferred to limited channel a-EEG, as regional and focal abnormalities, stages of sleep and the spectrum of abnormalities are better detected (Shellhaas et al. 2011). However background on an a-EEG has also been shown to be useful in prognostication (Zhang et al. 2013).

Continuity, amplitude, symmetry, synchrony, interburst intervals, sharps, sleep cycling, frequency, reactivity and maturational status are some of the features on EEG that are used to evaluate normalcy of the background patterns (Watanabe et al. 1980, Tharp et al. 1981, Shewmon 1990, Lombroso and Holmes 1993, Laroia et al. 1998, Nagarajan et al. 2010).

The Sarnat encephalopathy scale is used frequently in clinical practice and grades the severity of neonatal encephalopathy from 1 to 3 (Sarnat and Sarnat 1976). EEG background abnormalities parallel the clinical severity and are thought to be more specific and sensitive than the clinical grading in prognostication (El-Ayouty et al. 2007). The background on the EEG is often graded as normal, mildly abnormal, moderately abnormal or severely abnormal based on visual analysis, preferably by a well-trained neurologist/neurophysiologist.

Several studies have demonstrated the excellent prognostic value of the EEG background analysis to predict mortality and morbidity in infants with neonatal seizures and neonatal encephalopathy (Tharp et al. 1981, Clancy 2006, Volpe 2008, Nagarajan et al. 2010, Uria-Avellanal et al. 2013). Most infants (>90%) with neonatal encephalopathy who have a normal or mildly abnormal background on EEG do well, whereas those with severely abnormal backgrounds have a high incidence of mortality or adverse neurodevelopmental outcomes (90%). The outcomes in those infants with neonatal encephalopathy and moderate abnormalities is difficult to predict with approximately half doing reasonably well and half having significant problems as children and adults (Volpe 2008). We developed a numerical score to grade the background in infants with neonatal seizures, by assigning a numerical value for each of the parameters traditionally used to assess background and expressed the score as a percentage. Abnormalities in continuity and amplitude were given greater weight compared with the other parameters. Higher numerical scores reflecting a greater degree of background abnormality were associated with increasing incidence of neuroimaging abnormalities, neurodevelopmental impairment, cerebral palsy, vision and hearing impairment and epilepsy (Nagarajan et al. 2010). Numerical scores may be more objective, less prone to interpreter variability and easier to use in analysing neonatal EEGs. Further refinements and studies are required to assess inter-observer agreement and value in predicting specific deficits in the long term.

Infants with brain injury or impairment of function may not be able to demonstrate the sleep-wake patterns usually seen in a standard one-hour v-EEG (Janjarasjitt et al. 2008, Scher 2008). Antenatal neurological injury may have evolved to a subacute or chronic stage by the time the child is born. The EEG background soon after birth may not reflect the severity of the brain impairment. Newer techniques using frequency and time-dependant computer analysis may enhance the ability of the neonatal EEG background analysis to assess prenatally acquired injuries (Scher 2004, Guerit et al. 2009).

Standard v-EEG and a-EEG

Standard multichannel v-EEG is considered the optimal modality for the accurate diagnosis of neonatal seizures. V-EEG has been used to diagnose neonatal seizures for a long time and antedated the development of a-EEG. The recording of multiple channels in a standard EEG increases the amount of brain sampled and results in the detection of all electrographic seizures that project to the surface. The details on how to record a neonatal v-EEG are discussed in the chapter on recording of a neonatal EEG (Chapter 3). The standard v-EEG also allows us to accurately identify focus of seizure onset, and seizure propagation patterns.

Standard v-EEG requires a good technologist to record the study and an expert neurologist/neurophysiologist to interpret the study. Standard V-EEG is labour- and cost-intensive and not readily available, especially when it is required to be initiated after hours, on holidays, and so on. The a-EEG is a much simplified version of the standard EEG, with a reduced number of electrodes that provide a filtered, smoothened, rectified, time-compressed record of EEG amplitude. It is easy to apply, is relatively simple to interpret and has some efficacy for seizure detection – this has been improved further by having raw EEG data from the few channels displayed (Shellhaas et al. 2007, Rakshasbhuvankar et al. 2015). It provides the possibility of increasing the diagnosis of electrographic seizures in the neonate, especially when standard v-EEG is unavailable. The a-EEG is most often interpreted by the neonatal clinicians. Most neonatal intensive care units in developed countries have access to and use the a-EEG now.

It is important for the neurologists to have an understanding of the a-EEG and its role in clinical practice and for the neonatologists of the a-EEG's limitations in seizure detection and the value of the standard multichannel v-EEG. A complementary paradigm that incorporates and makes the best and most practical use of both modalities is necessary. When seizures are suspected (clinically or on a-EEG) we recommend at least one recording of an hour's duration of conventional v-EEG as soon as possible and preferably repeated intermittently (continuous v-EEG would be the ideal option) based on clinical need and practical constraints. A team approach to diagnosis and management with involvement of neurology and neonatology is essential to optimise care and outcomes in infants with neonatal seizures.

Recommendations for which neonates should have a v-EEG and for how long

- A standard one-hour multichannel v-EEG should be undertaken in all infants with neonatal encephalopathy, in those with clinically identified events that are thought to be seizures and in those at high risk for seizures.
- Those with a moderate to severely abnormal background and/or electrographic seizures on the standard v-EEG recording should ideally have continuous monitoring with v-EEG.
- Neonates at high risk for seizures, including those with HIE, intracranial haemorrhage, intracranial infections, or neonatal stroke, should ideally be monitored continuously for 24 hours to screen for seizures.
- In neonates with EEG seizures, v-EEG monitoring should ideally be continued for at least a 24-hour period of no seizures.

- In infants undergoing therapeutic hypothermia one may wish to monitor for 48–72 hours because of the risk of delayed seizures and seizures occurring during rewarming.
- V-EEG monitoring should be considered in infants with certain inborn errors of metabolism, infants undergoing cardiac surgery with cardiopulmonary bypass, and infants on extracorporeal membrane oxygenation.

Continuous monitoring in infants with seizures or suspected seizures or at high risk for seizures is best undertaken with conventional v-EEG as this has a higher specificity and sensitivity for seizure detection compared to a-EEG. If continuous v-EEG is not possible, then a-EEG with intermittent multichannel v-EEG should be done. If no form of continuous EEG monitoring is available, then repeated standard v-EEGs should be performed as clinically indicated and practical.

Conclusion

The unique pattern of the neonatal brain with rather prolific excitatory circuits and relatively sparse inhibitory circuits is thought to be important for activity-driven synaptogenesis, synaptic plasticity, and rapid growth, development and maturation of the brain. This heightened state of excitability also probably makes the neonate vulnerable to seizures. Neonatal seizures are difficult to recognise and accurate diagnosis is essential. The conventional multichannel v-EEG remains the best method of identifying, characterising, classifying and quantifying seizures. It also remains one of the best methods of prognosticating in early neonatal life. A routine one-hour v-EEG provides a 'snap shot' of brain activity, while a continuous v-EEG recording is likely to have even greater diagnostic and prognostic utility.

REFERENCES

Beal JC, Cherian K, Moshe SL (2012) Early-onset epileptic encephalopathies: Ohtahara syndrome and early myoclonic encephalopathy. *Pediatr Neurol* 47: 317–323. doi: http://dx.doi.org/10.1016/j.pediatrneurol. 2012.06.002.

Berg AT, Berkovic SF, Brodie MJ, et al. (2010) Revised terminology and concepts for organization of seizures and epilepsies: Report of the ILAE Commission on Classification and Terminology, 2005–2009. *Epilepsia* 51: 676–685. doi: http://dx.doi.org/10.1111/j.1528-1167.2010.02522.x.

Boylan GB (2011) EEG monitoring in the neonatal intensive care unit: A critical juncture. *Clin Neurophysiol: Official Journal of the International Federation of Clinical Neurophysiology* 122: 1905–1907. doi: http://dx.doi.org/10.1016/j.clinph.2011.03.015.

Boylan GB, Burgoyne L, Moore C, O'Flaherty B, Rennie, J (2010) An international survey of EEG use in the neonatal intensive care unit. *Acta Paediatr* 99: 1150–1155. doi: http://dx.doi.org/10.1111/j.1651-2227.2010.01809.x.

Boylan GB, Kharoshankaya L, Wusthoff CJ (2015) Seizures and hypothermia: Importance of electroencephalographic monitoring and considerations for treatment. *Semin Fetal Neonatal Med* 20: 103–108. doi: http://dx.doi.org/10.1016/j.siny.2015.01.001.

Bragatti JA (2011) Recognition of seizures in neonatal intensive care units. *Clinical Neurophysiol: Official Journal of the International Federation of Clinical Neurophysiology* 122: 1069–1070. doi: http://dx.doi.org/10.1016/j.clinph.2010.11.005.

Bye AM, Cunningham CA, Chee KY, Flanagan, D (1997) Outcome of neonates with electrographically identified seizures, or at risk of seizures. *Pediatr Neurol* 16: 225–231. doi: http://dx.doi.org/10.1016/S0887-8994(97)00019-2.

Bye A, Flanagan D (1995) Electroencephalograms, clinical observations and the monitoring of neonatal seizures. *J Paediatr Child Health* 31: 503–507. doi: http://dx.doi.org/10.1111/j.1440-1754.1995. tb00872.x.

Clancy RR (2006) Summary proceedings from the neurology group on neonatal seizures. *Pediatrics* 117: S23–S27.

Clancy RR, Legido A, Lewis, D (1988) Occult neonatal seizures. *Epilepsia* 29: 256–261. doi: http://dx.doi. org/10.1111/j.1528-1157.1988.tb03715.x.

Dichter MA (2009) Emerging concepts in the pathogenesis of epilepsy and epileptogenesis. *Arch Neurol* 66: 443–447. doi: http://dx.doi.org/10.1001/archneurol.2009.10.

Dzhala VI, Talos DM, Sdrulla DA, et al. (2005) NKCC1 transporter facilitates seizures in the developing brain. *Nature Med* 11: 1205–1213. doi: http://dx.doi.org/10.1038/nm1301.

El-Ayouty M, Abdel-Hady H, El-Mogy S, Zaghlol H, El-Beltagy M, Aly H (2007) Relationship between electroencephalography and magnetic resonance imaging findings after hypoxic-ischemic encephalopathy at term. *Am J Perinatol* 24: 467–473. doi: http://dx.doi.org/10.1055/s-2007-986686.

Engel J Jr. (2006) Report of the ILAE classification core group. *Epilepsia* 47: 1558–1568. doi: http://dx.doi. org/10.1111/j.1528-1167.2006.00215.x.

Garfinkle J, Shevell MI (2011) Prognostic factors and development of a scoring system for outcome of neonatal seizures in term infants. *Eur J Paediatr Neurol: EJPN: Official Journal of the European Paediatric Neurology Society* 15: 222–229. doi: http://dx.doi.org/10.1016/j.ejpn.2010.11.002.

Glass HC, Sullivan JE (2009) Neonatal seizures. *Curr Treat Options Neurol* 11: 405–413. doi: http://dx.doi. org/10.1007/s11940-009-0045-1.

Guerit JM, Amantini A, Amodio P, et al. (2009) Consensus on the use of neurophysiological tests in the intensive care unit (ICU): Electroencephalogram (EEG), evoked potentials (EP), and electroneuromyography (ENMG). *Neurophysiol Clin* 39; 71–83. doi: http://dx.doi.org/10.1016/j.neucli.2009.03.002.

ILAE Epigraph (Fall 2015) Classifying seizures in the very young: Initial plans of the neonatal seizure task force (part of ILAE Commission on Classification & Terminology). 17 (3).

Janjarasjitt S, Scher MS, Loparo KA (2008) Nonlinear dynamical analysis of the neonatal EEG time series: The relationship between neurodevelopment and complexity. *Clin Neurophysiol* 119: 822–836. doi: http://dx.doi.org/10.1016/j.clinph.2007.11.012.

Laroia N, Guillet R, Burchfiel J, Mcbride MC (1998) EEG background as predictor of electrographic seizures in high-risk neonates. *Epilepsia* 39: 545–551. doi: http://dx.doi.org/10.1111/j.1528-1157.1998.tb01418.x.

Legido A, Clancy RR, Berman PH (1991) Neurologic outcome after electroencephalographically proven neonatal seizures. *Pediatrics* 88: 583–596.

Lombroso CT, Holmes GL (1993) Value of the EEG in neonatal seizures. *Epilepsy* 6: 39–70. doi: http:// dx.doi.org/10.1016/S0896-6974(05)80010-6.

Malone A, Ryan CA, Fitzgerald A., Burgoyne L, Connolly S, Boylan GB (2009) Interobserver agreement in neonatal seizure identification. *Epilepsia* 50: 2097–2101. doi: http://dx.doi.org/10.1111/j.1528-1167. 2009.02132.x.

Mastrangelo M, Van Lierde A, Bray M, Pastorino G, Marini A, Mosca F (2005) Epileptic seizures, epilepsy and epileptic syndromes in newborns: A nosological approach to 94 new cases by the 2001 proposed diagnostic scheme for people with epileptic seizures and with epilepsy. *Seizure: The Journal of the British Epilepsy Association* 14: 304–311. doi: http://dx.doi.org/10.1016/j.seizure.2005.04.001.

Mcbride MC, Laroia N, Guillet R (2000) Electrographic seizures in neonates correlate with poor neurodevelopmental outcome. *Neurology* 55: 506–513. doi: http://dx.doi.org/10.1212/WNL.55.4.506.

Mccoy B, Hahn CD (2013) Continuous EEG monitoring in the neonatal intensive care unit. *J Clin Neurophysiol* 30: 106–114. doi: http://dx.doi.org/10.1097/WNP.0b013e3182872919.

Mizrahi EM, Kellaway P (1987) Characterization and classification of neonatal seizures. *Neurology* 37: 1837–1844. doi: http://dx.doi.org/10.1212/WNL.37.12.1837.

Murray DM, Boylan GB, Ali I, Ryan CA, Murphy BP, Connolly S (2008) Defining the gap between electrographic seizure burden, clinical expression and staff recognition of neonatal seizures. *Arch of Dis in Childhood. Fetal and Neonatal Ed* 93: F187–F191. doi: http://dx.doi.org/10.1136/adc.2005.086314.

Nagarajan L, Ghosh S, Palumbo L (2011a) Ictal electroencephalograms in neonatal seizures: Characteristics and associations. *Pediatr Neurol* 45: 11–16. doi: http://dx.doi.org/10.1016/j.pediatrneurol.2011.01.009.

Nagarajan L, Ghosh S, Palumbo L, Akiyama T, Otsubo H (2011b) Fast activity during EEG seizures in neonates. *Epilepsy Res* 97: 162–169. doi: http://dx.doi.org/10.1016/j.eplepsyres.2011.08.003.

Nagarajan L, Palumbo L, Ghosh S (2010) Neurodevelopmental outcomes in neonates with seizures: A numerical score of background encephalography to help prognosticate. *Journal of Child Neurology* 25: 961–968. doi: http://dx.doi.org/10.1177/0883073809355825.

Nagarajan L, Palumbo L, Ghosh S (2011c) Brief electroencephalography rhythmic discharges (BERDs) in the neonate with seizures: Their significance and prognostic implications. *J Child Neurol* 26: 1529–1533. doi: http://dx.doi.org/10.1177/0883073811409750.

Nagarajan L, Palumbo L, Ghosh S (2012) Classification of clinical semiology in epileptic seizures in neonates. *Eur J Paediatr Neurol* 16: 118–125. doi: http://dx.doi.org/10.1016/j.ejpn.2011.11.005.

O'Meara MW, Bye AM, Flanagan D (1995) Clinical features of neonatal seizures. *J Paediatr Child Health* 31: 237–240. doi: http://dx.doi.org/10.1111/j.1440-1754.1995.tb00793.x.

Oliveira AJ, Nunes ML, Da Costa JC (2000) Polysomnography in neonatal seizures. *Clin Neurophysiol* 111 (Suppl 2): S74–S80. doi: http://dx.doi.org/10.1016/S1388-2457(00)00405-3.

Pisani F, Cerminara C, Fusco C, Sisti L (2007) Neonatal status epilepticus vs recurrent neonatal seizures: Clinical findings and outcome. *Neurology* 69: 2177–2185. doi: http://dx.doi.org/10.1212/01.wnl.0000295674.34193.9e.

Pisani F, Copioli C, Di Gioia C, Turco E, Sisti L (2008) Neonatal seizures: Relation of ictal video-electroencephalography (EEG) findings with neurodevelopmental outcome. *J Child Neurol* 23: 394–398. doi: http://dx.doi.org/10.1177/0883073807309253.

Pressler RM, Mangum B (2013) Newly emerging therapies for neonatal seizures. *Semin Fetal Neonatal Med* 18: 216–223. doi: http://dx.doi.org/10.1016/j.siny.2013.04.005.

Rakshasbhuvankar A, Paul S, Nagarajan L, Ghosh S, Rao S. (2015) Amplitude-integrated EEG for detection of neonatal seizures: a systematic review, *Seizure*, 33:90-8. doi: 10.1016/j.seizure.2015.09.014. Epub 2015 Sep 26.

Sanchez RM, Jensen FE (2001) Maturational aspects of epilepsy mechanisms and consequences for the immature brain. *Epilepsia* 42: 577–585. doi: http://dx.doi.org/10.1046/j.1528-1157.2001.12000.x.

Sankar R, Painter MJ (2005) Neonatal seizures: After all these years we still love what doesn't work. *Neurology* 64: 776–777. doi: http://dx.doi.org/10.1212/01.WNL.0000157320.78071.6D.

Sarnat HB, Sarnat MS (1976) Neonatal encephalopathy following fetal distress. A clinical and electroencephalographic study. *Arch Neurol* 33: 696–705. doi: http://dx.doi.org/10.1001/archneur.1976.00500100030012.

Scher MS (2002) Controversies regarding neonatal seizure recognition. *Epileptic Disorders: International Epilepsy Journal with Videotape* 4: 139–158.

Scher MS (2003) Neonatal seizures and brain damage. *Pediatr Neurol* 29: 381–390. doi: http://dx.doi.org/10.1016/S0887-8994(03)00399-0.

Scher MS (2004) Automated EEG-sleep analyses and neonatal neurointensive care. *Sleep Med* 5: 533–540. doi: http://dx.doi.org/10.1016/j.sleep.2004.07.002.

Scher MS (2008) Ontogeny of EEG-sleep from neonatal through infancy periods. *Sleep Med* 9: 615–636. doi: http://dx.doi.org/10.1016/j.sleep.2007.08.014.

Scher MS, Hamid MY, Steppe DA, Beggarly ME, Painter MJ (1993) Ictal and interictal electrographic seizure durations in preterm and term neonates. *Epilepsia* 34: 284–288. doi: http://dx.doi.org/10.1111/j.1528-1157.1993.tb02412.x.

Schmutzler KM, Nunes ML, Da Costa JC (2005) The relationship between ictal activity and sleep stages in the newborn EEG. *Clin Neurophysiol: Official Journal of the International Federation of Clinical Neurophysiology* 116: 1520–1532. doi: http://dx.doi.org/10.1016/j.clinph.2005.02.024.

Shellhaas RA, Chang T, Tsuchida T, et al. (2011) The American clinical neurophysiology society's guideline on continuous electroencephalography monitoring in neonates. *Journal of Clinical Neurophysiology: Official Publication of the American Electroencephalographic Society* 28: 611–617. doi: http://dx.doi.org/10.1097/WNP.0b013e31823e96d7.

Shellhaas RA, Soaita AI, Clancy RR (2007) Sensitivity of amplitude-integrated electroencephalography for neonatal seizure detection. *Pediatrics* 120: 770–777. doi: http://dx.doi.org/10.1542/peds.2007-0514.

Shetty J (2015) Neonatal seizures in hypoxic-ischaemic encephalopathy – risks and benefits of anticonvulsant therapy. *Dev Med Child Neurol* 57 (Suppl 3): 40–43. doi: http://dx.doi.org/10.1111/dmcn.12724.

Shewmon DA (1990) What is a neonatal seizure? Problems in definition and quantification for investigative and clinical purposes. *Journal of Clinical Neurophysiology: Official Publication of the American Electroencephalographic Society* 7: 315–368. doi: http://dx.doi.org/10.1097/00004691-199007000-00003.

Tharp BR (2002) Neonatal seizures and syndromes. *Epilepsia* 43 (Suppl 3): 2–10. doi: http://dx.doi.org/10.1046/j.1528-1157.43.s.3.11.x.

Tharp BR, Cukier F, Monod N (1981) The prognostic value of the electroencephalogram in premature infants. *Electroencephalogr Clin Neurophysiol* 51: 219–236. doi: http://dx.doi.org/10.1016/0013-4694(81)90136-X.

Uria-Avellanal C, Marlow N, Rennie JM (2013) Outcome following neonatal seizures. *Semin Fetal Neonatal Med* 18: 224–232. doi: http://dx.doi.org/10.1016/j.siny.2013.01.002.

Volpe JJ (1981) Neurology of the newborn. *Major Prob Clin Pediatr* 22: 1–648.

Volpe JJ (1989) Neonatal seizures: Current concepts and revised classification. *Pediatrics* 84: 422–428.

Volpe, JJ (2008) Neurology of the newborn. In: Volpe JJ, editor. *Neonatal Seizures,* 5th ed. Philadelphia, PA: WB Saunders Elsevier.

Watanabe K, Miyazaki S, Hara K, Hakamada S (1980) Behavioral state cycles, background EEGs and prognosis of newborns with perinatal hypoxia. *Electroencephalogr Clin Neurophysiol* 49: 618–625. doi: http://dx.doi.org/10.1016/0013-4694(80)90402-2.

Wical BS (1994) Neonatal seizures and electrographic analysis: Evaluation and outcomes. *Pediatr Neurol* 10: 271–275. doi: http://dx.doi.org/10.1016/0887-8994(94)90121-X.

Wirrell EC (2005) Neonatal seizures: To treat or not to treat? *Semin Pediatr Neurol* 12: 97–105. doi: http://dx.doi.org/10.1016/j.spen.2005.03.004.

Wusthoff CJ (2013) Diagnosing neonatal seizures and status epilepticus. *J Clin Neurophysiol* 30: 115–121. doi: http://dx.doi.org/10.1097/WNP.0b013e3182872932.

Zangaladze A, Nei M, Liporace JD, Sperling MR (2008) Characteristics and clinical significance of subclinical seizures. *Epilepsia* 49; 2016–2021. doi: http://dx.doi.org/10.1111/j.1528-1167.2008.01672.x.

Zhang D, Ding H, Liu L, et al. (2013) The prognostic value of amplitude-integrated EEG in full-term neonates with seizures. *PLoS One* 8: e78960. doi: http://dx.doi.org/10.1371/journal.pone.0078960.

3
RECORDING A VIDEO-EEG STUDY IN A NEONATE

Linda Palumbo and Lakshmi Nagarajan

Neonatal seizures pose diagnostic and management challenges, even today, despite the many advances in neonatal intensive care. It is often not possible by clinical acumen or evaluation alone to distinguish between seizure-related and non-seizure-related movements and phenomena in the neonate. Electroclinical dissociation (ECD) adds to the complexity: many neonatal seizures have no clinical correlates and are only identified by electroencepahalography (EEG) (Scher 2002, Clancy 2006, Murray et al. 2008, Volpe 2008, Malone et al. 2009, Nagarajan et al. 2011a, 2012). An EEG, preferably conventional multichannel video-EEG (v-EEG), is essential to confirm, detect, characterise and quantify the seizure burden, as well as to assess response to therapy (Watanabe 2014). Evaluation of the background on the v-EEG (and the amplitude-integrated EEG [a-EEG]) also helps with prognostication for neurodevelopmental outcome (Holmes and Lombroso 1993, Hellstrom-Westas et al. 1995, Nagarajan et al. 2010, Merchant and Azzopardi 2015).

The execution of a good quality neonatal v-EEG recording by a neurophysiology technologist is an essential step to enable proficient interpretation of the v-EEG by a neurologist/neurophysiologist with expertise (Boylan et al. 2010, Neubauer et al. 2011). A neurophysiology technologist has to be skilled and be able to adapt his or her technique of acquiring a v-EEG study to many different conditions. These include the need for adequate infection control techniques (asepsis), the infant's age and size, the overall well-being of the neonate, the other interventions and monitoring that are in place, the environment (neonatal intensive care unit or neurophysiology laboratory), the family and health professionals milling around the infant and the noise and chaos (both physical and emotional) of a busy clinical setting (Kaminska et al. 2015). In this chapter we discuss the practical issues encountered in the recording of a conventional v-EEG. The principles would also apply to recording of a-EEG.

EEG electrode application
The technologist needs to be aware of the indication for the v-EEG and the planned duration of the recording, prior to embarking on application of the electrodes. An explanation of the procedure to the family and sometimes the neonatal staff is necessary. Liaison with the neonatal staff for optimal visualisation and recording is essential. The technologist has to be flexible; interruptions to electrode application and set-up may occur due to clinical care requirements.

It is essential to verify the name of the infant and ensure you have the right patient, prior to starting a study. The age of the infant (postmenstrual, chronological) should be documented. Perinatal history is useful to acquire. Other important information to be recorded includes the temperature of the infant before, during and after the EEG, anti-epileptic drugs (AEDs) administered before and during the recording, anti-epileptic drug levels when pertinent, administration of any drugs or alteration of parenteral or enteral regimes. Therapeutic interventions such as assisted ventilation, therapeutic hypothermia and ionotropic support may influence the recording and should be noted. Metabolic perturbations, infections, significant changes in clinical profile and other relevant clinical features (e.g. a cephalhaematoma, a surgical scar over the scalp, significant plagiocephaly) should be noted.

We use gold cup electrodes for recording. Other electrode options include silver/silver chloride electrodes, disposable cup electrodes, disposable flat surface electrodes, electrode caps and subdermal needle electrodes (Wallois et al. 2007, Neubauer et al. 2011, Lofhede et al. 2012, Lamblin and de Villepin-Touzery 2015, Lloyd et al. 2015). The most commonly used cup electrodes may cause abrasions or pressure points. Sterile disposable electrodes minimise the risk of infections. Needle electrodes are good for impedance and may result in better recordings but they increase the chance of infections. Innovations such as the textile electrodes (Lofhede et al. 2012) may minimise effects on the delicate neonatal scalp. Each neurology department should have a standard protocol that the staff is familiar with, and that can be adapted/modified for an individual infant.

Adequate skin preparation is the key for obtaining a good EEG. This can be obtained by wiping the skin on the scalp with an alcohol wipe, using an abrasive scrub such as Lemon Prep (if necessary) and use of a conduction paste (such as Elefix; Nihon Kodon, OM Canada). Gold cup electrodes are particularly useful as they can be purchased in different sizes and may be affixed to the scalp using squares of micropore tape (Fig. 3.1). Needle

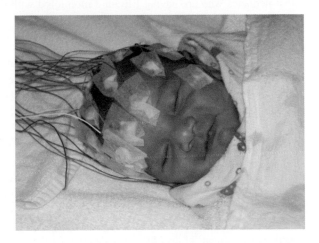

Figure 3.1. Electrodes affixed to the scalp using micropore tape for the 10–20 montage.

electrodes obviously do not need the scrub or the conduction paste. A bandage is sometimes helpful to keep the electrodes in place especially for prolonged recordings. Some centres routinely use electrode caps; we do not have personal experience with their use in neonates.

Number of electrodes

We apply the full array of electrodes in accordance with the international 10–20 system in most neonates (term and preterm), with some exceptions such as infants less than 25 weeks of age and infants with microcephaly (Figs. 3.1 and 3.2). A neonatal-trained technologist should be able to achieve this, with acceptable impedances (<5K Ohms), without producing bridging or other artefacts. The 10–20 system provides better coverage of the infant's cranium/brain and displays seizure onsets and propagation patterns more clearly than the modified neonatal 8–10 electrode array (Fig. 3.2) used in many centres (Shellhaas et al. 2008, Shellhaas et al. 2011). Increasing the electrode density improves neonatal seizure and source localisation, as well as information regarding spatial patterning that can be extracted from the EEG (Odabaee et al. 2013).

In addition to the scalp electrodes, several non-cerebral electrodes should be applied to record other physiological parameters. We routinely monitor the electromyography (EMG) over the submental region. This channel is useful to pick up sucking, tongue and mouthing type of movements (Fig. 3.3). We also apply additional EMG electrodes when clinically indicated (e.g. paroxysmal motor phenomenon involving limbs that are suspicious for seizures). Electrooculography (EOG) electrodes are necessary to detect eye movements. We place one close to and below the lateral canthus on one side and above the lateral canthus on the other side, with each EOG electrode referenced to the contralateral mastoid; other electrode combinations may be used for EOG. A single-channel ECG tracing is standard for a v-EEG recording. Respiratory movements may be monitored using a respiband or just EMG electrodes. EOGs and EMGs help identify the level of alertness of the infant and in staging of sleep. Most neonates who are having EEG are monitored with pulse oximetry.

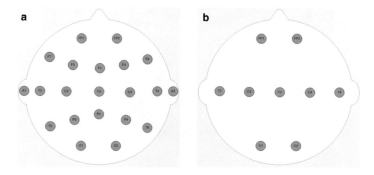

Figure 3.2. (a) Schematic representations of the EEG electrode array for the 10–20 system and (b) limited electrode array in a modified neonatal montage.

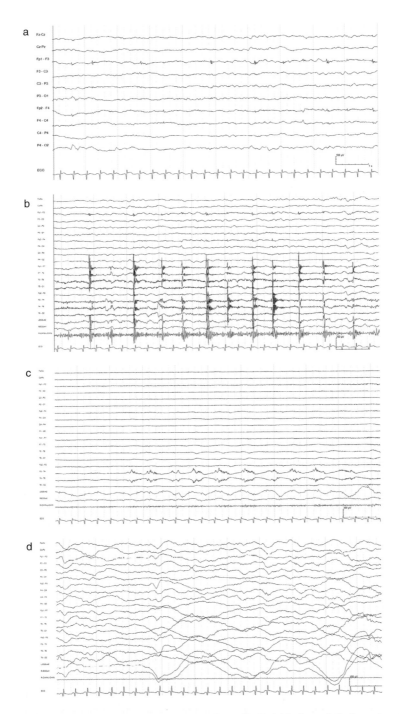

Figure 3.3. EEG epochs showing artefacts. In panel a, a limited 10-channel display raises the possibility of polyphasic sharps from the frontal leads. A full montage in panel b shows the obvious sucking artefact. Panel c shows mouthing artefact in an EEG with an abnormal background. Panel d demonstrates heat artefact.

This should also be recorded in the study, if possible. Annotations are entered in real time when the technologist is present. They may also be entered while reviewing the study. It is often useful to have a predetermined standard list of commonly used annotations. Intermittent photic stimulation can be undertaken during an EEG recording; however this is often difficult in a sick infant.

Recording systems for v-EEG

Digital recordings are the norm now in most parts of the world. We use the Compumedics system (Compumedics Limited, Vic Australia) with Profusion EEG software. Multiple systems (with relative merits and demerits) are available. Digital systems allow reformatting of montages, while analysing the EEG. Those who have used the analogue system previously and the digital system now will certainly vouch for the advantages of the digital recordings. Most standard v-EEG systems sample at rates of 256–512 Hz, while newer systems allow much higher rates. The availability of synchronised video recordings with EEG enables accurate assessment of clinical events of concern and the semiology of electroclinical seizures. Identification of suspicious rhythmic activity on EEG as artefact becomes easier when the synchronised video is viewed (see Figs. 3.3 and 3.4). Video also helps staging sleep and level of alertness of the infant.

Montages and filters for EEG

Our standard montages include bipolar double banana, transverse montages, source montage, average reference montage and referential montage to the mastoids, montage to the vertex and customised montages. Figure 3.5 shows an epoch of EEG displayed with different montages and number of channels. It is important to know about the montages, the relevance of inter-electrode distances and any modified electrode placement in order to correctly interpret the study. When electro-cerebral inactivity is seen, it is important to verify this by using montages with long inter-electrode distances. We routinely review the EEG with filter settings of 0.3–0.5 for the low frequency filter (LFF) and 70 for the high frequency filter (HFF). Filter settings for EMG (LFF: 1.5, HFF: 30–70), EOG (LFF: 0.5–1.5, HFF: 30–70) and ECG (LFF: 1.5, HFF: 30) need to be individualised. Filter settings and type of filters need to be modified to look at specific aspects of the EEG, for example use of a high-pass finite response filter to look for fast frequency activity and modification of LFF and HFF settings when looking at ultra-slow or very fast activity (Vanhatalo and Kaila 2006, Nagarajan et al. 2011b, Lamblin and de Villepin-Touzery 2015).

Artefacts on v-EEG recording

The environment in the neonatal intensive care unit is often hostile to obtaining good quality artefact free recordings. Artefacts may result from nearby electrical equipment (including those used to monitor or treat the neonate; see Fig. 3.6) and movements imposed by demands of clinical care in a busy nursery. Some artefacts are obvious, whereas some are quite subtle. It is useful for the neurologist to be cognizant of common artefacts on a v-EEG tracing. Figures 3.3, 3.4 and 3.6 are examples of some of the artefacts that are seen on EEG; the video is often useful to clarify their nature. An efficient technologist can pick

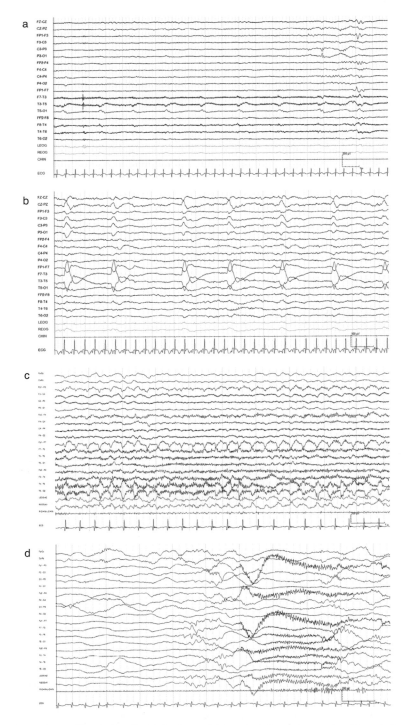

Figure 3.4. Panels a and b show artefacts due to hiccups. Panel c illustrates a patting artefact. Video recording or technologist's comment is useful to identify such artefacts. A chin tremor artefact is seen in panel d. Montages and calibration as in Figure 3.6.

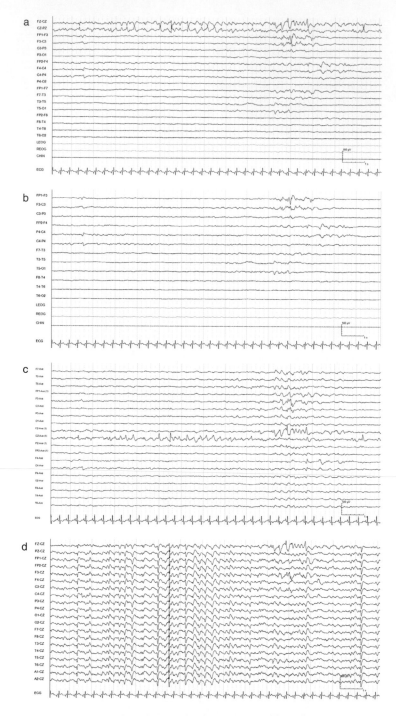

Figure 3.5. Panel a shows an electrographic discharge from Cz. Sharps are seen from either hemisphere. A limited channel recording or display (panel b) will miss the midline electrographic discharge. Referential montages have to be selected appropriately: the discharge is clearly seen in panel c (average reference), while a Cz reference is obviously unhelpful (panel d).

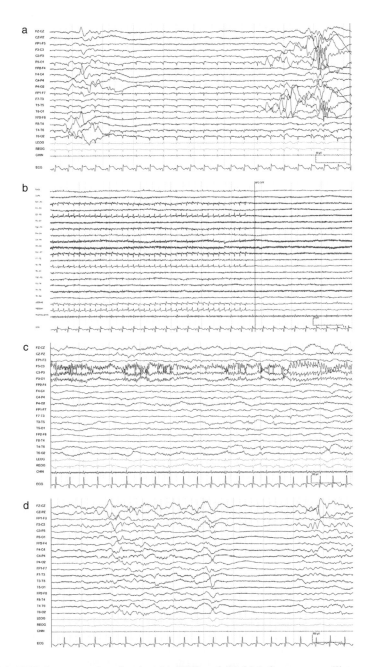

Figure 3.6. EEG from neonates showing (a) ECG and (b) high-frequency oscillatory ventilation (HFO) artefacts. Note that the HFO was turned off midway through the epoch. Panel c shows artefacts in a surface EEG recording (left parasagittal) due to a nearby needle electrode (C3) used for a-EEG recording; and (d) shows that the artefact disappeared when the needle was removed. The EEGs are shown in a double banana montage with top two channels (in black) showing midline derivations, the next four (in blue) left parasagittal, followed by four right parasagittal (in maroon), then four left temporal (in blue) and four right temporal (in maroon). The last four traces show electrooculography and electromyography and ECG. Calibration bars in the right lower part of each panel.

these up and alert the neurologist. The reporting neurologist should be vigilant to the possibility of an unusual looking, not easily explained, EEG pattern being artefactual.

Duration of recordings

Our standard v-EEG recordings are of at least an hour's duration. This usually enables capturing one sleep cycle. In neonates with brain impairment, longer studies or repeat studies may be required to assess background abnormalities and their severity.

To capture neonatal seizures, assess seizure burden and monitor response to therapy, continuous v-EEG monitoring is optimal and should be aimed for. Practical constraints often limit the availability of v-EEG monitoring for neonates at risk for seizures and those with confirmed seizures. A judicious combination of repeated v-EEG studies, with continuous a-EEG monitoring, maybe more feasible; this is undertaken in most centres, including ours.

Conclusion

A high standard neonatal v-EEG clinical service and research programme requires both excellent recordings and expertise in evaluation, interpretation and extraction of useful information. In this chapter we have discussed the practice in our department and offered some guidelines to ensure 'safe and sound' v-EEG recordings.

REFERENCES

Boylan G, Burgoyne L, Moore C, O'Flaherty B, Rennie J (2010) An international survey of EEG use in the neonatal intensive care unit. *Acta Paediatr* 99: 1150–1155. doi: http://dx.doi.org/10.1111/j.1651-2227.2010.01809.x.

Clancy RR (2006) Summary proceedings from the neurology group on neonatal seizures. *Pediatrics* 117: S23–S27.

Hellstrom-Westas L, Rosen I, Svenningsen NW (1995) Predictive value of early continuous amplitude integrated EEG recordings on outcome after severe birth asphyxia in full term infants. *Arch Dis Child Fetal Neonatal Ed* 72: F34–F38. doi: http://dx.doi.org/10.1136/fn.72.1.F34.

Holmes GL, Lombroso CT (1993) Prognostic value of background patterns in the neonatal EEG. *J Clin Neurophysiol* 10: 323–352. doi: http://dx.doi.org/10.1097/00004691-199307000-00008.

Kaminska A, Cheliout-Heraut F, Eisermann M, Touzery De Villepin A, Lamblin MD (2015) EEG in children, in the laboratory or at the patient's bedside. *Neurophysiol Clin* 45: 65–74. doi: http://dx.doi.org/10.1016/j.neucli.2014.11.008.

Lamblin MD, De Villepin-Touzery A (2015) EEG in the neonatal unit. *Neurophysiol Clin* 45: 87–95. doi: http://dx.doi.org/10.1016/j.neucli.2014.11.007.

Lloyd R, Goulding R, Filan P, Boylan G (2015) Overcoming the practical challenges of electroencephalography for very preterm infants in the neonatal intensive care unit. *Acta Paediatr* 104: 152–157. doi: http://dx.doi.org/10.1111/apa.12869.

Lofhede J, Seoane F, Thordstein M (2012) Textile electrodes for EEG recording–a pilot study. *Sensors (Basel)* 12: 16907–16919. doi: http://dx.doi.org/10.3390/s121216907.

Malone A, Ryan CA, Fitzgerald A, Burgoyne L, Connolly S, Boylan GB (2009) Interobserver agreement in neonatal seizure identification. *Epilepsia* 50: 2097–2101. doi: http://dx.doi.org/10.1111/j.1528-1167.2009.02132.x.

Merchant N, Azzopardi D (2015) Early predictors of outcome in infants treated with hypothermia for hypoxic-ischaemic encephalopathy. *Dev Med Child Neurol* 57 (Suppl 3): 8–16. doi: http://dx.doi.org/10.1111/dmcn.12726.

Murray DM, Boylan GB, Ali I, Ryan CA, Murphy BP, Connolly S (2008) Defining the gap between electrographic seizure burden, clinical expression and staff recognition of neonatal seizures. *Arch Dis Child. Fetal and Neonatal Edition* 93: F187–F191. doi: http://dx.doi.org/10.1136/adc.2005.086314.

Nagarajan L, Ghosh S, Palumbo L (2011a) Ictal electroencephalograms in neonatal seizures: Characteristics and associations. *Pediatric Neurology* 45: 11–16. doi: http://dx.doi.org/10.1016/j.pediatrneurol.2011.01.009.

Nagarajan L, Ghosh S, Palumbo L, Akiyama T, Otsubo H (2011b) Fast activity during EEG seizures in neonates. *Epilepsy Res* 97: 162–169. doi: http://dx.doi.org/10.1016/j.eplepsyres.2011.08.003.

Nagarajan L, Palumbo L, Ghosh S (2010) Neurodevelopmental outcomes in neonates with seizures: A numerical score of background encephalography to help prognosticate. *J Child Neurol* 25: 961–968. doi: http://dx.doi.org/10.1177/0883073809355825.

Nagarajan L, Palumbo L, Ghosh S (2012) Classification of clinical semiology in epileptic seizures in neonates. *Eur J Paediatr Neurol* 16: 118–125. doi: http://dx.doi.org/10.1016/j.ejpn.2011.11.005.

Neubauer D, Osredkar D, Paro-Panjan D, Skofljanec A, Derganc M (2011) Recording conventional and amplitude-integrated EEG in neonatal intensive care unit. *Eur J Paediatr Neurol* 15: 405–416. doi: http://dx.doi.org/10.1016/j.ejpn.2011.03.001.

Odabaee M, Freeman WJ, Colditz PB, Ramon C, Vanhatalo S (2013) Spatial patterning of the neonatal EEG suggests a need for a high number of electrodes. *Neuroimage* 68: 229–235. doi: http://dx.doi.org/10.1016/j.neuroimage.2012.11.062.

Scher MS (2002) Controversies regarding neonatal seizure recognition. *Epileptic Disord* 4: 139–158.

Shellhaas RA, Chang T, Tsuchida T, et al. (2011) The American clinical neurophysiology society's guideline on continuous electroencephalography monitoring in neonates. *J Clin Neurophysiol: Official Publication of the American Electroencephalographic Society* 28: 611–617. doi: http://dx.doi.org/10.1097/WNP.0b013e31823e96d7.

Shellhaas RA, Gallagher PR, Clancy RR (2008) Assessment of neonatal electroencephalography (EEG) background by conventional and two amplitude-integrated EEG classification systems. *J Pediatr* 153: 369–374. doi: http://dx.doi.org/10.1016/j.jpeds.2008.03.004.

Vanhatalo S, Kaila K (2006) Development of neonatal EEG activity: From phenomenology to physiology. *Semin Fetal Neonatal Med* 11: 471–478. doi: http://dx.doi.org/10.1016/j.siny.2006.07.008.

Volpe JJ (2008) Neurology of the newborn. In: Volpe JJ, editor. *Neonatal Seizures,* 5th ed. Philadelphia, PA: WB Saunders Elsevier.

Wallois F, Vecchierini MF, Heberle C, Walls-Esquivel E (2007) [Electroencephalography (EEG) recording techniques and artifact detection in early premature babies]. *Neurophysiol Clin* 37: 149–161. doi: http://dx.doi.org/10.1016/j.neucli.2007.07.001.

Watanabe K (2014) Neurophysiological aspects of neonatal seizures. *Brain Dev* 36: 363–371. doi: http://dx.doi.org/10.1016/j.braindev.2014.01.016.

4

THE ROLE OF AMPLITUDE-INTEGRATED EEG IN THE MANAGEMENT OF NEONATAL SEIZURES

Lena Hellström-Westas, Ingmar Rosén and Linda S. de Vries

A majority of infants with seizures in the neonatal period have had previous insults affecting cerebral blood flow, oxygenation and metabolism. Such insults frequently occur in the perinatal period, in conjunction with the delivery or as a result of conditions appearing after birth. This is also the reason why most seizures develop during the first three days after birth (Ronen et al. 1999). Less frequently, neonatal seizures are the results of congenital malformations, epileptic syndromes or metabolic diseases although seizures in infants affected by such conditions tend to be very severe and refractory to antiepileptic medications, and they also frequently appear during the first week after birth (Tekgul et al. 2006). Neonatal seizures are often recognized because infants develop abnormal clinical movements or behaviour. However, several studies utilizing video-EEG have shown that many suspected clinical seizures do not have corresponding EEG seizure activity (Mizrahi and Kellaway 1987, Murray et al. 2008). Furthermore, a majority of neonatal seizures have very subtle clinical symptoms or are entirely subclinical (Clancy et al. 1988, Bye and Flanagan 1995). During recent years it has become increasingly evident that the efficacy of antiepileptic medications cannot be judged by clinical responses only, since administration of these medications frequently is associated with a decrease in the amount of electroclinical seizures while subclinical may continue unchanged or even increase, a term called (ECD) or 'uncoupling' (Boylan et al. 2002, Scher et al. 2003).

Given the need for accurate diagnosis and management of neonatal seizures as mentioned above, the amplitude-integrated EEG (a-EEG) trend in combination with display of a limited-channel EEG (a-EEG/EEG) has been widely applied and proven to be very useful for the following:

* Detection of clinically silent or subtle seizures in infants at high risk,
* Diagnosis of electrographic seizures in infants with suspected seizures,
* Monitoring effects of antiepileptic treatment,
* Monitoring cerebral function (electrocortical activity and functional cerebral integrity such as sleep-wake cycling) in infants with seizures.

However, the a-EEG/EEG method also has the following limitations that users must be aware of:

• With the reduced number of electrodes, it is not possible to detect all seizures
• Several studies have shown the necessity of adequate training for accurate diagnosis of seizures
• Brief seizures may easily be overlooked in the time-compressed a-EEG trend
• Episodic appearance of artefacts of various sources may be mistaken for seizures

The a-EEG method

The a-EEG trend is a method for continuous long-term monitoring of brain function in infants at high risk infants during neonatal intensive care. The method has gained increasing popularity in neonatal intensive care units (NICUs) during the last two decades because it has repeatedly proven useful in the management of infants with hypoxic-ischaemic encephalopathy and in infants with suspected seizures (Hellström-Westas et al. 1995, Toet et al. 1999). Since the a-EEG is also very easy to apply, within minutes it can give immediate important information on cerebral activity. Although mainly used in NICUs, the a-EEG trend was not originally designed for use in neonates; it was created in the late 1960s for use in adult intensive care, for following cerebral recovery after cardiac arrest and for monitoring of patients with status epilepticus (Maynard et al. 1969).

The a-EEG trend is created from the EEG; the main features include an asymmetric filter, which attenuates low- and high-frequency activity (most activity below 2 Hz and above 15 Hz is filtered out), rectifying, and the display of maximum and minimum amplitudes with a semi-logarithmic scale on a time compressed record (Maynard et al. 1969). For many years, the a-EEG trend was only available in purpose-built monitors, so called cerebral function monitors (CFMs). In these monitors it was initially only possible to assess the a-EEG trend, which was usually printed on paper, but there was no display of the EEG. Furthermore, it was not possible to store or make offline analysis of the recording. Consequently, in the older CFMs, epileptic seizure activity could only be suspected, but not verified, unless a parallel recording displaying the EEG was performed.

Newborn infants of all gestational ages can be monitored with a-EEG/EEG. The normal development of the a-EEG pattern has been described in several publications (Thornberg and Thiringer 1990, Zhang D et al. 2011). The most prominent maturational feature in the a-EEG trend is a gradual rise in the amplitude of the lower border reflecting increasing EEG continuity. Sleep-wake cycling can also be seen in very preterm infants and is characterized by sinusoidal narrowing and broadening of the a-EEG trace. Quiet sleep can be discerned from active sleep and wakefulness by a more discontinuous background, resulting in broadening of the trace and a lower minimum amplitude (Fig. 4.1a). At 32–34 gestational weeks, these background patterns correspond to the clinical assessment of quiet and active sleep periods (Greisen et al. 1985). Maturation of a-EEG amplitudes is similar across the head, although amplitudes are slightly lower in occipital and frontal leads than in central and temporal areas (Niemarkt et al. 2012). In parallel with the

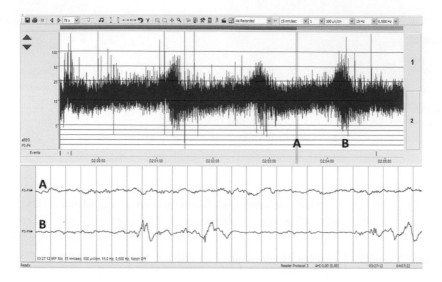

Figure 4.1a. This 6-hour a-EEG recording (corresponding EEG samples, duration 26 seconds) from a term infant shows a continuous normal voltage pattern with sleep-wake cycling with 'A' corresponding to wakefulness or active sleep and the more discontinuous activity in 'B' corresponding to the tracé alternant pattern during quiet sleep.

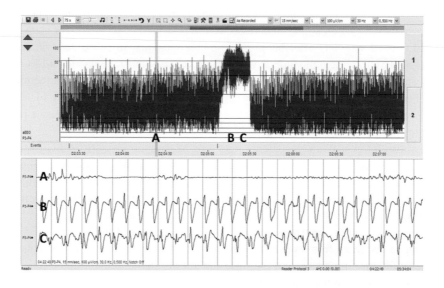

Figure 4.1b. A single seizure with duration 20 minutes is clearly visible on the discontinuous background in this 4-hour a-EEG recording with corresponding 26-second EEG samples in the lower half of the panel.

EEG, a-EEG amplitudes become higher if the distance between the electrodes is increased (Quigg and Leiner 2009).

Neonatal electrographic seizures are usually defined as sudden, repetitive and evolving (in frequency, morphology and amplitude) ictal patterns with a clear beginning, middle and end and with a duration of at least 10 seconds (Shellhaas et al. 2007a, Murray et al. 2008, Tsuchida et al. 2013). The matching seizure pattern in the a-EEG trend is usually characterized by a transient increase in a-EEG amplitude (both lower and upper margin) corresponding to the temporal behaviour of the epileptic seizure activity in the EEG (Fig. 4.1b). Since such activity differs from the overall background activity, it is usually easily discernible, and frequently recurring seizures and status epilepticus will resemble a saw-tooth pattern (Fig. 4.2a and Fig. 4.2b). Rarely, seizures result in transient depression of the a-EEG trace, although this pattern has been described in infants with infantile spasms and EEG showing high-voltage hypsarrhythmia with desynchronizations in conjunction with seizures.

Artefacts are common in neonatal long-term recordings of a-EEG/EEG and are due to mechanical ventilation, not least high-frequency oscillation ventilation, electrocardiogram, muscle activity and interference from electric equipment. Recordings from frontal and temporal areas may be especially susceptible to muscular activity. Movement artefacts and patting of the infant can be misinterpreted as seizures, since this may create rhythmic activity that can be mistaken for seizures (Evans et al. 2010). Another caveat regarding seizure detection in the a-EEG trend is that brief seizures may not be possible to detect in the compressed a-EEG trace. Furthermore, continuously ongoing seizures could also be missed since they do not create major frequency or amplitude changes in the EEG that will create

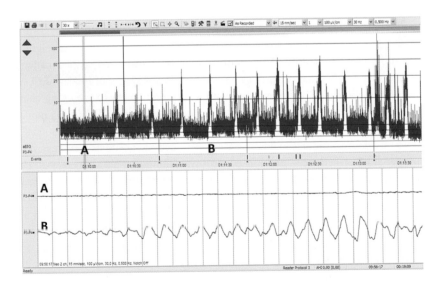

Figure 4.2a. Repeated electrographic seizures emerging on a very depressed a-EEG/EEG background pattern in a severely asphyxiated infant during the first hours after delivery. Single-channel a-EEG/ EEG recorded from P3–P4 with duration 4 hours (duration EEG samples is 26 seconds).

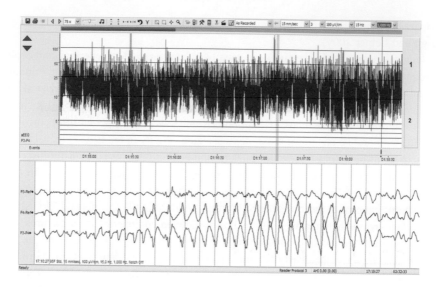

Figure 4.2b. Repetitive brief seizures appearing roughly every 10 minutes, each with a duration of 20–25 seconds and starting on the right side in a term infant with a right-sided stroke. The seizure (note EEG montage P3–Ref, P4–Ref, P3–P4) corresponds to the vertical blue line through the 4-hour a-EEG trend. The electrocortical background is slightly depressed and with less developed sleep-wake cycling than in Fig. 4.1a.

changes in the a-EEG amplitude (Fig. 4.3a). Because of the a-EEG filtering, seizures of very low frequency may not be possible to detect in the a-EEG trend (Fig. 4.3b).

During the last decade, most a-EEG monitors have introduced continuous display and digital storage of the EEG signal. Consequently, in these modern monitors the original EEG signal should always be addressed for confirmation of a suspected seizure pattern. The a-EEG trend, along with other trends, is also available in a majority of modern EEG equipment used for continuous EEG monitoring with a varying number of recording channels.

The limited number of recording electrodes is a major feature of a-EEG/EEG monitoring, and initially a single bi-parietal trace was recorded. Traditionally, P3–P4 (international 10–20 system) was used for recordings in adults since these electrode positions were regarded to be close to arterial watershed areas, and this concept was introduced also in neonates. Bilateral recordings are increasingly used, usually recorded from frontal-parietal or frontal-central leads, for example, F3–P3/C3 and F4–P4/C4, and such recordings may also include a cross-cerebral channel, P3–P4 or C3–C4. Having one or at most two channels is often considered a major limitation, as focal seizures may remain unnoticed. On the other hand, one should appreciate that the a-EEG was introduced into the NICU as a monitoring device, and at present, in some units 5–10 infants are being simultaneously monitored on a daily basis. To perform multichannel EEG monitoring in all such infants would probably be too demanding for many units. The use of a-EEG monitoring, in combination with a limited-channel or multichannel EEG, is increasing also in paediatric and adult intensive care, as a means for intensivists to be able to monitor bedside and immediately respond to changes in a patient's brain activity.

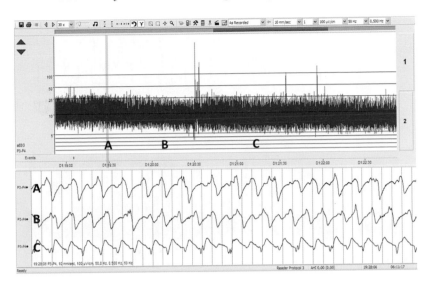

Figure 4.3a. At the first glance this a-EEG trend may look like a continuous pattern without sleep-wake cycling. The EEG in 'A', 'B' and 'C' reveals, however, that this asphyxiated infant had continuously ongoing seizures for many hours.

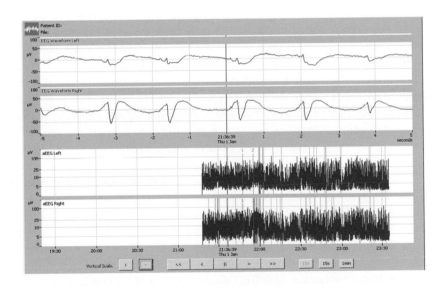

Figure 4.3b. Two-channel recording from an extremely preterm infant. The a-EEG/EEG background is discontinuous. The seizure detection alarm (yellow) has detected low-frequency (0.5 Hz) rhythmic activity originating from a suspected electrographic seizure, which is not possible to detect in the a-EEG trend.

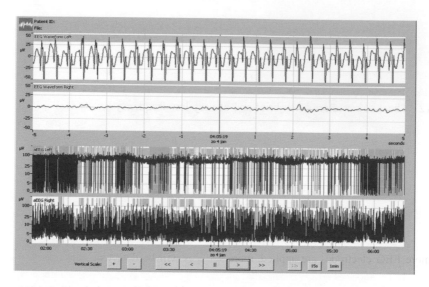

Figure 4.3c. The seizure detection alarm in this recording is marking rhythmic activity. The EEG on the left side shows suspected seizure activity but the a-EEG trends reveals that this is an artefact.

Detection of subclinical seizures in infants at high risk

The incidence of neonatal seizures is around 1–3 per 1000 newborn infants in the general population. However, newborn infants admitted for neonatal intensive care constitute a high-risk population and among these infants the risk for seizures is much higher. Early studies, using the CFM, revealed that subclinical electrographic seizures were common in high-risk NICU populations; in one study 16% of recorded infants experienced suspected status epilepticus with a seizure duration of at least 1 hour (Hellström-Westas et al. 1985). These findings were later verified by EEG studies, demonstrating that a majority of neonatal seizures are subclinical (Clancy et al. 1988). It is difficult to estimate the prevalence of seizures in modern NICU populations. Previous data indicate that probably at least 5% of NICU-treated infants may experience seizures, as estimated by studies using EEG and a-EEG (Scher et al. 1993, Hellström-Westas et al. 1995). The true figures are likely to be higher, since the study by Scher et al. only included infants with EEG-verified seizures, demonstrating a seizures incidence of 3.4% in NICU-treated infants, while a NICU using a-EEG monitoring (without EEG) reached a slightly higher number, 4.5%. In certain groups of patients at high risk the prevalence of seizures is higher, for example, neonates with moderate hypoxic-ischaemic encephalopathy and infants undergoing surgery for congenital heart disease. In these infants, a-EEG/EEG is currently part of the standard monitoring in many NICUs and commonly initiated soon after birth (Shah et al. 2014). Early seizures are also common in very preterm infants developing intraventricular haemorrhages (IVHs), and suspected seizures have been found in the a-EEGs of 50–70% of these infants (Greisen et al. 1987, Hellström-Westas et al. 1991, Olischar et al. 2007). Although it was known that IVH increased the risk for electrocortical background depression and seizures, the prevalence of seizures was not known before these infants had long-term monitoring. The risk for development of large IVHs has decreased during the last two decades and saw-tooth patterns indicating recurrent seizures in the a-EEG are more rarely seen now, compared with before. However, recent data indicate that electrographic seizures may still be prevalent among very preterm and extremely preterm infants (Shah et al. 2010, Wikström et al. 2012). These seizures are often brief and of very low frequency (0.5–1 Hz), which means that they may not be possible to detect in the a-EEG trace because of the time-compressed trend and the high-pass a-EEG filter (Fig. 4.3c). These seizures seem to be associated with development of IVH but there is no clear relation with long-term outcome, as shown in a few small study populations (Shah et al. 2010, Wikström et al. 2012, Vesoulis et al. 2013).

Performance of a-EEG/EEG for seizure detection

Although the a-EEG/EEG will reveal many clinically undetected seizures, it cannot be expected that the limited-channel recording will detect all seizures. A general principle is that if more EEG electrodes are applied, more seizures will be detected. This was shown very clearly in two studies assessing conventional and video-EEGs in newborn infants. Bye and Flanagan (1995) demonstrated, in a study using video-EEG recorded with a 12-electrode modification of the 10–20 system compared with EEG recorded from 4 electrodes, that neonatal seizures are frequent and that 85% of seizures have no clinical manifestations. In total, 1420 seizures were recorded in 32 infants (26 term and 6 preterm). When the reduced electrode montage was used, the number of seizures was underestimated in 19 infants, and in 2 infants no seizures were detected. Tekgul et al. (2005) compared a 19-electrode full montage EEG with a 9-electrode reduced montage EEG in 151 EEGs from 139 preterm and term infants. In total 187 seizures were identified in 31 EEGs from 30 infants using the full montage while the reduced 9-electrode montage identified 166 seizures (89%) in 30 EEGs from 29 of the infants. The reduced montage had a sensitivity of 96.8% and a specificity of 100% for detecting electrographic seizures as compared to the full EEG. The investigators also assessed the reduced montage capability for grading background abnormalities and found a specificity and sensitivity of 87% and 80%, respectively, as compared with the full montage.

Several comparisons regarding seizure detection have been made between the a-EEG and either a limited-channel EEG or full EEG. In an early comparison of a-EEG with simultaneously recorded EEG including single-channel a-EEG/EEG from 5 infants and five-channel a-EEG/EEG from 10 infants (in total 227 hours of monitoring), 48 seizures were found in the single-channel EEG, corresponding to only 15 detectable seizures in the corresponding a-EEG (and 4 clinical seizures). In contrast, in the five-channel a-EEGs, all six infants with seizures were identified by the a-EEG traces (five infants had only single seizures, and one infant had repetitive seizures); four of the infants did not have clinical seizures. These results indicate that seizures may be easier to identify in the a-EEG when more channels are used. Seizures that were not possible to detect with the single-channel a-EEG were either of brief duration (<30 seconds) or, as in one infant, continuously ongoing (Hellström-Westas 1992).

In a later study, a single-channel a-EEG (P3–P4) was compared to a 30-minute recording of a 19-channel EEG in 33 infants at high risk. The 19-channel EEG detected seizures in 10 infants, while seizures were only detected by the a-EEG in 8 infants although both of the 2 infants with seizures that were 'missed' by the a-EEGs had received antiepileptic treatment for previously suspected seizures in the a-EEG. Seizures that were not detected by the a-EEG were of either very short duration or low amplitude or focal occipital (Toet et al. 2002). In another investigation, comparing 351 hours of two-channel a-EEG/EEG (F3–C3, F4–C4) with simultaneously recorded conventional EEG from 11 leads in 21 term infants, seizures were identified in 7 infants, one of whom had status epilepticus. The two-channel a-EEG/EEG detected 31 of the 41 (76%) non-status epilepticus seizures in six out of the seven infants with seizures. Also in this study the seizures missed were predominantly of occipital origin. False positive identification in the a-EEG/EEG was the result of muscle, electrode and patting artefacts (one false positive per 39 hours) (Shah et al. 2008).

Two studies compared the performance of single-channel a-EEG/EEG and two- or multichannel a-EEG/EEG. Bourez-Swart et al. (2009) compared seizure detection rates by single- and multichannel a-EEGs created from nine-channel conventional EEGs recorded in 12 infants with 121 seizures. The sensitivity of a single-channel a-EEG without simultaneous EEG for seizure-detection was low (30%) and improved to 39% when multichannel a-EEGs, created from the conventional EEG, were assessed. Single-channel a-EEG identified 11 out of 12 patients with seizures, and multichannel a-EEG identified all patients.

Van Rooij et al. (2010) compared seizure detection rates from single- and two-channel a-EEG/EEG recordings (F3–P3, F4–P4 and P3–P4) in 34 infants, 14 with unilateral brain injury, 18 with diffuse injury and 2 infants without signs of brain injury on MRI. In total 18% more seizures were detected by the two-channel recordings, but there were no major differences in seizure detection rates between single- and two-channel a-EEG recordings. In infants with unilateral lesions, some seizures also appeared on the contralateral side or in the cross-cerebral recording that did not appear on the ipsilateral side. Comparably, in infants with diffuse lesions, some seizures appeared in the cross-cerebral recording that did not appear in the bilateral recordings.

One of the most comprehensive comparisons between a-EEG/EEG and conventional EEG was presented by Shellhaas et al. (2007a). These investigators evaluated 125 conventional EEGs recorded from 121 term infants using a 11-electrode system according to the international 10–20 system modified for neonatal 10–20 system. In total, the 125 EEGs contained 851 seizures. When the EEG from a single lead (C3–C4) was used, 78% of the seizures in the conventional EEG were possible to detect. Since more than one seizure appeared in many recordings, 94% of EEGs containing seizures were detected by the single-channel EEG in C3–C4. These figures should be compared with 26% of seizures (in 40% of EEGs) that were detected when only the a-EEG trend was assessed without possibility of assessing the corresponding single-channel EEG in the same EEGs as above and clearly showing that inspection of the a-EEG trend only is not sufficient for clinical monitoring (Shellhaas et al. 2007b). Wusthoff et al. (2009) further demonstrated that with electrodes on the forehead (Fp3 and Fp4) less than 70% of EEGs with seizures were identified.

In another study, including 62 term infants with clinical seizures verified by conventional EEG, a single-channel a-EEG with and without the corresponding EEG was compared with the conventional EEG (Zhang L et al. 2011). When only the single-channel a-EEG was assessed, 44% of seizures could be identified, while 86% of seizures were detected when the single-channel a-EEG with corresponding EEG was visible. Increased seizure detection with both the a-EEG and the a-EEG/EEG was associated with more frequent seizures (>5 seizures/hour), prolonged seizures (>60 seconds) and seizures of central origin.

In another study, Frenkel et al. (2011) compared the ability by different professionals (student, fellow, neonatologist) to detect seizures in single-channel a-EEG/EEG (as compared to 41 seizures identified in eight-channel EEG). The sensitivity for detecting seizures in the a-EEG/EEG ranged from 71% to 84% and the specificity from 36% to 96%, and was highest for the more experienced assessors.

The results of these studies are summarized in Table 4.1. The topographic distribution of neonatal seizures, with the majority of seizures present in central and temporal leads, is probably the main reason why it is possible to detect at least 80–90% of seizures in a conventional EEG by a single- or two-channel a-EEG/EEG (Bye and Flanagan 1995, Patrizi et al. 2003, Shellhaas et al. 2007b, Bourez-Swart et al. 2009). It should be stressed that such a high seizure detection rate requires that the whole limited-channel EEG is evaluated in detail, and not only the a-EEG trend (Wikström et al. 2012).

TABLE 4.1

Summary of studies comparing a-EEG (with or without corresponding EEG, i.e. a-EEG/EEG) with single or multiple channels of EEG for seizure detection

Study	Characteristics	Main findings
Hellström-Westas, 1992	a) 1-ch a-EEG vs. 1-ch EEG (N=10 infants) b) 5-ch a-EEG vs. 5-ch EEG (N=5 infants)	1-ch a-EEG: 15/48 (31%) seizures detected 5-ch a-EEG: all seizures detected
Toet et al. 2002	1-ch a-EEG vs. 30 min 19-ch EEG (N=33 monitored infants, 10 had seizures on EEG)	1-ch a-EEG: detected seizures in 8 of the 10 infants and suspected seizures in 1 infant
Shellhaas et al. 2007b	1-ch a-EEG (C3–C4) vs. cEEG (125 EEGs from 121 infants with 851 seizures, 6 assessors)	1-ch a-EEG: detected median 26% of seizures and median 40% of recordings containing seizures; experienced assessors detected more seizures
Shellhaas et al. 2007a	1-ch EEG (C3–C4) vs. cEEG (125 EEGs from 121 infants with 851 seizures)	1-ch EEG: detected 78% of seizures and 94% of recordings containing seizures, underestimated duration of seizures
Shah et al. 2008	2-ch a-EEG/EEG vs. cEEG (N=41 seizures in 7 out of 21 monitored infants)	2-ch a-EEG/EEG: detected 31/41 seizures, i.e. sensitivity 76%; specificity 78%; positive predictive value 78%; negative predictive value 78%

(continued)

TABLE 4.1

Summary of studies comparing a-EEG (with or without corresponding EEG, i.e. a-EEG/EEG) with single or multiple channels of EEG for seizure detection *(continued)*

Study	Characteristics	Main findings
Wusthoff et al. 2009	1-ch EEG (Fp3-Fp4) vs. cEEG (125 EEGs with 330 seizures)	1-ch EEG (Fp3-Fp4): detected 46% of seizures, and 66% of recordings containing seizures
Bourez-Swart et al. 2009	1-ch a-EEG or 9-ch a-EEG vs. 9-ch EEG (*N*=12 infants with 121 seizures)	1-ch a-EEG: detected 30% of seizures (95% CI: 0.22, 0.38) in 11 infants. C3–C4 optimal electrode derivation. 9-ch a-EEG: detected 39% of seizures (95% CI: 0.31, 0.48) and all 12 infants with seizures
van Rooij et al. 2010	2-ch a-EEG/EEG vs. 1-ch a-EEG/EEG (*N*=34 infants with seizures; 18 with unilateral injury, 14 with bilateral injury, and 2 with no injury	2-ch a-EEG/EEG: 18% more seizures detected; detected more seizures on ipsilateral side in 79% of infants with unilateral injury; and, detected 39% more seizures in infants with diffuse brain damage
Evans et al. 2010	2-ch a-EEG vs. 12-ch EEG (44 infants).	EEG: seizures present in 20 infants (45.5%) 2-ch a-EEG: suspected seizures in 28 (63.6% seizures overdiagnosed, most frequently due to movement artefacts): sensitivity 80%, specificity 50%
Frenkel et al. 2011	1-ch a-EEG/EEG vs. 8-ch EEG (10 infants with 41 seizures). More experienced vs. less experienced interpreter	1-ch a-EEG/EEG detection of individual seizures: sensitivity 71–84%, specificity 36–96%; neonatologist/ neurologist higher detection rate than student/fellow
Zhang L et al. 2011	1-ch a-EEG or a-EEG/EEG vs. cEEG (62 infants with 876 seizures)	1-ch a-EEG: detected 44% of seizures 1-ch a-EEG/EEG: detected 86% of seizures Factors associated with higher detection rate: >5 seizures/hour, seizure duration >60 seconds, central origin of seizures

ch, channel; cEEG, conventional EEG as defined by investigator.

Several studies have shown that staff training and experience are essential prerequisites for the optimal use of a-EEG/EEG in the NICU, both for seizure detection and also for assessment of background activity. Development of seizure detection alarms does help to recognize more seizures, especially brief seizures that repeatedly have been proven to be more difficult to identify and low-frequency seizures in very preterm infants (Fig. 4.3b and c). The question whether more recording electrodes will result in improved seizure management remains to be answered, as well as the question how many electrodes are optimal.

Monitoring infants at high risk

An increasing number of NICUs are currently monitoring electrocortical activity in infants at high risk with limited-channel a-EEG/EEG, conventional EEG or video-EEG. All methods have well-known advantages and limitations. Shellhaas and Barks (2012) assessed the value of introducing a-EEG monitoring in encephalopathic term infants, and found that the use of a-EEG was associated with a significantly shorter duration to seizure diagnosis and with a lower proportion of infants receiving a seizure diagnosis without electrographic verification of the seizures. The use of a-EEG was not associated with less recorded conventional EEGs, with administration of more antiepileptic medications or with more imaging studies.

Two randomized studies assessed the value of continuous a-EEG/EEG monitoring (Lawrence et al. 2009, van Rooij et al. 2010). One of the studies included 40 infants with high risk randomized to a two-channel a-EEG/EEG with a visible screen or video-EEG with a blinded screen (Lawrence et al. 2009). In total 1116 seizures (>90% clinically silent) were detected in 12 infants, with no difference between the two groups. This study also evaluated a seizure event detector, which detected 615 (55%) of the seizures in 11 of the 12 infants. However, the NICU staff only responded to the alarm in 7 of the 11 infants. The other study included 33 infants randomized to a visible or a blank a-EEG/EEG monitor screen (van Rooij et al. 2010). Consequently, clinical seizures were treated in the group with a blank screen, while also electrographic seizures could be treated in the group with a visible a-EEG/EEG screen. There was a non-significant trend towards shorter seizure duration in the group randomized to a visible screen. In the group randomized to a blank screen (treating clinical seizures), there was a correlation between total seizure duration and severity of brain injury on MRI. This correlation was not present in the group randomized to a visible screen, indicating that antiepileptic treatment may interrupt this association and therefore could be beneficial. There was no difference between the two groups in the number of administered antiepileptic drugs (AEDs).

Conclusion

The a-EEG/EEG is increasingly used for monitoring of newborn infants in NICUs worldwide. The simplicity by which the method can be applied and the easy basic interpretation, which can be made bedside by the neonatal staff, are contributing factors besides the fact that the method has repeatedly proven to be of clinical value. Continuous cerebral monitoring with a-EEG/EEG or EEG is more and more becoming part of clinical standard monitoring of vital functions in neonates with high risk. The success of neonatal a-EEG/EEG monitoring is probably a major reason behind the emerging practice of continuous EEG monitoring with an increasing number of channels and evaluation of new EEG-based trends to improve recognition of adverse cerebral events during long-term monitoring. The clinical use of a-EEG/EEG is associated with earlier diagnosis of seizures in encephalopathic infants, and fewer infants with a seizure diagnosis without EEG verification. The increased use of a-EEG/EEG has not been associated with an increased use of AEDs (Shellhaas and Barks 2012, Wietstock et al. 2015). The information from the a-EEG/EEG (Fig. 4.4) is much more accurate than clinical observation for evaluation of antiepileptic treatment, and

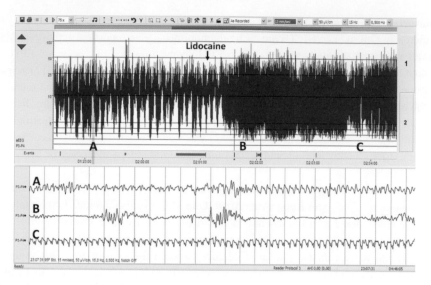

Figure 4.4. This 6-hour a-EEG/EEG recording shows a saw-tooth pattern, indicating an electrographic status epilepticus which is verified by the corresponding EEG (A). Lidocaine infusion was started during the recording and 30 minutes later seizures were abolished (B). However, 2.5 hours later a seizure reappears (C) and is the beginning of a new status epilepticus (not shown).

more effective antiepileptic treatment may also be the reason why two observational studies using a-EEG/EEG reported lower rates of postnatal epilepsy than other studies (Hellström-Westas et al. 1995, Toet et al. 2005).

The a-EEG/EEG differs from the conventional/video-EEG in several aspects. The temporal resolution of the time-compressed a-EEG trend makes it easy to overview long-term trends in brain activity but also makes minor deviations, for example, single short seizures, difficult to identify. Recording from a limited number of electrodes makes the a-EEG/EEG easy to apply and interpret but makes it less sensitive than the conventional EEG for detecting seizures. However, the possibility to perform long-term recordings is an advantage and also allows for easy assessment of seizure burden and responses to antiepileptic treatment. Another advantage is the easy application that allows for many high-risk infants without evident cerebral symptoms to be monitored and screened for seizures. In this context it should also be stressed that it is necessary to perform conventional EEGs in infants who are monitored with a-EEG/EEG. In 2013, the American Clinical Neurophysiology Society published the first guidelines for continuous EEG monitoring in neonates (Tsuchida et al. 2013).

Recent studies have shown that when monitoring is performed, not only the a-EEG trend but also the corresponding limited-channel EEG should be assessed since it has been clearly demonstrated that the a-EEG trend alone, without visible EEG, is not very precise for seizure detection. However, with a single channel a-EEG and a visible EEG, it may be possible to detect up to 90% of seizures in a conventional EEG. Whether at least one or two channels should be monitored is difficult to decide; however, when more than one channel is used it is easier to assess possible artefacts and it is also possible to assess on which side abnormalities such as seizures or background depression appear. Automated seizure detection alarms are being developed and tested and are available on some devices, and they appear to improve seizure detection. However, the technical aspects of such alarms are challenging since rhythmic activity of non-cerebral origin is common in NICUs, for example, from high-frequency oscillation ventilation, and may result in a high proportion of false positive alarms. Several studies have pointed out the importance of accurate training for correct interpretation of a-EEG/EEG recordings. We recommend that all EEG-based monitoring is conducted in close collaboration with neurologists and clinical neurophysiologists.

REFERENCES

Bourez-Swart MD, van Rooij L, Rizzo C, et al. (2009) Detection of subclinical electroencephalographic seizure patterns with multichannel amplitude-integrated EEG in full-term neonates. *Clin Neurophysiol* 120: 1916. doi: http://dx.doi.org/10.1016/j.clinph.2009.08.015.

Boylan GB, Rennie JM, Pressler RM, Wilson G, Morton M, Binnie CD (2002) Phenobarbitone, neonatal seizures, and video-EEG. *Arch Dis Child Fetal Neonatal Ed* 86: F165. doi: http://dx.doi.org/10.1136/fn.86.3.f165.

Bye AM, Flanagan D (1995) Spatial and temporal characteristics of neonatal seizures. *Epilepsia* 36: 1009. doi: http://dx.doi.org/10.1111/j.1528-1157.1995.tb00960.x.

Clancy RR, Legido A, Lewis D (1988) Occult neonatal seizures. *Epilepsia* 29: 256. doi: http://dx.doi.org/10.1111/j.1528-1157.1988.tb03715.x.

Evans E, Koh S, Lerner JT, Sankar R, Garg M (2010) Accuracy of amplitude integrated EEG in a neonatal cohort. *Arch Dis Child Fetal Neonatal Ed* 95: F169. doi: http://dx.doi.org/10.1136/adc.2009.165969.

Frenkel N, Friger M, Meledin I, et al. (2011) Neonatal seizure recognition-comparative study of continuous-amplitude integrated EEG versus short conventional EEG recordings. *Clin Neurophysiol* 122: 1091. doi: http://dx.doi.org/10.1016/j.clinph.2010.09.028.

Greisen G, Hellström-Vestas L, Lou H, Rosen I, Svenningsen N (1985) Sleep-waking shifts and cerebral blood flow in stable preterm infants. *Pediatr Res* 19: 1156. doi: http://dx.doi.org/10.1203/00006450-198511000-00008.

Greisen G, Hellström-Westas L, Lou H, Rosén I, Svenningsen NW (1987) EEG depression and germinal layer haemorrhage in the newborn. *Acta Paediatr Scand* 76: 519. doi: http://dx.doi.org/10.1111/j.1651-2227.1987.tb10509.x.

Hellström-Westas L (1992) Comparison between tape-recorded and amplitude-integrated EEG monitoring in sick newborn infants. *Acta Paediatr* 81: 812. doi: http://dx.doi.org/10.1111/j.1651-2227.1992.tb12109.x.

Hellström-Westas L, Blennow G, Lindroth M, Rosén I, Svenningsen NW (1995) Low risk of seizure recurrence after early withdrawal of antiepileptic treatment in the neonatal period. *Arch Dis Child Fetal Neonatal Ed* 72: F97. doi: http://dx.doi.org/10.1136/fn.72.2.f97.

Hellström-Westas L, Rosén I, Swenningsen NW (1985) Silent seizures in sick infants in early life. Diagnosis by continuous cerebral function monitoring. *Acta Paediatr Scand* 74: 741. doi: http://dx.doi.org/10.1111/j.1651-2227.1985.tb10024.x.

Hellström-Westas L, Rosén I, Svenningsen NW (1991) Cerebral function monitoring during the first week of life in extremely small low birthweight (ESLBW) infants. *Neuropediatrics* 22: 27. doi: http://dx.doi.org/10.1055/s-2008-1071411.

Lawrence R, Mathur A, Nguyen The Tich S, Zempel J, Inder T (2009) A pilot study of continuous limited-channel aEEG in term infants with encephalopathy. *J Pediatr* 154: 835. doi: http://dx.doi.org/10.1016/j.jpeds.2009.01.002.

Maynard D, Prior PF, Scott DF (1969) Device for continuous monitoring of cerebral activity in resuscitated patients. *Br Med J* 29: 545. doi: http://dx.doi.org/10.1136/bmj.4.5682.545-a.

Mizrahi EM, Kellaway P (1987) Characterization and classification of neonatal seizures. *Neurology* 37: 1837. doi: http://dx.doi.org/10.1212/WNL.37.12.1837.

Murray DM, Boylan GB, Ali I, Ryan CA, Murphy BP, Connolly S (2008) Defining the gap between electrographic seizure burden, clinical expression and staff recognition of neonatal seizures. *Arch Dis Child Fetal Neonatal Ed* 93: F187. doi: http://dx.doi.org/10.1136/adc.2005.086314.

Niemarkt HJ, Jennekens W, Maartens IA, et al. (2012) Multi-channel amplitude-integrated EEG characteristics in preterm infants with a normal neurodevelopment at two years of corrected age. *Early Hum Dev* 88: 209. doi: http://dx.doi.org/10.1016/j.earlhumdev.2011.08.008.

Olischar M, Klebermass K, Waldhoer T, Pollak A, Weninger M (2007) Background patterns and sleep-wake cycles on amplitude-integrated electroencephalography in preterms younger than 30 weeks gestational age with peri-/intraventricular haemorrhage. *Acta Paediatr* 96: 1743. doi: http://dx.doi.org/10.1111/j.1651-2227.2007.00462.x.

Patrizi S, Holmes GL, Orzalesi M, Allemand F (2003) Neonatal seizures: Characteristics of EEG ictal activity in preterm and fullterm infants. *Brain Dev* 25: 427. doi: http://dx.doi.org/10.1016/S0387-7604(03)00031-7.

Quigg M, Leiner D (2009) Engineering aspects of the quantified amplitude-integrated electroencephalogram in neonatal cerebral monitoring. *J Clin Neurophysiol* 26: 145. doi: http://dx.doi.org/10.1097/WNP.0b013e3181a18711.

Ronen GM, Penney S, Andrews W (1999) The epidemiology of clinical neonatal seizures in Newfoundland: A population-based study. *J Pediatr* 134: 71. doi: http://dx.doi.org/10.1016/S0022-3476(99)70374-4.

Scher MS, Alvin J, Gaus L, Minnigh B, Painter MJ (2003) Uncoupling of EEG-clinical neonatal seizures after antiepileptic drug use. *Pediatr Neurol* 28: 277. doi: http://dx.doi.org/10.1016/S0887-8994(02)00621-5.

Scher MS, Aso K, Beggarly ME, Hamid MY, Steppe DA, Painter MJ (1993) Electrographic seizures in preterm and full-term neonates: Clinical correlates, associated brain lesions, and risk for neurologic sequelae. *Pediatrics* 91: 128.

Shah DK, Mackay MT, Lavery S, et al. (2008) Accuracy of bedside electroencephalographic monitoring in comparison with simultaneous continuous conventional electroencephalography for seizure detection in term infants. *Pediatrics* 121: 1146. doi: http://dx.doi.org/10.1542/peds.2007-1839.

Shah DK, Wusthoff CJ, Clarke P, et al. (2014) Electrographic seizures are associated with brain injury in newborns undergoing therapeutic hypothermia. *Arch Dis Child Fetal Neonatal Ed*, Jan 17 [Epub ahead of print]. doi: http://dx.doi.org/10.1136/archdischild-2013-305206.

Shah DK, Zempel J, Barton T, Lukas K, Inder TE (2010) Electrographic seizures in preterm infants during the first week of life are associated with cerebral injury. *Pediatr Res* 67: 102. doi: http://dx.doi.org/10.1203/PDR.0b013e3181bf5914.

Shellhaas RA, Barks AK (2012) Impact of amplitude-integrated electroencephalograms on clinical care for neonates with seizures. *Pediatr Neurol* 46: 32. doi: http://dx.doi.org/10.1016/j.pediatrneurol.2011.11.004.

Shellhaas RA, Clancy RR (2007a) Characterization of neonatal seizures by conventional EEG and single-channel EEG. *Clin Neurophysiol* 118: 2156. doi: http://dx.doi.org/10.1016/j.clinph.2007.06.061.

Shellhaas RA, Soaita AI, Clancy RR (2007b) Sensitivity of amplitude-integrated electroencephalography for neonatal seizure detection. *Pediatrics* 120: 770. doi: http://dx.doi.org/10.1542/peds.2007-0514.

Tekgul H, Bourgeois BF, Gauvreau K, et al. (2005) Electroencephalography in neonatal seizures: Comparison of a reduced and a full 10/20 montage. *Pediatric Neurol* 32: 155. doi: http://dx.doi.org/10.1016/j.pediatrneurol.2004.09.014.

Tekgul H, Gauvreau K, Soul J, et al. (2006) The current etiologic profile and neurodevelopmental outcome of seizures in term newborn infants. *Pediatrics* 117: 1270. doi: http://dx.doi.org/10.1542/peds.2005-1178.

Thornberg E, Thiringer K (1990) Normal patterns of cerebral function monitor traces in term and preterm neonates. *Acta Paediatr Scand* 79: 20. doi: http://dx.doi.org/10.1111/j.1651-2227.1990.tb11324.x.

Toet MC, Groenendaal F, Osredkar D, van Huffelen AC, de Vries LS (2005) Postneonatal epilepsy following amplitude-integrated EEG-detected neonatal seizures. *Pediatr Neurol* 32: 241. doi: http://dx.doi.org/10.1016/j.pediatrneurol.2004.11.005.

Toet MC, Hellström-Westas L, Groenendaal F, Eken P, de Vries LS (1999) Amplitude integrated EEG 3 and 6 hours after birth in full term neonates with hypoxic-ischaemic encephalopathy. *Arch Dis Child Fetal Neonatal Ed* 81: F19. doi: http://dx.doi.org/10.1136/fn.81.1.f19.

Toet MC, van der Meij W, de Vries LS, Uiterwaal CS, van Huffelen KC (2002) Comparison between simultaneously recorded amplitude integrated EEG (cerebral function monitor (CFM) and standard EEG in neonates. *Pediatrics* 109: 772. doi: http://dx.doi.org/10.1542/peds.109.5.772.

Tsuchida TN, Wusthoff CJ, Shellhaas RA, et al. (2013) American clinical neurophysiology society standardized EEG terminology and categorization for the description of continuous EEG monitoring in neonates: Report of the American Clinical Neurophysiology Society critical care monitoring committee. *J Clin Neurophysiol* 30: 161. doi: http://dx.doi.org/10.1097/WNP.0b013e3182872b24.

van Rooij LG, de Vries LS, van Huffelen AC, Toet MC (2010) Additional value of two-channel amplitude integrated EEG recording in full-term infants with unilateral brain injury. *Arch Dis Child Fetal Neonatal Ed* 95: F160. doi: http://dx.doi.org/10.1136/adc.2008.156711.

van Rooij LG, Toet MC, van Huffelen AC, et al. (2010) Effect of treatment of subclinical neonatal seizures detected with aEEG: Randomized, controlled trial. *Pediatrics* 125: e358. doi: http://dx.doi.org/10.1542/peds.2009-0136.

Vesoulis ZA, Inder TE, Woodward LJ, Buse B, Vavasseur C, Mathur AM (2013) Early electrographic seizures, brain injury, and neurodevelopmental risk in the very preterm infant. *Pediatr Res Dec* 23. doi: 10.1038/pr.2013.245. [Epub ahead of print] doi: http://dx.doi.org/10.1038/pr.2013.245.

Wietstock SO, Bonifacio SL, Sullivan JE, Nash KB, Glass HC (2015) Continuous Video Electroencephalographic (EEG) Monitoring for Electrographic Seizure Diagnosis in Neonates: A Single-Center Study. *J Child Neurol*. Jun 30. pii: 0883073815592224. [Epub ahead of print]

Wikström S, Pupp IH, Rosén I, et al. (2012) Early single-channel aEEG/EEG predicts outcome in very preterm infants. *Acta Paediatr* 101: 719. doi: http://dx.doi.org/10.1111/j.1651-2227.2012.02677.x.

Wusthoff CJ, Shellhaas RA, Clancy RR (2009) Limitations of single-channel EEG on the forehead for neonatal seizure detection. *J Perinatol* 29: 237. doi: http://dx.doi.org/10.1038/jp.2008.195.

Zhang D, Liu Y, Hou X, et al. (2011) Reference values for amplitude-integrated EEGs in infants from preterm to 3.5 months of age. *Pediatrics* 127: e1280. doi: http://dx.doi.org/10.1542/peds.2010-2833.

Zhang L, Zhou YX, Chang LW, Luo XP (2011) Diagnostic value of amplitude-integrated electroencephalogram in neonatal seizures. *Neurosci Bull* 27: 251. doi: http://dx.doi.org/10.1007/s12264-011-1413-x.

5

ADVANCES IN NEUROPHYSIOLOGY AND NEONATAL SEIZURES: AUTOMATED SEIZURE DETECTION

Nathan J. Stevenson and Geraldine B. Boylan

Seizures are the most common neurological emergency in the neonatal intensive care unit (NICU) and require prompt identification and treatment. Neonatal seizures are acute events, occur in 1–5 per 1000 live births (Vasudevan and Levene 2013), and seizure onset is primarily in the first week of life. Neonatal seizures are intermittent events, although status epilepticus is common, and their number and duration can vary significantly both within and across aetiologies (Lynch et al. 2012, Lynch et al. 2015, Low et al. 2014). Mortality following seizure in term neonates ranges from 7% to 16% with the prevalence of adverse outcomes ranging from 27% to 55% (Uria-Avellanal et al. 2013). The quest to establish if seizures exacerbate brain injury or are merely a symptom of the underlying problem is still an active area of research. Nevertheless, there is universal agreement that seizures must be treated urgently despite the fact that they present a considerable diagnostic and therapeutic challenge. Because of their subtle nature, clinical diagnosis is challenging, and up to 80% of seizures may be missed without continuous electroencephalography (EEG) monitoring (Murray et al. 2008). In addition, interpretation of neonatal EEG is a highly specialised skill that is rarely available out of hours in the NICU, if at all. Consequently, many neonates with seizures go undiagnosed and untreated.

The current gold standard for neonatal seizure detection is the visual interpretation of multichannel EEG by the human expert (Boylan et al. 2013). The interpretation of multichannel neonatal EEG is challenging and requires specific expertise in neurophysiology for reliable interpretation. A range of evolving patterns from multiple cortical sources must be identified and interpreted in the context of the clinical scenario and in combination with information from other physiological parameters such as heart rate and oxygenation. Nevertheless, the visual interpretation of multichannel EEG has high reliability (Shah et al. 2008, Stevenson et al. 2015).

If the aim of neurocritical care is to reduce the overall seizure burden in a neonate, then the early detection of seizures and subsequent intervention are vital. The difficulties in clinical recognition and the delays associated with expert analysis of the EEG have resulted in the uptake of the amplitude-integrated EEG (a-EEG) within the NICU for seizure detection. The a-EEG is a simplified version of the EEG recorded from a reduced number of electrodes that provides a filtered, time-compressed measurement of EEG amplitude. It is based on the cerebral function monitor developed by Maynard et al. (1969) for the monitoring of coma patients. The a-EEG is easy to apply (3–5 electrodes are usually required), is relatively simple to interpret and can significantly accelerate clinical decision making, with some efficacy for seizure detection. As with any compromise solution, its advantages are offset by its limitations: a single- or two-channel recording montage can only potentially detect 80% of seizures compared to an eight-channel montage, over-diagnosis is high due to artefact, seizures with short duration (<30 s) and low amplitude are not well recognised and inter-observer agreement is significantly lower than multichannel EEG (Shellhaas et al. 2007, Shah et al. 2008). Interpretation is further complicated by the lack of standardisation for a-EEG algorithms implemented in many currently available a-EEG devices from different manufacturers, resulting in differences in the a-EEG signals displayed (Quigg and Leiner 2009). Modern a-EEG machines have attempted to overcome the problem of over-diagnosis by displaying two channels of a-EEG (Fig. 5.1) in combination with the corresponding raw EEG channels; this has resulted in improved seizure detection and inter-observer agreement in the hands of experienced users (Shah et al. 2008). An alternate solution would be the introduction of a seizure detection algorithm that generates an output based on analysis of the multichannel EEG, which could be visualised in a similar manner to the a-EEG.

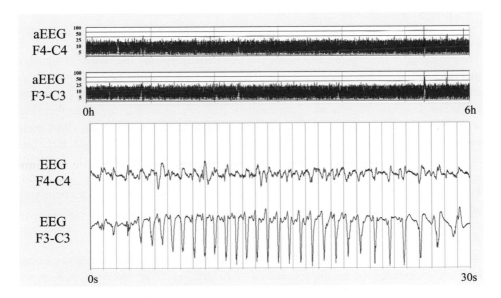

Figure 5.1. A typical a-EEG display – two-channel a-EEG and raw EEG display.

This chapter outlines recent developments in neonatal seizure detection algorithms (NSDAs) from algorithm details and performance analysis, to visualisations of algorithm outputs for clinicians and scope for large-scale application.

Neonatal seizure detection algorithms

The aim of a neonatal seizure detection algorithm (NSDA) is to determine the presence or absence of seizure activity in the EEG using computer-based analysis. Such algorithms are now possible because of the advent of digital EEG machines, which allow computers to readily process this digital data, in real time. The general structure of all NSDAs is similar. This structure can be simplified into a four-stage process: *pre-processing, feature extraction, classification* and *post-processing*. The pre-processing stage involves the application of filters, resampling and segmentation of the EEG into short duration epochs. Feature extraction involves the estimation of a series of summary statistics from each EEG epoch. These summary statistics are designed to represent signal characteristics that are maximally divergent between EEG epochs of seizure and non-seizure. The classification stage converts the series of summary statistics into single datum that represents the likelihood of seizure being present in the EEG epoch under analysis. The post-processing stage involves additional filtering or smoothing, the combination of information from multiple EEG channels, a determination if the likelihood is sufficient to annotate the presence of a seizure followed by a collaring operation that extends the duration of the detected seizure. Each stage can be considered as a further simplification of the EEG signal towards a binary seizure or non-seizure annotation. This process is shown for a multiple-channel EEG recording in Figure 5.2.

PRE-PROCESSING

The recording of the digital EEG signal requires initially passing the raw EEG signal, a measurement of voltage over time, through a low-pass anti-aliasing filter and then to an analogue to digital converter. This samples the EEG signal at 200–256 times per second (Hz). The dominant frequencies of the neonatal EEG are focused in the delta, theta and alpha bands. Several NSDAs filter the incoming signal to pass frequencies within these bands and then resample the signal at lower sampling frequency (32 or 64 Hz). This resampling process reduces the number of samples required to represent the EEG and subsequently accelerates computation. NSDAs can also use fixed duration EEG epochs for analysis. In this case the EEG is typically divided into epochs of 2 to 64 seconds with an overlap, in time, of 50% to 75%.

FEATURE EXTRACTION

According to Clancy and Legido (1987) neonatal seizures manifest on the EEG as a clear ictal event characterised by the appearance of sudden, repetitive, evolving, stereotyped waveforms that have a definite beginning, middle and end, and last for a minimum of 10 seconds. These seizures emerge from a background pattern that displays both stochastic and chaotic characteristics with notable modulations of amplitude apparent over minutes and hours (Notley and Elliot 2003, Stevenson et al. 2013). In many cases, this background

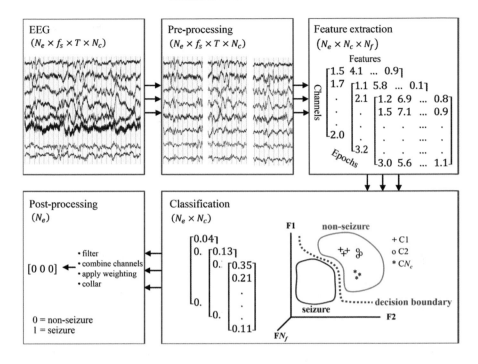

Figure 5.2. Analysis of the neonatal EEG for the detection of seizures. Each equation relates to how much information is output at each stage. N_e, the number of epochs under analysis; N_c, the number of channels under analysis; N_f, the number of features extracted from each epoch; T, the duration of each epoch in seconds; f_s, sampling frequency in Hz; F, feature extracted from each epoch of EEG; C, the EEG channel under analysis.

EEG activity exhibits significant signs of abnormality reflecting the underlying pathology. It is also commonly contaminated by artefacts (electrical activity not generated by the brain) resulting from movements, muscle, pulse, respiration and external sources of electrical activity such as ventilators, infusion pumps or the electrical supply (see Fig. 5.3).

Features extracted from the EEG are, therefore, typically designed to be responsive to one or more seizure characteristics while non-responsive to a variety of background and artefact activities (see Fig. 5.4). The process is complicated by the fact that occasional periods of background EEG may display some of the characteristics of seizure and the prevalence of these seizure-like patterns may be equivalent to true seizure activity.

The characteristic of a seizure that is most informative, but difficult to automatically extract from the EEG, is the evolving repetition. Periodic repetition is a highly discriminatory characteristic of a signal and it can be easily extracted using Fourier analysis. The evolution of seizure, however, results in a repetition that is not strictly periodic, resulting in frequency content that changes over time. The morphology of the seizure discharge is also not purely sinusoidal (see Fig. 5.5). The pseudo-periodic and non-sinusoidal nature of EEG seizure reduces the effectiveness of detection via peaks in the frequency domain

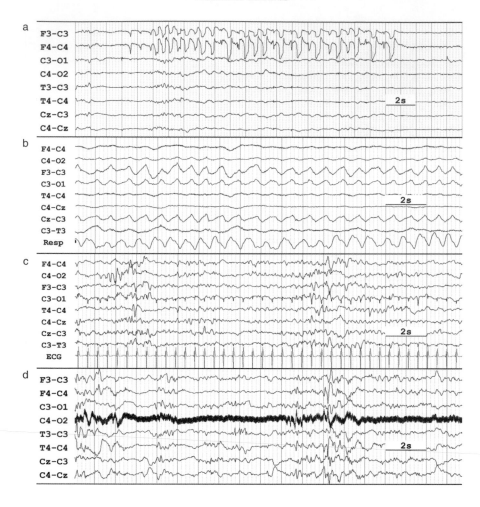

Figure 5.3. Examples of neonatal EEG artefacts: (a) repeated blinking on the frontal channels; (b) respiratory artefact on F3–C3, C3–O1, Cz–C3 that is clearly synchronized with the respiratory movement channel; (c) ECG artefact on C3–O1 that is clearly synchronized with the ECG and (d) 50 Hz interference from the electrical supply on C4–O2.

estimated by Fourier analysis (see Fig. 5.6). This is further complicated by the fact that repetition is also manifested in several artefactual EEG patterns such as respiration and electrocardiogram (ECG)/pulse artefacts and even short periods of background EEG can appear periodic.

The original paper on neonatal seizure detection attempted to overcome this time variation in the periodicity by scoring the autocorrelation function in such a fashion that slight deviation of peaks could be accounted for (Liu et al. 1992). Gotman et al. (1997a) took a different approach that utilised the area in a band of the EEG spectrum

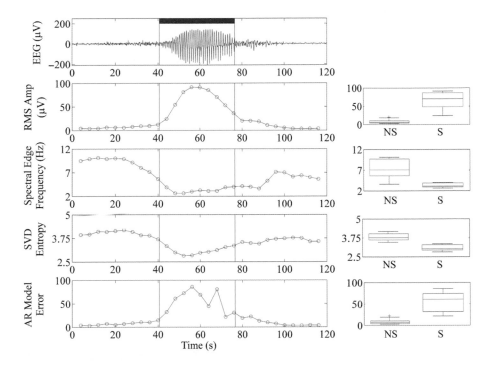

Figure 5.4. Features that respond to the presence of seizure in the EEG. The red bar in the top plot denotes the annotation of the EEG by the human expert. S, seizure; NS, non-seizure. Features are defined in Greene et al. (2008a). RMS Amp, root mean square amplitude; SVD, singular value decompositionm; AR, autoregressive.

rather than the peak value. This resulted in a feature that was robust to some smearing of the spectrum caused by pseudo-periodicity. This method was further developed by Karayiannis et al. in their Type A detector (Karayiannis et al. 2006). An interesting solution to the detection of pseudo-periodicity was applied to neonatal seizure detection by Celka and Colditz (2002). The authors used a multidimensional phase plane to represent the EEG signal. Pseudo-periodicity in the phase plane will manifest as a hyper-ellipse assuming a stable waveform morphology. Details of the hyper-ellipse can be extracted using singular value decomposition and used as a feature for seizure detection. More recent methods such as those of Navakatikyan et al. (2006) and Deburchgraeve et al. (2008) have attempted to identify time-varying repetition using the short-term correlation of wave sequences or spikes extracted from the EEG under analysis, respectively. An advantage of such methods was that by defining the characteristics of the wave sequence/spike the authors were also able to detect waveforms with a specific morphology, improving the robustness of these measures in the presence of repetitive non-seizure waveforms. Methods based on the analysis in the joint time-frequency domain (see Fig. 5.6) such as the time-frequency matched filter and non-

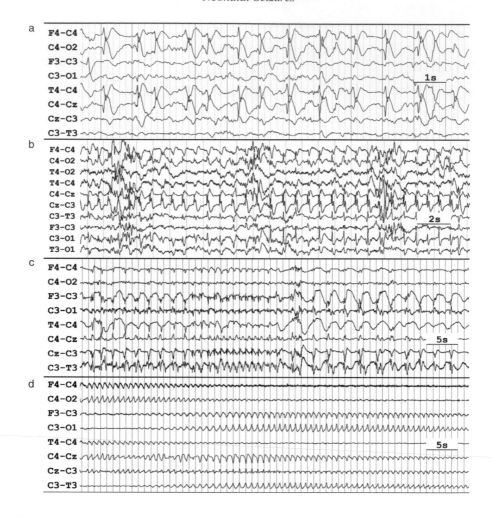

Figure 5.5. Examples of neonatal seizures: (a) right-sided 1–2 Hz seizure discharge; (b) 1–2 Hz biphasic seizure over the central region; (c) multifocal seizure discharges showing evolving morphology and frequency characteristics and (d) seizure that starts on the right side at 1 Hz and wanes as the seizure spreads and evolves to the left hemisphere.

stationary frequency marginal have also been employed to detect pseudo-periodicity in the EEG (Stevenson et al. 2012, Khlif et al. 2013).

Features of pseudo-periodicity in the EEG are useful source of information for seizure detection. Roessgen et al. (1998) outlined a model-based method for the detection of neonatal seizures. The model of EEG generation initially outlined by Lopes Da Silva et al. (1974) was used to form the basis of the detection method (see Fig. 5.7). The model was driven by white Gaussian noise to simulate the presence of non-seizure and a saw-tooth

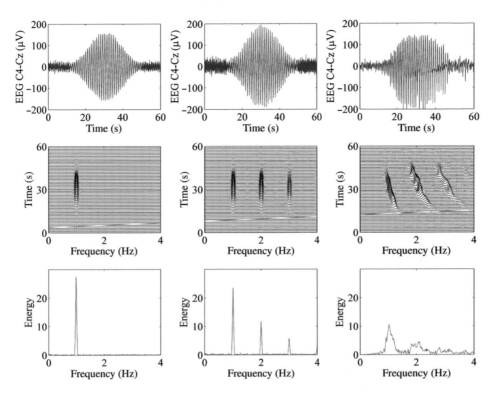

Figure 5.6. The difficulties of using Fourier analysis to detect seizure caused by non-sinusoidal waveforms and pseudo-periodicity. The first column shows a simulated EEG with a purely sinusoidal signal with a constant period of repetition, the second column shows a simulated EEG with a non-sinusoidal signal and the third column shows an epoch of real EEG seizure. Shown from top to bottom are the time domain, joint time–frequency domain and frequency domain representation of a waveform. Note the effective reduction in the peak at around 1 Hz – it is the ratio of this peak to the background or residual level that is typically used to detect periodicity in a signal. The energy is conserved between signals.

waveform to simulate the presence of seizure. The relative energy in the seizure and non-seizure spectrum was estimated directly from an epoch of EEG with Whittle's approximation and used as a detection statistic. Analysis of the quality of fit of autoregressive and Gaussian process models has also been used to generate features (Faul et al. 2007, Greene et al. 2008a).

An elegant feature for seizure detection was proposed by Altenburg et al. (2003). This feature, the synchronisation likelihood, provides an estimate of the mutual information or synchronisation between EEG channels. As neonatal seizures tend to generalise on the EEG an increase in the synchronization of the EEG between channels can be used to detect seizures. This is one of the few features that take into account the multiple-channel nature of the EEG recording.

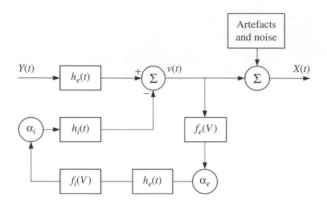

Figure 5.7. A model of EEG generation. The input $Y(t)$ is typically assumed to be white Gaussian noise, $X(t)$ is the resultant EEG, transfer functions $h(t)$ are typically decaying exponentials, functions $f(V)$ are nonlinearities and subscript indices e and i denote excitatory and inhibitory influences respectively.

More generic features have also been used to support seizure detection. Measures of signal amplitude such as the root mean square of the EEG, the mean of the absolute value of the EEG or the output of the nonlinear energy operator provide some measures of discrimination between seizure and non-seizure epochs. The main problem with amplitude is that several normal, abnormal and artefactual patterns in the EEG also have increased amplitude (see Fig. 5.3). Some of these problems can be overcome by pre-filtering the EEG in specific frequency bands such as delta or theta, which reflect a general increase in amplitude while rejecting several artefactual characteristics generated by muscle, movement, ECG or respiration. This filtering can be performed in the frequency (Fourier analysis) or scale domains (Wavelet analysis). By estimating power in a frequency band, the amplitude and frequency content of a signal can be analysed concurrently. This is the case in the a-EEG, which is commonly used to assist seizure detection in the NICU.

Several other features such as Hjorth parameters, line length, fractal dimension and spectral entropy and features extracted from a joint time-frequency representation have all been used for neonatal seizure detection (Greene et al. 2008a, Motamedi-Fakhr et al. 2014).

Information from other physiological signals can also provide useful information when attempting to determine the presence of seizure. Measures of heart rate variability have been shown to be able to identify seizure (Malarvili and Mesbah 2009, Doyle et al. 2010). The recording of respiration and the ECG can be used to reject periods of EEG repetition that may be detected as seizure but are in fact artefacts. Methods such as correlation analysis or independent component analysis have been used for this task and have resulted in improved NSDA accuracy (DeVos et al. 2011).

CLASSIFICATION

There is currently no perfect single feature for the identification of EEG seizures; the patterns within the EEG are too complex and the variability between neonates is too high for a simple solution. A classifier is a mathematical construct that can combine many features to improve the detection of seizures. Classifiers that have been used in NSDAs include decision trees with heuristically chosen thresholds, artificial neural networks, linear discriminant analysis, Gaussian mixture models and support vector machines (Aarabi et al. 2006, Greene 2008b, Mitra et al. 2009, Thomas et al. 2010, Temko et al. 2011a). The concept of a classifier is relatively simple, although its implementation can be more complex. The core components of a classifier are the feature space and the decision boundary; an example is shown in Figure 5.2. The feature space is a multidimensional space (the dimension is the number of features) that spans the possible values for the features (seizure and non-seizure). The decision boundary provides an efficient separation of the feature space into regions of seizure and non-seizure. Each classifier uses a different form of decision boundary and this decision boundary must be estimated or trained using a small feature set containing examples from seizure and non-seizure EEG epochs. Once the decision boundary is estimated via a training process, features of an incoming epoch of EEG can be assigned as seizure or non-seizure, depending on the region it falls into.

The classifier output can essentially be considered as a combination of features that result in a super-feature optimised for the detection of seizure. The disadvantage of such a black box approach is that the exact mechanics of the combination is often difficult to relate to EEG activity.

POST-PROCESSING

The post-processing stage converts the classifier outputs into a final decision. Post-processing stages can include methods to combine decisions from multiple EEG channels, smoothing filtering outputs (mean or median filters) and collaring (a process of extending the detection). Spatial or temporal weighting functions can also be applied based on *a priori* knowledge of neonatal seizures (Temko et al. 2012a, Temko et al. 2012b). Post-processing can also include secondary decision stages that take into account the results of separate EEG classification systems such as artefact detection or EEG grading (Stevenson et al. 2013, Stevenson et al. 2014). The visualisation of the NSDA output is also performed at this stage.

Performance assessment

Assessing the performance of an NSDA and comparing the performance of NSDAs from different research groups are not trivial tasks. There is an inherent trade-off in any NSDA between the ability of an NSDA to recognise seizure and its ability to recognise non-seizure. The inherent imbalance in the amount of seizure with respect to non-seizure in a recording and the various requirements of a typical end user require the use of a number of performance measures to define the quality of an NSDA (see Fig. 5.8). The performance assessment must also be performed with a clear separation between training and testing data, particularly when multiple features are used, or when multiple thresholds are set, within the NSDA.

Ideally, the NSDA annotation of an EEG recording should be compared directly with the gold standard, that is, the annotation of the human expert. A second-by-second comparison (integral-overlap comparison; Wilson et al. 2003; see Fig. 5.9) will result

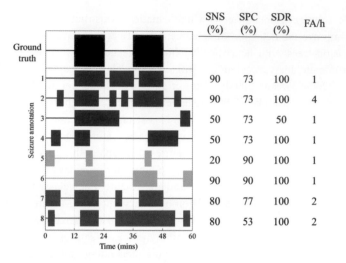

Figure 5.8. The comparison of several simulated neonatal seizure detection algorithm (NSDA) anno-tations to the ground truth – human expert annotation. NSDA annotation 6 best matches the ground truth. SNS, temporal sensitivity; SPC, temporal specificity; SDR, event-based sensitivity (seizure detection rate); FA/h, false positives (alarms) per hour.

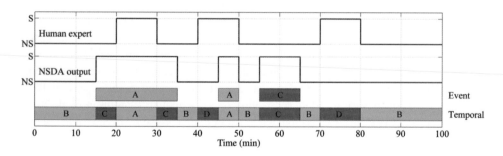

Figure 5.9. Comparing the annotations of the human expert and neonatal seizure detection algorithm (NSDA) in a temporal and event-based framework. A, true positive; B, true negative; C, false positive; D, false negative. An event-based assessment results in a sensitivity of 66.6% (2/3 events) and 0.6 false positives per hour (1 false positive in 100 minutes). A temporal assessment results in a sensitivity of 50% (15/30 minutes) and a specificity of 71.4% (50/70 minutes).

in measures of sensitivity and specificity, which can be used to generate receiver opera-tor characteristics (ROC). The ROC is a useful measure of performance as it can visu-alise the sensitivity and specificity of an NSDA over a range of detection thresholds. This is particularly useful as an NSDA implemented to assist review of an EEG by a neurophysiologist may require high sensitivity while an NSDA implemented as a decision support device in the NICU may require high specificity. Measures of sensitivity and specificity can be, however, biased towards the detection of long duration seizures. They can also be unevenly affected when there is an imbalance in the prevalence of seizure and non-seizure, which is typically 1:100 in long duration neonatal EEG recordings. This means that correct re-classification of short periods of seizure will increase the sensitivity more than the corresponding decrease in specificity; this is particularly relevant for NSDAs that use collaring as a post-processing stage. These biases can be partially overcome by including the results from an event-based comparison (any overlap comparison; Wilson et al. 2003; see Fig. 5.9), resulting in a seizure detection rate and a number of false alarms per hour. Event-based assessment is, however, only an assessment of seizure events as non-seizure cannot be construed as an event and collaring may reduce the number of false alarms. Further performance metrics such as the number of seizure detections per annotated seizure, precision and recall can be used to support a claim of NSDA performance.

While the combination of these metrics provides useful information when comparing the NSDA output to the annotation of the human expert (the gold standard), such measures do not provide information on the potential improvements in the clinical recognition of seizures due to the translation of an NSDA to the clinical setting. In other words, we do not know the level of NSDA performance that is required to see a significant improvement in the clinical recognition of seizures in the NICU. This requires alternate measures that can be compared to clinical recognition (as real time annotation of the EEG is not performed in the NICU). Measures such as the time of seizure onset (initially and after anticonvulsant administration in the case of recurrent seizures) or the number of anticonvulsants administered in the presence of EEG-confirmed seizures provide the possibility of reliably comparing clinical recognition of seizure with and without the support of an NSDA.

Comparing NSDAs from different research groups based on these various performance values is complicated by significant differences in the data sets used to develop each algorithm. The majority of NSDAs are developed on data from a limited number of short, high-quality recordings that are attended by the EEG technologist. While this amount of data is sufficient to show the potential efficacy of some NSDAs, it is not sufficient to estimate the performance for real-world application, which will be on long duration monitoring in excess of 72 hours with minimal, if any, involvement from the EEG technologist. The development of public domain long duration data sets can solve the majority of problems associated with NSDA comparison.

The reported accuracy of several NSDAs and the data sets used in development are shown in Table 5.1.

Challenges
There are three current challenges for NSDAs: their performance is still below the level of inter-observer agreement between visual interpretation of the neonatal EEG, the applicability of an NSDA in the NICU is unknown and the robustness of the NSDA across a range of recording environments is unknown.

TABLE 5.1
A summary of NSDAs and their performance

Algorithm	Continued development	Method	DB length h (N)	S:NS Dur	NS neonates	AUC	SNS (%)	SPC (%)	SDR (%)	FA/h (N/h)
Lui et al. 1992		Correlation based	1.0 (14)	1 : 1	Yes		84	98		
Gotman et al. 1997a		Spectrum based	282 (55)		No				71	1.7
	Gotman et al. 1997b	Validation	237 (54)		Yes				66	2.3
Roessgen et al. 1998		EEG modelling	2.3 (2)	1 : 42.1	No		89	73	97	
	Celka et al. 2001	Singular spectrum analysis	0.5 (4)	1 : 1	No		93	96		
	Hassanpour et al. 2004	Low and high frequency signatures	0.8 (5)		No		100	93		
	Mesbah et al. 2012	EEG and HRV	2.8 (8)	1 : 5.1	No		95	94		
	Boashash et al. 2012	Time-frequency features	0.4 (9)	1 : 1	No		98	94		
	Khlif et al. 2013	Time-frequency matched filter	13.9	1 : 2.3			82	97	85	0.36
Altenburg et al. 2003		Spatial synchronization (excl. artefact)	0.3 (21)	1 : 1	No		85	75		
	Smit et al. 2004	Spatial synchronization (incl. artefact)	10.4 (19)		No		66	90		
Navakatikyan et al. 2006		Wave sequence analysis	24 (55)	1 : 6.8	Yes		83	87	90	2
	Lawrence et al. 2009	Clinical validation	2708 (40)		Yes				55	0.09

Reference	Method	DB (Dur)	S : NS		AUC	SNS	SPC	SDR	FA/h
Aarabi et al. 2006	Multistage system	5.1 (6)	1 : 3.2	No		91	95	100	1.17
Aarabi et al. 2007	Multistage knowledge-based system	110 (10)	1 : 5.9	No		74	86	80	1.55
Karayiannis et al. 2006	Pseudo-sinusoidal	2 (15)	1 : 1	No		84	80		
Mitra et al. 2009	Multistage system	120 (76)	1 : 11.0	Yes				80	0.78
Greene et al. 2007	EEG + ECG features	154 (10)	1 : 3.7	No	0.77	72	71	81	3.15
Greene et al. 2008b	Classification architectures	252 (17)	1 : 9.6	No	0.82	33	96	81	
Thomas et al. 2010	Gaussian mixtures	268 (17)	1 : 5.9	No	0.96			79	0.5
Temko et al. 2011a/b	Support vector machines	268 (17)	1 : 5.9	No	0.96	90	90	89	1
Temko et al. 2012a	Spatial weighting	268 (17)	1 : 5.9	No	0.97			87	0.5
Temko et al. 2012b	Temporal weighting	816 (18)	1 : 10.9	No	0.97	70		65	0.24
Temko et al. 2013	Adaptive post-processing	2540 (51)		Yes	0.96			71	0.25
Stevenson et al. 2012	Pseudo-periodicity	826 (18)	1 : 11.0	No	0.91	71	93	78	0.97
Deburchgraeve et al. 2008	Spike train + oscillatory detection	218 (26)		Yes				85	0.66
Cherian et al. 2011	Clinical validation	756 (24)	1 : 27.9	No		59		66	0.58
DeVos et al. 2011	Artefact rejection (ICA)	104 (13)		No				87	0.29

(DB, database, S, seizure, NS, non-seizure, Dur, duration, AUC, area under the receiver operator characteristic, SNS, sensitivity, SPC, specificity, SDR, seizure detection rate, FA/h, false alarms per hour)

69

The inter-observer agreement between visual interpretations of the neonatal EEG by human experts is high. A recent study of inter-observer agreement on a large data set of neonatal EEG marked by three international experts resulted in a kappa value of 0.827 (95% CI: 0.769–0.865), a temporal based assessment resulted in a median seizure agreement rate of 83.0% (IQR: 76.6–89.5%) and a median non-seizure agreement rate of 99.7% (IQR: 98.9–99.8%), while an eventbased assessment resulted in a median seizure agreement rate of 83.0% (IQR: 72.9–86.6%) at a median of 0.018 (IQR: 0.000–0.090) disagreements per hour (Stevenson et al. 2015). These values represent the benchmark performance an NSDA should achieve to be comparable with the annotation of the human expert and are currently not met by any NSDA (see Table 5.1). In fact, the decision threshold where the majority of NSDAs performance was evaluated has been overly sensitive.

Current NDSAs, however, may still provide sufficient accuracy to be used in the NICU as a decision support device. The ability of an NSDA to operate universally in the NICU has yet to be thoroughly examined. The stability of NSDA performance due to variations in recording electrodes, montages and impedances as well as EEG machines must be investigated to support a large-scale roll-out of NSDAs. Such a roll-out also requires useful visualisations of the NSDA output for interpretation by the clinician. Several possible visualisations are shown in Figure 5.10, and an important measure of seizure activity, the hourly seizure burden, is shown in Figure 5.11. Only clinical trials can determine if visualisation of the NSDA output can improve the clinical recognition of seizures. One such trial is currently under way in Europe (https://clinicaltrials.gov/ct2/show/NCT02160171).

Future prospects

Advances in computing and networking within NICUs mean that the implementation of an NSDA does not have to be restricted to the cot-side EEG machine. Most modern NICUs are now fully networked and it is possible to stream EEG data in real time to a central server for processing (see Fig. 5.12). Central servers have the advantage of a large data handling capacity with the ability to allow real-time processing of ano-nymised physiological data that EEG experts can log into and review in real time, irrespective of location. This central server can also run the NSDA and then forward both the EEG data and the NSDA output to the human expert for review. The resultant annotation can then be sent back to the NICU for display on the EEG machine. The link between the external server and the neurophysiologist will become more diffuse over time as the detection performance of the NSDA improves. There is also potential for additional analyses of the EEG and other physiological signals to be performed on the external server.

This method has several advantages such as the facility to provide continuous automated seizure detection support for several hospitals, the capability to store large amounts of data for review by several experts and the ability to provide access to continuous EEG expertise to geographically remote sites.

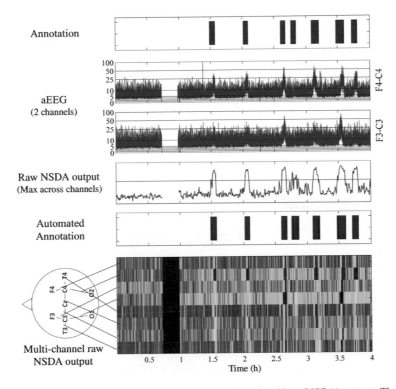

Figure 5.10. Visualisation of the neonatal seizure detection algorithm (NSDA) output. The single-channel NSDA output can be considered as an a-EEG type output that has been optimised to represent the presence of seizure rather than the amplitude of the EEG. If spatial information is required, then a multichannel visualisation permits localisation of the seizure; the example shows several generalised seizures with predominate activity on the occipital region of the right hemisphere.

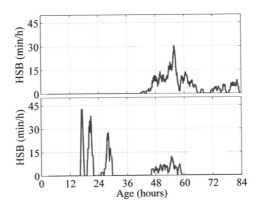

Figure 5.11. The hourly seizure burden (HSB) trend estimated from the seizure annotations of two neonates. This trend, which is based on the neonatal seizure detection algorithm output, provides useful information to the clinician on the time course of seizures in a neonate.

71

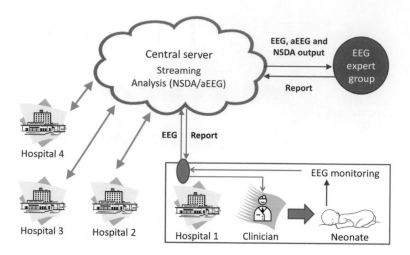

Figure 5.12. The information flow of EEG interpretation from the neonate to the clinician in a streaming-based assessment of neonatal seizures. NSDA, neonatal seizure detection algorithm.

Conclusion

Neonatal seizure detection in the NICU is challenging and 24-hour expert surveillance is required. Monitoring the neonatal EEG using the a-EEG has filled the gap for many years but it is now clear that a-EEG has limitations for neonatal seizure detection. Multichannel EEG monitoring is the gold standard for the accurate detection of all neonatal seizures but caregivers at the cot-side rarely have the expertise to interpret the EEG. We believe that efforts should be focused on providing help for cot-side caregivers to interpret the neonatal EEG and aid in decision support. Automated neonatal seizure detection research is advancing at a considerable pace but efforts have still not been made to incorporate it into routine clinical practice. Clearly there is an unmet clinical need for this type of technology in the NICU and clinical validation is required before any algorithm can be used routinely. An algorithm that reaches the required performance standards as a research tool may not be entirely suitable for routine clinical use. User interface design for decision support in the NICU will also need considerable effort in the future in order to ensure widespread adoption of this technology.

REFERENCES

Aarabi A, Grebe R, Wallois F (2007) A multistage knowledge-based system for EEG seizure detection in newborn infants. *Clin Neurophysiol* 118 (12): 2781–2797. doi: http://dx.doi.org/10.1016/j.clinph.2007.08.012.

Aarabi A, Wallois F, Grebe R (2006) Automated neonatal seizure detection: A multistage classification system through feature selection based on relevance and redundancy analysis. *Clin Neurophysiol* 117 (2): 328–340. doi: http://dx.doi.org/10.1016/j.clinph.2005.10.006.

Altenburg J, Vermeulen RJ, Strijers RL, Fetter WP, Stam CJ (2003) Seizure detection in the neonatal EEG with synchronization likelihood. *Clin Neurophysiol* 114 (1): 50–55. PubMed PMID: 12495763. doi: http://dx.doi.org/10.1016/S1388-2457(02)00322-X.

Boylan GB, Stevenson NJ, Vanhatalo S (2013) Monitoring neonatal seizures. *Semin Fetal Neonatal Med* 18: 202–208. doi: http://dx.doi.org/10.1016/j.siny.2013.04.004.

Celka P, Colditz P (2002) A computer-aided detection of EEG seizures in infants: A singular-spectrum approach and performance comparison. *IEEE T Bio-med Eng* 49 (5): 455–462. doi: http://dx.doi.org/10.1109/10.995684.

Cherian PJ, Deburchgraeve W, Swarte RM, et al. (2011) Validation of a new automated neonatal seizure detection system: A clinician's perspective. *Clin Neurophysiol* 122 (8): 1490–1499. doi: http://dx.doi.org/10.1016/j.clinph.2011.01.043.

Clancy RR, Legido A (1987). The exact ictal and interictal duration of electroencephalographic neonatal seizures. *Epilepsia* 28: 537–541. doi: http://dx.doi.org/10.1111/j.1528-1157.1987.tb03685.x.

De Vos M, Deburchgraeve W, Cherian PJ (2011) Automated artifact removal as preprocessing refines neonatal seizure detection. *Clin Neurophysiol* 122 (12): 2345–2354. doi: http://dx.doi.org/10.1016/j.clinph.2011.04.026.

Deburchgraeve W, Cherian PJ, De Vos M (2008) Automated neonatal seizure detection mimicking a human observer reading EEG. *Clin Neurophysiol* 119 (11): 2447–2454. doi: http://dx.doi.org/10.1016/j.clinph.2008.07.281.

Doyle OM, Temko A, Marnane W, Lightbody G, Boylan GB (2010) Heart rate based automatic seizure detection in the newborn. *Med Eng Phys* 32: 829–839. doi: http://dx.doi.org/10.1016/j.medengphy.2010.05.010.

Faul S, Gregorcic G, Boylan G, Marnane W, Lightbody G, Connolly S (2007) Gaussian process modeling of EEG for the detection of neonatal seizures. *IEEE T Bio-med Eng,* 54: 2151–2162, doi: http://dx.doi.org/10.1109/TBME.2007.895745.

Gotman J, Flanagan D, Rosenblatt B, Bye A, Mizrahi EM (1997a) Evaluation of an automatic seizure detection method for the newborn EEG. *Electroencephalogr Clin Neurophysiol* 103 (3): 363–369. doi: http://dx.doi.org/10.1016/S0013-4694(97)00005-2.

Gotman J, Flanagan D, Zhang J, Rosenblatt B (1997b) Automatic seizure detection in the newborn: Methods and initial evaluation. *Electroencephalogr Clin Neurophysiol* 103 (3): 356–362. doi: http://dx.doi.org/10.1016/S0013-4694(97)00003-9.

Greene BR, Faul S, Marnane WP, Lightbody G, Korotchikova I, Boylan GB (2008a) A comparison of quantitative EEG features for neonatal seizure detection. *Clin Neurophysiol* 119 (6): 1248–1261. doi: http://dx.doi.org/10.1016/j.clinph.2008.02.001.

Greene BR, Marnane WP, Lightbody G, Reilly RB, Boylan GB (2008b) Classifier models and architectures for EEG-based neonatal seizure detection. *Physiol Meas* 29 (10): 1157–1178. doi: http://dx.doi.org/10.1088/0967-3334/29/10/002.

Hassanpour H, Mesbah M, Boashash B (2004) Time-frequency based newborn EEG seizure detection using low and high frequency signatures. *Physiol Meas* 25 (4): 935–944. doi: http://dx.doi.org/10.1088/0967-3334/25/4/012.

Karayiannis NB, Mukherjee A, Glover JR (2006) Detection of pseudosinusoidal epileptic seizure segments in the neonatal EEG by cascading a rule-based algorithm with a neural network. *IEEE T Bio-med Eng* 53 (4): 633–641. doi: http://dx.doi.org/10.1109/TBME.2006.870249.

Khlif MS, Colditz PB, Boashash B (2013) Effective implementation of time-frequency matched filter with adapted pre and postprocessing for data-dependent detection of newborn seizures. *Med Eng Phys* 35 (12): 1762–1769. doi: http://dx.doi.org/10.1016/j.medengphy.2013.07.005.

Lawrence R, Mathur A, Nguyen The Tich S, Zempel J, Inder T (2009) A pilot study of continuous limited-channel a-EEG in term infants with encephalopathy. *J Pediatr* 154 (6): 835–841.e1. doi: http://dx.doi.org/10.1016/j.jpeds.2009.01.002.

Liu A, Hahn JS, Heldt GP, Coen RW (1992) Detection of neonatal seizures through computerized EEG analysis. *Electroencephalogr Clin Neurophysiol* 82 (1): 30–37. doi: http://dx.doi.org/10.1016/0013-4694(92)90179-L.

Lopes Da Silva FH, Hoeks A, Smits H, Zetterberg LH (1974) Model of brain rhythmic activity: The alpha-rhythm of the thalamus. *Kybernetik* 15: 27–37. doi: http://dx.doi.org/10.1007/BF00270757.

Low E, Mathieson SR, Stevenson NJ, et al. (2014) Early postnatal EEG features of perinatal arterial ischaemic stroke with seizures. *PLoS ONE* 9: e100973. doi: 10.1371/journal.pone.0100973. doi: http://dx.doi.org/10.1371/journal.pone.0100973.

Lynch NE, Stevenson NJ, Livingstone V, Murphy BP, Rennie JM, Boylan GB (2012) The temporal evolution of electrographic seizure burden in neonatal hypoxic ischemic encephalopathy. *Epilepsia* 53: 549–557. doi: http://dx.doi.org/10.1111/j.1528-1167.2011.03401.x.

Lynch NE, Stevenson NJ, Livingstone V, Mathieson S, Murphy BP, Rennie JM, Boylan GB (2015) The temporal characteristics of seizures in neonatal hypoxic ischemic encephalopathy treated with hypothermia. *Seizure* 33: 60–65, http://dx.doi.org/10.1016/j.seizure.2015.10.007.

Malarvili MB, Mesbah M (2009) Newborn seizure detection based on heart rate variability. *IEEE T Bio-Med Eng* 56: 2594–2603. doi: http://dx.doi.org/10.1109/TBME.2009.2026908.

Maynard D, Prior PF, Scott DF (1969) Device for continuous monitoring of cerebral activity in resuscitated patients. *Br Med J* 4: 545–546. doi: http://dx.doi.org/10.1136/bmj.4.5682.545-a.

Mitra J, Glover JR, Ktonas PY, et al. (2009) A multistage system for the automated detection of epileptic seizures in neonatal electroencephalography. *J Clin Neurophysiol* 26 (4): 218–226. doi: http://dx.doi.org/10.1097/WNP.0b013e3181b2f29d.

Motamedi-Fakhr S, Moshrefi-Torbati M, Hill M, Hill CM, White PR (2014) Signal processing techniques applied to human sleep EEG signals – A review. *Biomed Signal Proces* 10: 21–33. doi: http://dx.doi.org/10.1016/j.bspc.2013.12.003.

Murray DM, Boylan GB, Ali I, Ryan CA, Murphy BP, Connolly S (2008) Defining the gap between electrographic seizure burden, clinical expression and staff recognition of neonatal seizures. *Arch Dis Child Fetal Neonatal Ed* 93 (3): F187–F191. doi: http://dx.doi.org/10.1136/adc.2005.086314.

Navakatikyan MA, Colditz PB, Burke CJ, Inder TE, Richmond J, Williams CE (2006) Seizure detection algorithm for neonates based on wave-sequence analysis. *Clin Neurophysiol* 117 (6): 1190–1203. doi: http://dx.doi.org/10.1016/j.clinph.2006.02.016.

Notley SV, Elliot SJ (2003) Efficient estimation of a time-varying dimension parameter and its application to EEG analysis. *IEEE T Bio-med Eng* 50: 594–602.

Quigg M, Leiner D (2009) Engineering aspects of the quantified amplitude-integrated electroencephalogram in neonatal cerebral monitoring. *J Clin Neurophysiol* 26: 145–149. doi: http://dx.doi.org/10.1097/WNP.0b013e3181a18711.

Roessgen M, Zoubir AM, Boashash B (1998) Seizure detection of newborn EEG using a model-based approach. *IEEE T Bio-med Eng* 45 (6): 673–685. doi: http://dx.doi.org/10.1109/10.678601.

Shah DK, Mackay MT, Lavery S, et al. (2008) Accuracy of bedside electroencephalographic monitoring in comparison with simultaneous continuous conventional electroencephalography for seizure detection in term infants. *Pediatrics* 121 (6): 1146–1154. doi: http://dx.doi.org/10.1542/peds.2007-1839.

Shellhaas RA, Soaita AI, Clancy RR (2007) Sensitivity of amplitude-integrated electroencephalography for neonatal seizure detection. *Pediatrics* 120 (4): 770–777. doi: http://dx.doi.org/10.1542/peds.2007-0514.

Smit LS, Vermeulen RJ, Fetter WP, Strijers RL, Stam CJ (2004) Neonatal seizure monitoring using nonlinear EEG analysis. *Neuropediatrics* 35 (6): 329–335. doi: http://dx.doi.org/10.1055/s-2004-830367.

Stevenson NJ, Clancy RR, Vanhatalo S, Rosén I, Boylan GB (2015) Inter-observer agreement for neonatal seizure detection using multi-channel EEG. *Ann Clin Transl Neurol* 2 (11): 1002–1011. doi: http://dx.doi.org/10.1002/acn3.249; 10 pages.

Stevenson NJ, Korotchikova I, Temko A, Lightbody G, Marnane WP, Boylan GB (2013) An automated system for grading EEG abnormalities in term neonates with hypoxic ischaemic encephalopathy, *Ann Biomed Eng* 41: 775–785. doi: http://dx.doi.org/10.1007/s10439-012-0710-5.

Stevenson NJ, O'Toole JM, Korotchikova I, Boylan GB (2014) Artefact detection in neonatal EEG. *Proc. 36th Annual International Conference of the IEEE EMBS* 99: 926–929. doi: http://dx.doi.org/10.1109/embc.2014.6943743.

Stevenson NJ, O'Toole JM, Rankine LJ, Boylan GB, Boashash B (2012) A nonparametric feature for neonatal EEG seizure detection based on a representation of pseudo-periodicity. *Med Eng Phys* 34 (4): 437–446. doi: http://dx.doi.org/10.1016/j.medengphy.2011.08.001.

Temko A, Boylan G, Marnane W, Lightbody G (2013) Robust neonatal EEG seizure detection through adaptive background modeling. *Int J Neural Syst* 23 (4): 1350018. doi: 10.1142/S0129065713500184. doi: http://dx.doi.org/10.1142/S0129065713500184.

Temko A, Lightbody G, Thomas EM, Boylan GB, Marnane W (2012a) Instantaneous measure of EEG channel importance for improved patient-adaptive neonatal seizure detection. *IEEE T Bio-med Eng* 59 (3): 717–727. doi: http://dx.doi.org/10.1109/TBME.2011.2178411.

Temko A, Stevenson N, Marnane W, Boylan G, Lightbody G (2012b) Inclusion of temporal priors for automated neonatal EEG classification. *J Neural Eng* 9 (4): 046002. doi: 10.1088/1741-2560/9/4/046002. doi: http://dx.doi.org/10.1088/1741-2560/9/4/046002.

Temko A, Thomas E, Marnane W, Lightbody G, Boylan G (2011a) EEG-based neonatal seizure detection with Support Vector Machines. *Clin Neurophysiol* 122 (3): 464–473. doi: http://dx.doi.org/10.1016/j.clinph.2010.06.034.

Temko A, Thomas E, Marnane W, Lightbody G, Boylan GB (2011b) Performance assessment for EEG-based neonatal seizure detectors. *Clin Neurophysiol* 122 (3): 474–482. doi: http://dx.doi.org/10.1016/j.clinph.2010.06.035.

Thomas EM, Temko A, Lightbody G, Marnane WP, Boylan GB (2010) Gaussian mixture models for classification of neonatal seizures using EEG. *Physiol Meas* 31 (7): 1047–1064. doi: http://dx.doi.org/10.1088/0967-3334/31/7/013.

Uria-Avellanal C, Marlow N, Rennie JM (2013) Outcome following neonatal seizures. *Semin Fetal Neonatal Med* 224–232. doi: http://dx.doi.org/10.1016/j.siny.2013.01.002.

Vasudevan C, Levene M (2013) Epidemiology and aetiology of neonatal seizures. *Semin Fetal Neonatal Med* 18: 185–191. doi: http://dx.doi.org/10.1016/j.siny.2013.05.008.

Wilson SB, Scheuer ML, Plummer C, Young B, Pacia S (2003) Seizure detection: correlation of human experts. *Clin Neurophysiol* 114: 2156–2164.

6
NEUROIMAGING IN NEONATAL SEIZURES

Camilo Jaimes, Christos Papadelis and P. Ellen Grant

The primary goal of neuroimaging is to help determine the etiology of neonatal seizures, which in turn helps to guide clinical management and prognosis. Neuroimaging serves as a complement to the clinical examination, electroencepahalography (EEG) evaluation and laboratory investigations, and must be interpreted in this context.

The most common neuroimaging modalities used in the evaluation of neonatal seizures are ultrasound and magnetic resonance imaging (MRI). Ultrasound is a non-invasive, inexpensive, bedside screening tool typically used to search for hemorrhage or hydrocephalus when a neonate, especially a preterm or unstable neonate, presents with seizures. Computed tomography (CT) may be performed to provide an urgent assessment when there is concern for fractures or hemorrhage. Otherwise, CT is rarely performed unless MRI is unavailable because of the exposure to ionizing radiation as well as the lower sensitivity and specificity for diagnosing brain disorders associated with seizures compared to MRI. MRI is the modality of choice when seizures are identified because of the multiple contrast mechanisms and rich physiological information it provides. In most institutions, neonatal MRI can be performed without sedation or anesthesia, making it an insignificant risk study. In this chapter, we will provide an overview of ultrasound and MRI technologies as well as imaging findings in the most common disorders associated with neonatal seizures. We conclude with a brief discussion on the emerging role of near infrared spectroscopy (NIRS) and magnetoencephalography (MEG).

Ultrasound

The newborn infant's brain is especially well suited for ultrasound imaging as the small head size allows adequate penetration of sound waves to deep structures and the open fontanels and sutures provide acoustic windows. Ultrasound has high sensitivity for the detection of parenchymal hemorrhage (Raets et al. 2015) and can also provide indirect physiological information on cerebral blood flow by evaluation of resistive indices with Doppler imaging. Normal neonatal resistive indices vary between 0.6 and 0.8 (Lowe and Bailey 2011). In states associated with hyperperfusion, the resistive index decreases as a result of increased diastolic flow. Color Doppler can also be used to establish the patency of the major intracranial arteries, the deep venous system and the dural venous sinuses

(Lowe and Bailey 2011). Head ultrasound has high sensitivity for abnormalities in newborn infants with seizures. A recent study reported that cranial ultrasound demonstrated abnormalities in close to 90% of term newborn infants with seizures (Weeke et al. 2015). However, MRI was often needed to determine the nature of the findings or the full extent of abnormality, with MRI contributing additional information in 40% of cases and demonstrating findings not apparent in ultrasound in 12% of cases (Weeke et al. 2015). Thus, although ultrasound can serve as a useful bedside screening tool, MRI is still required for a complete assessment.

Magnetic resonance imaging

By virtue of its multiple types of image contrast, multiplanar capabilities, and lack of ionizing radiation, MRI is the modality of choice to examine neonates with suspected brain pathology (Barkovich et al. 1988, Girard and Raybaud 2011). In addition to anatomical information, various sequences can be used to assess microstructure, metabolism, vascular patency, and perfusion, providing a comprehensive evaluation of the brain (Izbudak and Grant 2011). In clinical practice, MRI is often used to characterize abnormalities detected on ultrasound or to exclude sonographically occult pathology in a newborn infant with a normal head ultrasound (Epelman et al. 2012). It can also be used as a first-line modality in patients with high clinical suspicion of a brain abnormality who are stable for transport to the MRI department. Sedation is rarely required in neonates; with appropriate preparation neonates can typically be imaged after a feed, during natural sleep with vacuum pillows to reduce head movements (van Wezel-Meijler et al. 2009).

MRI at 3.0 tesla (3T) is preferred as 3T results in a near twofold increase in signal to noise ratio compared to 1.5T, which can be used to increase spatial resolution and/or contrast to noise and/or to decrease scan times (Dahmoush et al. 2012). Better anatomic detail is advantageous when imaging the small structures of newborn infants and for characterization of subtle abnormalities such as focal cortical dysplasias (FCD) (Knake et al. 2005, Dahmoush et al. 2012). Magnetic resonance spectroscopy (MRS) as well as magnetic resonance angiography, susceptibility, blood-oxygen-level-dependent, and perfusion imaging with arterial spin labeling (ASL) also benefit from increased field strength (Gruetter et al. 1998, Franke et al. 2000, Haacke et al. 2009, Malamateniou et al. 2009, Dahmoush et al. 2012, Nowinski et al. 2013).

Imaging findings in common causes of neonatal seizures

Neonatal brains appear quite different from mature brains; therefore, it is important to be familiar with the appearance of the normal neonatal brain (Fig. 6.1). The broad categories of abnormalities that should be considered when imaging a neonate with seizures are cerebrovascular injury, trauma, infection, inborn errors of metabolism (IEMs), cerebral dysgenesis and phakomatoses associated with early seizures. Timing of presentation helps prioritize the differential diagnosis (Table 6.1; Sujansky and Conradi 1995, Miller et al. 1998, Volpe 2008, Greiner et al. 2012). Also note that hyperperfusion with or without cortical/subcortical decreases in apparent diffusion coefficient (ADC) can be a consequence, not a cause of persistent seizure activity. Finally, MRI may be normal in neonatal electrolyte

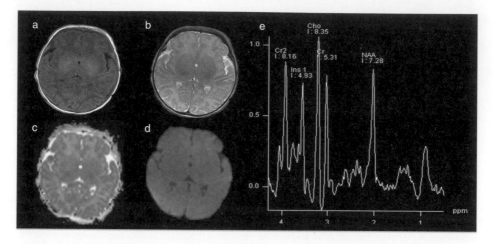

Figure 6.1. Normal brain MRI in a three-day-old term newborn infant. The MRI was obtained because of increased irritability and did not show any abnormalities. Symptoms resolved and the infant was normal on clinical follow-up. (a) Axial T1-weighted MRI demonstrates hypointense signal of the white matter with relative hyperintense signal in the cortical gray matter and deep gray nuclei. Note high signal intensity in the posterior limb of the internal capsule and in the ventrolateral thalamus, reflecting early myelination. (b) Axial T2-weighted image demonstrates normal hyperintense signal of the unmyelinated white matter, with low signal intensity in areas with early myelination. Normal appearance of (c) ADC and (d) DWI, with low signal intensity in the posterior limb of the internal capsule in the ADC map reflecting lower diffusion in myelinated white matter tracts. (e) Normal MRS obtained in the basal ganglia using a TE of 35 ms. The major peaks are labeled including NAA at 2 parts per million (ppm), creatine (Cr) at 3.0 ppm, Choline (Cho) at 3.2 ppm, and myo-inositol (Ins) at 3.5 ppm.

disorders such as hypoparathyroidism and is typically normal in direct drug effects, drug withdrawal, pyridoxine responsive seizures, and KCNQ 2/3 encephalopathy. A summary of abnormal imaging findings that help determine the etiology of neonatal seizures is provided in Table 6.1.

CEREBROVASCULAR INJURY

Brain injury can be arterial, because of focal arterial ischemic strokes or global lack of arterial supply of blood and oxygen (hypoxic ischemic injury) or venous because of venous ischemia, hemorrhage or edema.

Hypoxic ischemic injury

Hypoxic ischemic injury (HII) due to perinatal hypoxia or hypoperfusion is by far the most common cause of neonatal seizures, accounting for 40–60% of seizures in term neonates (Badawi et al. 1998, Pierrat et al. 2005, Vasudevan and Levene 2013, Weeke et al. 2015). Prompt initiation of therapeutic hypothermia significantly improves outcomes in neonates who meet clinical criteria for HII and is now the standard of care (Shankaran et al. 2005, Jacobs et al. 2007). Even with therapeutic hypothermia, seizure incidence is high but initial studies suggest seizures are less likely as hypothermia is induced (Wusthoff et al. 2011a, Low et al. 2012).

TABLE 6.1
Typical timing of presentation for common causes of neonatal seizures

<1 day	1–3 days	3 days–1 week	1–4 weeks	>4 weeks
Hypoxic ischemic encephalopathy IVH in term	Hypoxic ischemic injury arterial ischemic stroke venous thrombosis parenchymal hemorrhage IVH in term IVH in preterm	Arterial ischemic stroke venous thrombosis parenchymal hemorrhage		
SAH	SAH contusion SDH			
Intrauterine infection bacterial meningitis sepsis	Bacterial meningitis sepsis	Herpes simplex virus		
Hypoglycemia Pyridoxine dependency	Hypoparathyroidism glycine encephalopathy urea cycle disturbances pyridoxine dependency	Hypoparathyroidism Metabolic disorders	Metabolic disorders	
	Cerebral malformation	Cerebral malformation	Cerebral malformation	
				Sturge weber syndrome tuberous sclerosis complex
	KCNQ2/3 encephalopathy	KCNQ2/3 encephalopathy		
Drug effect	Drug withdrawal			

IVH: intraventricular haemorrhage; SAH, subarachnoid haemorrhage; SDH: subdural haemorrhage; KCNQ2/3: potassium channel Q2/3.

Sujansky and Conradi 1995, Miller et al. 1998, Volpe 2008, Greiner et al. 2012.

Most patients undergo head ultrasound prior to cooling to exclude hemorrhage. Ultrasound may demonstrate nonspecific findings of brain edema including sulcal swelling, accentuated differentiation of the gray-white matter, and a slit like configuration of the ventricles. Increased echogenicity in the thalami, basal ganglia, and white matter may also be seen (Epelman et al. 2010). Resistive indices on Doppler ultrasound may be decreased because of increased diastolic flow (Stark and Seibert 1994). Hyperemia can be seen on ultrasound, a finding that correlates well with reports of increased flow on NIRS and perfusion MRI (Epelman et al. 2010, Wintermark et al. 2011, Pienaar et al. 2012). Although this hyperemic response may be due to loss of autoregulation, advanced NIRS shows that increased perfusion is associated with increased oxygen consumption arguing that increased perfusion is due to increased neuronal activity (Grant et al. 2009).

MRI is not routinely performed prior to cooling, as there is a narrow 6-hour window to initiate hypothermia. However, the role of MRI to demonstrate and characterize evolving brain injury is well accepted (Izbudak and Grant 2011, Ghei et al. 2014). The pattern of injury varies with the severity and duration of the insult. Short and severe episodes of hypoxia and hypoperfusion preferentially injure areas with high metabolic demand such as the posterior limb internal capsule (PLIC), ventral lateral thalamus, and dorsal lateral putamen (Fig. 6.2; Izbudak and Grant 2011). The corona radiata, perirolandic cortex, hippocampi, midbrain, dorsal brainstem, and superior vermis may also be involved. Injury

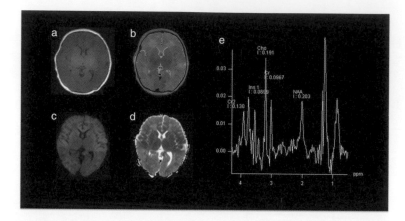

Figure 6.2. Newborn infant admitted to the NICU after prolonged and difficult delivery at home; the infant emerged limp and required resuscitation. The MRI shown was performed at day 5 of life and showed evidence of HII. (a) Axial T1-weighted image shows loss of normal hyperintense signal in the PLIC. (b) Axial T2-weighted image shows diffuse increase in signal in the basal ganglia, and patchy areas of edema involving the cortex and subcortical white matter. (c) DWI and (d) ADC images show areas of decreased diffusion affecting predominantly the deep gray nuclei and the internal capsules. Decreased diffusion also is noted involving portions of the frontal and parietal lobes, including the perirolandic cortices. (e) MRS acquired with a TE of 30 msec shows a large lactate peak (1.3 ppm). This constellation of findings is consistent with a central pattern of hypoxic-ischemic injury, commonly associated with a short and profound insult. The patient developed disseminated intravascular coagulopathy and multiorgan failure, which led to demise.

typically appears first as areas of decreased ADC often within 24 hours, with ADC thought to reach a nadir between the second and third day. Between 7 and 10 days after the insult, the ADC may pseudo-normalize (Boichot et al. 2006, Sagar and Grant 2006). In the first few days, the normal T1 hyperintense signal in the PLIC, ventral lateral thalami, and globus pallidus may be decreased or absent. On T2-weighted imaging, the basal ganglia may appear indistinct with loss of the expected hypointense signal in the PLIC. On MRS, lactate may be evident as a double peak at 1.3 ppm, which inverts on intermediate echo times (135–144 ms). Elevated lactate in the basal ganglia has been reported to correlate with poor long-term outcomes (Hanrahan et al. 1996, Zarifi et al. 2002, Boichot et al. 2006), but these studies predate hypothermia. Some evidence suggests that hypothermia may delay the time course of imaging findings (Chu 2008, Gano et al. 2013), and should be considered when interpreting images. As the injury evolves, abnormally decreased T1 and increased T2 signal evolve to abnormally increased T1 and decreased T2 signals. If the ventral lateral thalamus, PLIC, and ventrolateral putamen are acutely spared, with preferential injury to the cortex and subcortical white matter, disproportionately at the depths of the sulci, less severe but more prolonged HII is hypothesized (Izbudak and Grant 2011, Ghei et al. 2014). As both patterns of HII are often bilateral symmetric, abnormalities may be hard to identify without knowledge of the appearance of the normal neonatal brain.

Arterial ischemic stroke

Perinatal arterial ischemic stroke (PAIS) can be thrombotic or embolic (Raju et al. 2007). PAIS occurs in 1/2,300 to 1/2,500 live births and is the second leading cause of neonatal seizures in term infants (Kirton et al. 2011. Vasudevan and Levene 2013). An area of decreased ADC in a major arterial distribution is the hallmark of PAIS (Sagar and Grant 2006). PAIS also demonstrates increased T2 and decreased T1 signal intensity (Fig. 6.3). A great majority of strokes are unilateral (87%) and involve the middle cerebral artery (MCA) territory (74%). Multifocality has been described in 10% to 30% of infants (Kirton et al. 2011). The pattern of MCA stroke is related to postconceptional age, with term newborn infants demonstrating preferential cortical branch involvement and preterm infants having a higher incidence of lenticulostriate infarcts. Magnetic resonance angiography can help characterize dissection-type vascular injuries or identify a vessel cutoff related to a clot (Lequin et al. 2004). Susceptibility weighted imaging (SWI) sequences can help identify associated hemorrhage within the infarct bed but this is rare in the neonate. Literature suggests that increased cerebral perfusion results in lower venous deoxyhemoglobin concentration in the veins on SWI (Kitamura et al. 2011). ASL techniques also suggest that many ischemic strokes are associated with hyperperfusion at diagnosis (Pienaar et al. 2012, De Vis et al. 2013). The volume of the infarct on diffusion-weighted imaging (DWI) is an important predictor of outcome and correlates with the risk of seizures later in childhood (Wusthoff et al. 2011b).

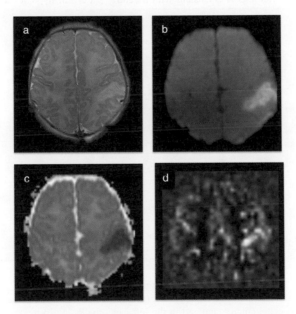

Figure 6.3. Perinatal arterial ischemic stroke in a newborn infant with twitching in the upper extremities, worse in the right arm. (a) Axial T2-weighted image shows increased signal in the left parietal lobe that corresponds with an area of decreased diffusivity on (b) DWI and (c) ADC, consistent with an infarct of distal MCA branches. (d) ASL perfusion image demonstrates elevated perfusion in the infarcted territory. Clinical follow up at two years of age did not reveal any focal neurologic deficits.

Venous infarct and hemorrhage

Preterm infants: In preterm infants, grade III intraventricular hemorrhage and periventricular hemorrhagic infarctions originating in the germinal matrix are the most common causes of seizures in the first few days of life (Volpe 2008). Head ultrasound is often the study of choice, and has demonstrated sensitivity up to 100% and specificity up to 91% for detection of hemorrhage greater than 5 mm, compared to MRI as a criterion standard (Intrapiromkul et al. 2013; Fig. 6.4).

Term infants: Hemorrhagic venous infarcts (Fig. 6.5) in infants born at term are typically caused by dural venous sinus or deep vein thrombosis, as opposed to germinal matrix hemorrhage in preterm infants. Up to two-thirds of patients with thrombosis present with seizures (Raets et al. 2015). The most commonly involved venous structures are the superior sagittal sinus, transverse sinus, internal cerebral veins, and basal vein of Rosenthal. Magnetic resonance venography can show absence of flow in an obstructed vessel. Clots will show increased blooming on SWI. At times, precontrast T1 images can be helpful, with clots appearing as a high T1 signal if greater than approximately three days old. If these results are inconclusive, postcontrast volumetric T1 images can be used to detect clots, which appear as intraluminal filling defects.

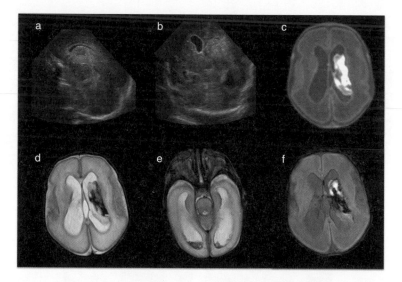

Figure 6.4. Grade III intraventricular hemorrhage in a 26-week old preterm newborn infant that appeared lethargic and had a drop in hemoglobin. (a) Sagittal and (b) coronal head ultrasound images show heterogeneous echogenicity centered in the left caudothalamic groove, consistent with hemorrhage in the germinal matrix. Axial (c) T1- and (d) T2-weighted images demonstrate a clot in the left germinal matrix. Note the smooth appearance of the cortex, which is a normal finding in preterm newborn infants. (e) Axial T2-weighted image at the level of the pons demonstrates blood products layering in the dependent portions of the lateral ventricles and mild hydrocephalus. (f) Susceptibility weighted images re-demonstrates the clot in the left germinal matrix.

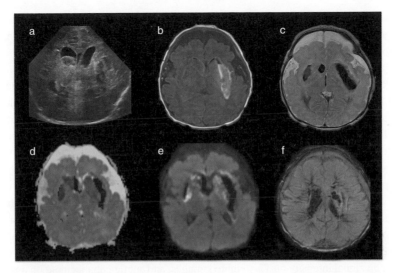

Figure 6.5. Venous infarction in a 1-day-old term neonate with history of preterm rupture of membranes, who developed cyanosis and required resuscitation. Multiple tonic-clonic seizures developed thereafter. (a) Coronal ultrasound image demonstrates heterogeneously increased echogenicity in the basal ganglia bilaterally. There is echogenic material in the lateral ventricles consistent with clot. Enlargement of the lateral ventricles is consistent with hydrocephalus. Axial (b) T1-weighted and (c) T2-weighted images demonstrate blood products in the bilateral basal ganglia, external capsules, and peri-insular regions, greater on the left. Blood also is present in the dependent portion of the lateral ventricles. (d) DWI and (e) ADC show areas of decreased diffusion in the caudate and lentiform nuclei bilaterally. (f) Axial SWI demonstrates low signal in multiple prominent medullary veins throughout both cerebral hemispheres, consistent with deep medullary vein thrombosis. A magnetic resonance venogram showed patent medullary veins, which can occur as the thrombosed vein gets recanalized.

TRAUMA

Although infrequent, parenchymal hemorrhage can be the result of parturitional injury and may be associated with skull fractures, instrumented delivery and/or coagulopathy. ultrasound can demonstrate the presence of most intraparenchymal hematomas, but MRI better characterizes the extent of the injury and can detect associated ischemic changes with DWI (Huisman et al. 2015). Frequently, intraparenchymal hematomas are associated with hemorrhage in other intracranial compartments, including subarachnoid hemorrhage, subdural hemorrhage, and epidural hemorrhage (Pollina et al. 2001). CT may be useful in this context; as compared to ultrasound and MRI, CT better characterizes calvarial fractures.

INFECTION

Perinatal infection

Central nervous system (CNS) infection should be considered in infants with seizures, especially if risk factors are present since up to 10% of neonatal seizures are due to infection (Vasudevan and Levene 2013).

The majority of acquired infections affecting the CNS in newborn infants result from hematogenous seeding of bacteria (Schneider et al. 2011). The most common causative agents include Group B streptococcus, *Escherichia coli*, and coagulase negative *Staphylococcus* (Gaschignard et al. 2011). The definitive diagnosis of CNS infection requires cerebrospinal fluid sampling to isolate the causative organism. However, imaging can identify associated findings and exclude complications such as abscess or hydrocephalus. Head ultrasound can screen ventricular size and detect intraventricular debris, look for large collections, and examine the majority of the brain parenchyma. If abnormalities are identified on ultrasound or clinical concern is high, a contrast enhanced MRI should be obtained (Schneider et al. 2011). The findings on MRI are dependent on the stage of infection. Prominent extra-axial spaces, including the subdural and subarachnoid spaces, are the earliest signs of meningeal inflammation (Schneider et al. 2011). At times, proteinaceous or purulent material fills the cerebrospinal fluid spaces and ventricles, appearing hyperintense on diffusion weighted imaging and fluid attenuated inverted recovery imaging (Fujikawa et al. 2006, Han et al. 2007). As the infection extends to involve the leptomeninges, abnormal contrast enhancement may be seen outlining the inflamed meninges and the ventricular walls. Meningitis can rapidly progress to frank encephalitis, which demonstrates low signal intensity on T1-weighted images, high signal intensity on T2-weighted images, and subtle enhancement on postcontrast images. Encephalitis can evolve to frank necrosis with bright DWI signal and low ADC or cause focal ischemic necrosis indirectly secondary to involvement of arteries or veins.

Viral CNS infections are less common, with the leading etiological agent being *Herpes simplex virus* (HSV). HSV encephalitis usually demonstrates decreased diffusion in cortical and subcortical areas (Okanishi et al. 2015). The pattern of involvement can be variable and can mimic global HII or stroke. As a result, HSV should always be considered in a neonate presenting with seizures and diffusion abnormalities, especially when the typical history for perinatal HII is lacking. As with HII, findings on DWI can precede those on anatomical images, and at times can be the only imaging evidence of infection (Fig. 6.6; Okanishi et al. 2015).

Congenital infection

Infections that occur prenatally can disrupt normal neuronal migration, myelination, and cortical development. Because of the more widespread access to prenatal care and immunizations, rubella and syphilis are now rare. However, congenital cytomegalovirus (CMV) and toxoplasmosis infections still result in significant morbidity. The severity of cerebral abnormalities in congenital CMV infection is related to the timing of the infection (Gaytant et al. 2005, Engman et al. 2008). CMV can affect the germinal zones and therefore early infections can result in microcephaly and severe diffuse polymicrogyria (PMG) whereas later infections result in a milder phenotype (Fink et al. 2010). MRI may also demonstrate edematous white matter with periventricular cysts in the anterior temporal or occipital lobes, parenchymal calcifications, and cerebellar hypoplasia (Barkovich and Lindan 1994, Fink et al. 2010). Congenital toxoplasmosis acquired prior to the 20th postconceptional week results in sequelae that are catastrophic, including microcephaly with severe cognitive impairment, hydrocephalus, micropthalmia, and blindness. Infections that occur later in pregnancy have milder manifestations. Parenchymal calcifications involving the cortex, periventricular white matter, and basal ganglia are readily appreciated on ultrasound and to a lesser degree on MRI (Nickerson et al. 2012).

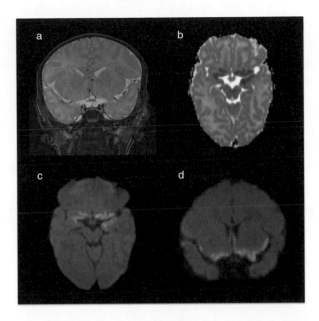

Figure 6.6. Herpes encephalitis in a 12-day-old neonate presenting with poor feeding, lethargy, and a rash. (a) Coronal T2-weighted and other anatomical imaging (not shown) demonstrated no acute abnormalities. (b) Axial ADC: (c) axial DWI and (d) and coronal reformation of the DWI data showed decreased diffusion in the posterior-inferior frontal, anteromedial temporal and insular cortices with involvement of fornices and left subinsular white matter. Clinical follow-up four months after the MRI revealed increased tone in the appendicular skeleton, predominantly in the lower extremities.

Metabolic Abnormalities

Transient

Transient decreases in glucose and sodium have been associated with specific imaging findings noted below. Other transient disturbances such as hypocalcaemia, hypomagnesae-mia, and hypernatremia may cause seizures but have not been associated with specific imaging features to date.

Hypoglycemia: In the first hours and days after delivery, newborn infants are at risk of developing hypoglycemia (Cornblath and Ichord 2000). In most instances, neonatal hypoglycemia is the result of insufficient oral intake to match the increased metabolic demands of extrauterine life. Less frequently, hypoglycemia can be the result of IEMs or endocrine disturbances, such as congenital hyperinsulinism (Deshpande and Ward Platt 2005). DWI provides the best diagnostic clue, demonstrating increased signal intensity preferentially in the occipital and parietal lobes. If the injury is severe or hypoglycemia persists, more significant decreases in ADC develop, indicating a more severe parenchymal injury (Fig. 6.7; Burns et al. 2008). Increased signal on T2-weighted images in the parietal and occipital lobes also can be seen, but it tends to be more subtle than the diffusion abnormalities. In the subacute phase, increased

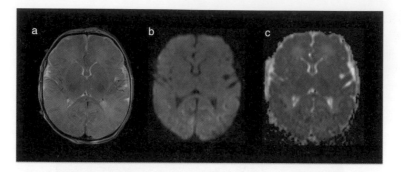

Figure 6.7. A 2-day-old infant with recurrent episodes of severe hypoglycemia (20 mg/dl) who was subsequently diagnosed with congenital hyperinsulinism. At the time of this MRI the newborn infant was encephalopatic. (a) T2-weighted image demonstrates high SI in the white matter in the parietal, temporal, and occipital regions. (b) DWI and (c) ADC show areas of decreased diffusion involving the temporal and occipital regions. These areas resolved on follow-up MRI obtained four days later, and findings were attributed to hypoglycemia. Diazoxide therapy was instituted, which resulted in normoglycemia and resolution of seizures.

T1-signal in areas of the cortex and in the deep gray nuclei can become apparent (Kim et al. 2006).

Hyponatremia: Neonatal seizures due to hyponatremia have been associated with transient elevation in myo-inositol and excitatory amino acids combined with decreased n-acetyl aspartate (NAA) on MRS (Lee et al. 1994). In addition, rapid correction of hyponatremia may result in changes as well: although no neonatal reports were identified, osmotic myelinosis should be considered in the appropriate clinical context if increased T2 signal and decreased diffusion are noted in the central pons with sparing of the corticospinal tract or in the bilateral basal ganglia, thalami, and white matter (Chua et al. 2002).

Inborn errors of metabolism
Defects in enzymatic activity result in metabolic derangements that can involve the CNS. Many of these diseases present as seizures in the neonatal period since maternal metabolism can partly supplement the deficient metabolic pathways of the fetus prior to birth. IEMs that present early in life often have potentially devastating consequences. When an IEM is suspected, an MRI should always be obtained. While many IEMs have nonspecific findings early in the course of disease, a combination of anatomical imaging and MRS can estimate the severity of the disease and guide the clinician. DWI also can be useful in the assessment of metabolic compromise or spongiform change. However, caution must be used when trying to determine the prognosis based on DWI, as regions of decreased diffusion may not represent evolving ischemic injury and may resolve without sequelae especially when the abnormality is limited to the white matter (Sagar and Grant 2006). In such reversible cases, the transient DWI abnormalities are thought to be due to transient metabolic compromise or vacuolar changes (Grant et al. 2001).

Metabolic disorders associated with neonatal epilepsy can be classified into: (1) disturbances in neurotransmitter metabolism, (2) disorders of energy production, and (3) biosynthetic defects (Van Hove and Lohr 2011). The most common disorders with imaging
findings are discussed below. In addition we describe imaging findings in four urea cycle
disorders.

1. *Disturbances in neurotransmitter metabolism:*
   (a) Non-Ketotic Hyperglycinaemia
Defects of the glycine decarboxylase P protein and amino-methyltransferase T protein are
the most common mutations associated with hyperglycinaemia in the newborn infant population (Patay 2011). Glycine elevation occurs in many biological fluids including the brain
parenchyma. Anatomical MRI often reveals diffuse swelling and edema. DWI may demonstrate decreased diffusion in the ventral lateral thalamus and corticospinal tract, similar to
HII. Findings progress rapidly to atrophy with abnormal myelination. MRS can be used to
demonstrate elevated glycine. However, as myo-inositol and glycine both resonate at 3.56
ppm, reliable identification of glycine requires acquisition of MRS with intermediate echo
time TE (135 ms). At this longer TE myo-inositol signal has decayed, and any residual peak
would be reflective of glycine content (Patay 2011).

2. *Disorders of energy production:*
   (a) Pyruvate dehydrogenase deficiency
MRI may be unrevealing, especially early on. Areas of edema demonstrated as swelling and
elevated signal on T2-weighted images have been described, but are usually subtle and
diffuse (van der Knaap et al. 1996). Partial agenesis of the corpus callosum is the most
common structural abnormality but germinolytic cysts and neuronal migration disorders
may be present (Soares-Fernandes et al. 2008, Ah Mew et al. 2011, Sofou et al. 2013). MRS
often provides the most definitive evidence of abnormality by demonstrating persistently
elevated lactate concentrations. A case report also described *in vivo* pyruvate detection as
a singlet at 2.37 ppm (Zand et al. 2003).
   (b) Respiratory chain disorders
Leigh syndrome or subacute necrotizing encephalomyopathy often presents in infancy with
poor suck and motor skills, often with seizures. Imaging findings consist of bilateral sym-
metrical increased T2 signal and decreased ADC involving the basal ganglia, thalami,
sustantia nigra, periaqueductal gray, dorsal pons, and/or dentate nuclei. Increased lactate
may also be present. These lesions may disappear on follow-up or progress to atrophy
(Sofou et al. 2013).
   Alpers syndrome, also known as progressive neuronal degeneration of childhood, is
characterized by regression and intractable epilepsy. When liver disease is also present, it
is called Alpers-Huttenlocher syndrome. In contrast to Leigh syndrome, where basal ganglia
lesions dominate, cortical lesions are more common in Alpers syndrome, although thalamic
lesions have been reported. Lactate may be present and there may be progressive volume
loss particularly in the posterior regions (Smith et al. 1996, Sofou et al. 2013). In severe
cases, neonates may present with diffuse cortical atrophy (de Laveaucoupet et al. 2005).

(c) Menkes disease

Menkes disease is an x-linked disorder of copper metabolism that results in deficient activity of copper-containing enzymes (Leventer et al. 1997). Infants present with seizures and encephalopathy often within the first weeks of life; however, the characteristic phenotypic features, in particular the 'coarse' or 'kinky' hair, may not be apparent until a few months of age (Jacobs et al. 1993, Verrotti et al. 2014). MRI shows patchy increased T2 signals. As the disease progresses, there is severe atrophy of the brain with development of extra-axial hygromas that are prone to bleed. Magnetic resonance angiogram shows tortuosity of the vessels, which appears to be related to progressive volume loss and is more subtle in the neonate (Jacobs et al. 1993, Takahashi et al. 1993).

(d) Sulfite oxidase deficiency

Sulfite oxidase is responsible for degradation of sulfur-containing amino acids. It can present as an isolated enzymatic defect or in association with xanthine oxidase deficiency (molybdenum cofactor deficiency). The enzyme is responsible for degradation of sulfur-containing amino acids. MRI reveals diffuse brain swelling in the acute stages. Areas of decreased diffusion also can be identified, affecting the cortex and deep gray nuclei. As injury progresses it leads to cystic encephalomalacia and diffuse brain atrophy later in infancy (Hoffmann et al. 2007, Girard and Raybaud, 2011).

3. *Biosynthetic defects: brain malformation and dysfunction:*

(a) Peroxisomal disorders

Zellweger syndrome results from near complete absence of peroxisomal function. Brain MRI shows a thick cortex with abnormal gyration, similar to PMG, with preferential involvement of the temporal and parietal lobes. Additional features include delayed myelination, subependymal cysts, malformations of the corpus callosum, incomplete opercularization and brain atrophy (Unay et al. 2005, Weller et al. 2008). MRS shows nonspecific findings reflective of severe and long-standing injury, including decreased NAA in the gray and white matter, decreased myo-inositol in the gray matter and increased lactate and lipids (Groenendaal et al. 2001, Patay 2011).

Neonatal adrenoleukodystrophy is an intermediate severity phenotype in the spectrum of peroxisomal enzymatic defects (Weller et al. 2008). MRI shows abnormalities in neuronal migration and myelination. Abnormal enhancement can be identified at times and is thought to represent active inflammation or demyelination (Weller et al. 2008, Patay 2011). Infantile refsum disease is perhaps the mildest form of peroxisomal enzyme deficiency. MRI shows a symmetric increase in T2 signal in the dentate cerebellar nuclei, periventricular white matter and occasionally the corpus callosum (Dubois et al. 1991, Choksi et al. 2003). Occasionally PMG may be observed.

(b) Neuronal ceroid lipofuscinosis

Neuronal ceroid lipofuscinosis is an autosomal recessive lysosomal storage disorder. Several forms have been described, with the infantile variant being diagnosed in the first weeks to months of life often with symptoms including seizures. Increased T2 signal is present throughout the white matter in all stages of the infantile form most marked in the periventricular region (Vanhanen et al. 1995, Knaap et al. 2005). As the disease progresses diffuse cerebral greater than cerebellar atrophy develops (Vanhanen et al. 1994). The thalami also develop a progressively hypointense signal on T2-weighted images, followed by the other deep gray nuclei (Vanhanen et al. 1994).

4. *Urea cycle disorders:*
Urea cycle enzymatic defects impair the ability of the organism to excrete ammonia. The most common mutations presenting in early neonatal life are ornithine transcarbamylase deficiency, carbamoyl phosphate synthase, and citrulinemia (Patay 2011). Elevated levels of ammonia exert direct toxicity in the CNS, and also lead to an imbalance between excitatory (glutamate) and inhibitory (gamma aminobutiric acid) neurotransmitters (Patay 2011). The deleterious effects of ammonia result in diffuse and severe vasogenic edema affecting preferentially brain regions that are unmyelinated. MRI shows low signal on T1-weighted images, high signal on T2-weighted images, and decreased diffusivity in the basal ganglia. High signal in the globi pallidi can also be seen (Gunz et al. 2013). Development of diffusely low ADC portends a poor prognosis (Bireley et al. 2012). MRS demonstrates an increase in glutamate and glutamine, a nonspecific increase in lactate, and decrease in myo-inositol (Choi and Yoo 2001).

A defective branched-chain alpha keto acid dehydrogenase results in an entity known as maple syrup urine disease, which affects energy supply, protein and myelin synthesis (Patay 2011). MRI shows diffuse cerebral edema, involving preferentially myelinated structures such as the cerebellar peduncles and white matter, and the PLIC. A vacuolating myelinopathy is responsible for the development of decreased diffusivity within these myelinated tracts (Ha et al. 2004). MRS demonstrates a positive peak at 0.9 ppm representative of the methyl groups of branch chained fatty acids, and 1.3 ppm representative of lactate (Jan et al. 2003).

MALFORMATIONS OF CORTICAL DEVELOPMENT
Overall, brain malformations are an uncommon cause of neonatal seizures, ranging from 3% to 17% (Vasudevan and Levene 2013). However, some malformations can be difficult to detect and therefore the true incidence is unclear. To maximize detection and fully characterize these lesions, the higher soft tissue contrast of MRI is required.

Focal cortical dysplasia
FCD is a term used to described a localized abnormality in the number and/or location of neurons, laminar architecture of the cortex, or histologic appearance of the neurons. The most recent classification of FCD was proposed by Blumcke and collaborators, which divides them into three categories: type I corresponds to abnormal laminar architecture of the cortex, type II corresponds to disrupted cortical lamination in association with specific cytological abnormalities including dysmorphic neurons and balloon cells, and type III represents abnormalities in architecture associated with focal lesions such as hippocampal sclerosis, tumors, or vascular malformations (Blumcke et al. 2011). FCD lesions can be very small and require thin slices with no skip to detect the low T1 and high T2 signal that identifies these lesions in neonates (Fig. 6.8).

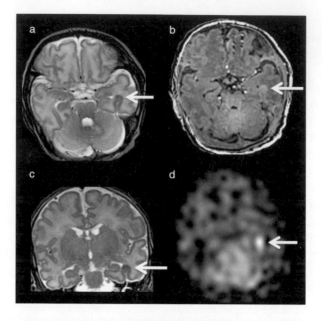

Figure 6.8. A 33-week gestation neonate presenting with intractable seizures, refractory to multiple antiepileptic medications. (a) Axial T2-weighted, (b) axial reformation of a coronal T1-weighted spoiled gradient echo image, and (c) coronal T2-weighted image show a small focus of cortical thickening (arrows) that on pathology was a Type IIB focal cortical dysplasia. (d) Axial pseudo-continuous ASL shows hyperperfusion in the region of the FCD (arrow) likely secondary to ongoing seizure activity. The patient underwent left anterior temporal lobectomy and became seizure-free.

Hemimegalencephaly

Hemimegalencephaly (HME) is characterized by asymmetric and hamartomatous enlargement of a hemisphere or a large part of a hemisphere. Histologically, HME is considered a hemispheric variant of FCD type II. HME can occur as an isolated diagnosis, or in association with syndromes including proteus, tuberous sclerosis, neurofibromatosis type I, and Klippel-Trenaunau-Webber (Griffiths et al. 1998, Abdel Razek et al. 2009). MRI shows asymmetry between the cerebral hemispheres, enlargement of the lateral ventricle on the affected side, abnormally low T2 signal throughout the involved white matter in neonates, and cortical abnormalities such as PMG, lissencephaly, or nodular heterotopia, amongst others (Fig. 6.9; Kalifa et al. 1987, Wolpert et al. 1994).

Polymicrogyria

PMG is a term used to describe a thick dysplastic cortex that demonstrates multiple shallow sulci with fine undulating gyri (Abdel Razek et al. 2009). PMG can be focal or diffuse, can be symmetric or asymmetric, and can involve one or both hemispheres. A majority of cases of PMG are idiopathic and involve the perisylvian regions (Raybaud and Widjaja 2011). In addition to the cortical abnormality, the overall white matter volume is decreased (Fig. 6.10).

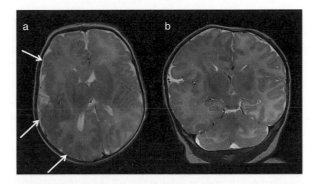

Figure 6.9. A 20-day-old infant with episodes of twitching in the left side of the body, which were confirmed to be seizures on admission EEG. (a) Axial and (b) coronal T2-weighted images demonstrate asymmetric enlargement of the right cerebral hemisphere consistent with hemimegalencephaly. The cortex of the right cerebral hemisphere shows diffuse polymicrogyria (arrows in figure part a). The patient underwent right functional hemispherectomy, with resolution of seizures. Moderate cognitive delays were noted on follow-up.

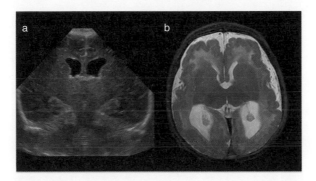

Figure 6.10. Diffuse PMG in a 4-week-old infant with an episode of respiratory arrest at home, presumed to be related to seizures. EEG performed on admission to the hospital confirmed the presence of seizures. No cause for PMG was identified, including metabolic, infectious, or toxic causes. (a) Coronal ultrasound image of the brain performed to exclude hemorrhage or hydrocephalus was interpreted as unremarkable. (b) Axial T2-weighted image demonstrates diffuse and severe PMG. There is prominence of the lateral ventricles and reduced white matter volume. The patient developed severe cognitive and motor deficits, requiring tracheostomy and gastrostomy.

When noted in a female with retinal lacunae and associated with heterotopia, agenesis, or partial agenesis of the corpus callosum and cysts, Aicardi syndrome should be considered (Hopkins et al. 2008). PMG can also be secondary to a multitude of insults including in utero vascular events, congenital infections such as CMV, or metabolic disorders (notably peroxisomal disorders; Patay 2011).

PHACOMATOSES

Tuberous sclerosis complex

Tuberous sclerosis complex (TSC) is an autosomal dominant disease with multisystem manifestations, including CNS lesions that can lead to seizures in the neonatal period (Grajkowska et al. 2010). One of the major diagnostic features of TSC is the presence of cortical tubers, which represent areas of FCD (Roach et al. 1998). Histologically, the tubers correspond to a disorganized cortex associated with dysplastic glia and neurons (Grajkowska et al. 2010). In newborn and young infants, tubers appear hyperintense on T1-weighted images and hypointense on T2-weighted images, because of the lack of surrounding myelination, with radial tracks that extend from the cortical malformation to the ependymal surface (Fig. 6.11a and b; Baskin 2008). Additional lesions in the brain of patients with TSC include sub-ependymal nodules, which are additional aggregates of dysplastic neurons and glia. Later in life subependymal giant cell astrocytoma can be identified as subependymal lesions that continue to grow over time (Grajkowska et al. 2010).

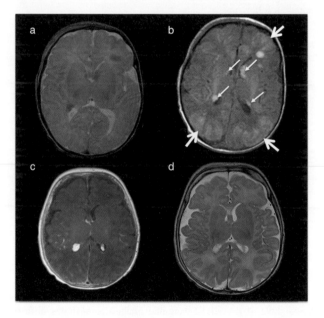

Figure 6.11. Phacomatoses in two different neonates. The top row shows findings of tuberous sclerosis complex in a 6-day-old neonate with seizures. Axial (a) T2-weighted MRI demonstrate foci of abnormally low SI involving the white matter and the cortex, that demonstrate high SI on (b) T1-weighted images, consistent with tubers (for examples, see thick arrows). In addition subependymal nodules, also low SI on T2 and high SI on T2, are evident (thin arrows). Cardiac tumors and renal angiomyolipomas also were present (not shown). The bottom row (parts c and d) show findings of Sturge Webber syndrome in a 4-week-old infant with bilateral port wine stains in the face, larger on the right side. (c) Axial T1-weighted image with IV gadolinium shows an enlarged choroid plexus in the right lateral ventricle and enhancement of multiple collaterals along the pial surface of the right temporal and parietal cerebral hemisphere, consistent with pial angiomatosis. (d) Axial T2-weighted MR image shows early evidence of right hemisphere atrophy.

Sturge–Weber syndrome

Sturge–Weber syndrome (SWS) is a sporadic venocapillary malformation affecting the leptomeninges, choroid, and skin, that usually follows the distribution of the first and second branches of the trigeminal nerve (Wheless et al. 2009). The venocapillary malformations of SWS are best assessed on gadolinium enhanced MRI, which demonstrates extensive enhancement of the abnormal leptomeningeal vessels. The choroid is frequently secondarily engorged. Over time and as a result of continuous seizure activity, volume loss and advanced myelination in the affected hemisphere are observed (Fig. 6.11c and d). SWI can show punctate microhaemorrhages and calcification due to chronic ischemia (Hu et al. 2008, Cagneaux et al. 2013).

Emerging role of near infrared spectroscopy and magnetoencephalography

NEAR INFRARED SPECTROSCOPY

The development of the NIRS method of diffuse correlation spectroscopy (DCS) has enabled bedside measurement of cerebral parenchymal blood flow (CBF) (Buckley et al. 2014). These DCS measures, when combined with frequency domain NIRS measures of cerebral oxygen saturation (SO_2) and pulse oximeter measures of arterial oxygen saturation (SaO_2), provide bedside estimates of the cerebral metabolic rate of oxygen consumption ($CMRO_2$) (Lin et al. 2013a, Buckley et al. 2014, Dehaes et al. 2014). Both DCS CBF measures and frequency domain NIRS-DCS measures of $CMRO_2$ show great potential as a complement to a-EEG and EEG to screen for abnormal neuronal activity with the potential to detect incoherent increases in neuronal activity that are difficult to detect with EEG (Franceschini et al. 2007, Grant et al. 2009, Lin et al. 2013b, Buckley et al. 2014, Dehaes et al. 2014). These initial studies show potential to localize the abnormal activity to a hemisphere but the presence of hair and the inherent ~ centimeter resolution currently limits localization potential (Dehaes et al. 2011).

MAGNETOENCEPHALOGRAPHY

We predict that the use of MEG in basic and clinical studies of neonatal and pediatric epilepsy will accelerate during the next decade as new neonatal and pediatric-sized MEG instruments are approved by the Food and Drugs Administration in the United States, as helium costs decrease because of the introduction of helium recyclers, and as software tools improve our ability to localize activity in real time (Papadelis et al. 2013). For example, a pediatric whole-head MEG system based on the BabySQUID partial coverage MEG system (Okada et al., 2006), has been installed at Children's Hospital of Philadelphia, called Artemis 123 (Roberts et al. 2014). A next-generation 0- to 3-year-old whole-head MEG system, the babyMEG, developed by Yoshio Okada PhD in collaboration with Tristan Inc. is now installed at Boston Children's Hospital Boston and includes a 100% recycling system (Cryomech Inc., Syracuse, NY). Additional hardware advances on the horizon include the possible development of room temperature whole-head MEG systems based on atomic magnetometers that are small enough to be used like an array of EEG electrodes fit to the head size (Sander et al. 2012). In parallel with these hardware advances are ongoing efforts to improve MEG software analysis to provide real-time magnetic source imaging.

Such advances would display cerebral activities in real time not at the detector level but projected onto the brain surface or specific brain regions, potentially expediting clinical decision making (Sudre et al. 2011). Thus we are poised at a critical time point in our ability to detect and monitor abnormal neuronal activity in neonates with the potential to transform our understanding of neonatal seizures in many disorders.

REFERENCES

Abdel Razek AA, Kandell AY, Elsorogy LG, Elmongy A, Basett AA (2009) Disorders of cortical formation: MR imaging features. *AJNR Am J Neuroradiol* 30: 4–11. doi: http://dx.doi.org/10.3174/ajnr.A1223.

Ah Mew N, Loewenstein JB, Kadom N et al. (2011). MRI features of 4 female patients with pyruvate dehydrogenase E1 alpha deficiency. *Pediatr Neurol* 45: 57–59. doi: http://dx.doi.org/10.1016/j.pediatrneurol.2011.02.003.

Badawi N, Kurinczuk JJ, Keogh JM et al. (1998) Antepartum risk factors for newborn encephalopathy: The Western Australian case-control study. *BMJ* 317: 1549–1553. doi: http://dx.doi.org/10.1136/bmj.317.7172.1549.

Barkovich AJ, Kjos BO, Jackson DE Jr, Norman D (1988) Normal maturation of the neonatal and infant brain: MR imaging at 1.5 T. *Radiology* 166: 173–180. doi: http://dx.doi.org/10.1148/radiology.166.1.3336675.

Barkovich AJ, Lindan CE (1994) Congenital cytomegalovirus infection of the brain: Imaging analysis and embryologic considerations. *AJNR Am J Neuroradiol* 15: 703–715.

Baskin HJ Jr. (2008) The pathogenesis and imaging of the tuberous sclerosis complex. *Pediatr Radiol* 38: 936–952. doi: http://dx.doi.org/10.1007/s00247-008-0832-y.

Bireley WR, Van Hove JL, Gallagher RC, Fenton LZ (2012) Urea cycle disorders: Brain MRI and neurological outcome. *Pediatr Radiol* 42: 455–462. doi: http://dx.doi.org/10.1007/s00247-011-2253-6.

Blumcke I, Thom M, Aronica E et al. (2011) The clinicopathologic spectrum of focal cortical dysplasias: A consensus classification proposed by an ad hoc task force of the ILAE diagnostic methods commission. *Epilepsia* 52: 158–174. doi: http://dx.doi.org/10.1111/j.1528-1167.2010.02777.x.

Boichot C, Walker PM, Durand C et al. (2006) Term neonate prognoses after perinatal asphyxia: Contributions of MR imaging, MR spectroscopy, relaxation times, and apparent diffusion coefficients. *Radiology* 239: 839–848. doi: http://dx.doi.org/10.1148/radiol.2393050027.

Buckley EM, Parthasarathy AB, Grant PE, Yodh AG, Franceschini MA (2014) Diffuse correlation spectroscopy for measurement of cerebral blood flow: Future prospects. *Neurophotonics* 1. doi: http://dx.doi.org/10.1117/1.nph.1.1.011009.

Burns CM, Rutherford MA, Boardman JP, Cowan FM (2008) Patterns of cerebral injury and neurodevelopmental outcomes after symptomatic neonatal hypoglycemia. *Pediatrics* 122: 65–74. doi: http://dx.doi.org/10.1542/peds.2007-2822.

Cagneaux M, Paoli V, Blanchard G, Ville D, Guibaud L (2013) Pre- and postnatal imaging of early cerebral damage in Sturge-Weber syndrome. *Pediatr Radiol* 43: 1536–1539. doi: http://dx.doi.org/10.1007/s00247-013-2743-9.

Choi CG, Yoo HW (2001) Localized proton MR spectroscopy in infants with urea cycle defect. *AJNR Am J Neuroradiol* 22: 834–837.

Choksi V, Hoeffner E, Karaarslan E, Yalcinkaya C, Cakirer S (2003) Infantile refsum disease: Case report. *AJNR Am J Neuroradiol* 24: 2082–2084.

Chu CT (2008) Eaten alive: Autophagy and neuronal cell death after hypoxia-ischemia. *Am J Pathol* 172: 284–247. doi: http://dx.doi.org/10.2353/ajpath.2008.071064.

Chua GC, Sitoh YY, Lim CC, Chua HC, Ng PY (2002) MRI findings in osmotic myelinolysis. *Clin Radiol* 57: 800–806. doi: http://dx.doi.org/10.1016/S0009-9260(02)90977-3.

Cornblath M, Ichord R (2000) Hypoglycemia in the neonate. *Semin Perinatol* 24: 136–149. doi: http://dx.doi.org/10.1053/sp.2000.6364.

Dahmoush HM, Vossough A, Roberts TP (2012) Pediatric high-field magnetic resonance imaging. *Neuroimaging Clin N Am* 22: 297–313, xi. doi: http://dx.doi.org/10.1016/j.nic.2012.02.009.

De Laveaucoupet J, Roffi F, Audibert F et al. (2005) Progressive neuronal degeneration of childhood: Prenatal diagnosis by MRI. *Prenat Diagn* 25: 307–310. doi: http://dx.doi.org/10.1002/pd.1128.

De Vis JB, Petersen ET, Kersbergen KJ et al. (2013) Evaluation of perinatal arterial ischemic stroke using noninvasive arterial spin labeling perfusion MRI. *Pediatr Res* 74: 307–313. doi: http://dx.doi.org/10.1038/pr.2013.111.

Dehaes M, Aggarwal A, Lin PY et al. (2014) Cerebral oxygen metabolism in neonatal hypoxic ischemic encephalopathy during and after therapeutic hypothermia. *J Cereb Blood Flow Metab* 34: 87–94. doi: http://dx.doi.org/10.1038/jcbfm.2013.165.

Dehaes M, Grant PE, Sliva DD et al. (2011) Assessment of the frequency-domain multi-distance method to evaluate the brain optical properties: Monte Carlo simulations from neonate to adult. *Biomed Opt Express* 2: 552–567. doi: http://dx.doi.org/10.1364/BOE.2.000552.

Deshpande S, Ward Platt M (2005) The investigation and management of neonatal hypoglycaemia. *Semin Fetal Neonatal Med* 10: 351–361. doi: http://dx.doi.org/10.1016/j.siny.2005.04.002.

Dubois J, Sebag G, Argyropoulou M, Brunelle F (1991) MR findings in infantile Refsum disease: Case report of two family members. *AJNR Am J Neuroradiol* 12: 1159–1160.

Engman ML, Malm G, Engstrom L et al. (2008) Congenital CMV infection: prevalence in newborns and the impact on hearing deficit. *Scand J Infect Dis* 40: 935–942. doi: http://dx.doi.org/10.1080/00365540802308431.

Epelman M, Daneman A, Chauvin N, Hirsch W (2012) Head ultrasound and MR imaging in the evaluation of neonatal encephalopathy: Competitive or complementary imaging studies? *Magn Reson Imaging Clin N Am* 20: 93–115. doi: http://dx.doi.org/10.1016/j.mric.2011.08.012.

Epelman M, Daneman A, Kellenberger CJ et al. (2010) Neonatal encephalopathy: A prospective comparison of head US and MRI. *Pediatr Radiol* 40: 1640–1650. doi: http://dx.doi.org/10.1007/s00247-010-1634-6.

Fink KR, Thapa MM, Ishak GE, Pruthi S (2010) Neuroimaging of pediatric central nervous system cytomegalovirus infection. *Radiographics* 30: 1779–1796. doi: http://dx.doi.org/10.1148/rg.307105043.

Franceschini MA, Thaker S, Themelis G et al. (2007) Assessment of infant brain development with frequency-domain near-infrared spectroscopy. *Pediatr Res* 61: 546–551. doi: http://dx.doi.org/10.1203/pdr.0b013e318045be99.

Franke C, Van Dorsten FA, Olah L, Schwindt W, Hoehn M (2000) Arterial spin tagging perfusion imaging of rat brain: Dependency on magnetic field strength. *Magn Reson Imaging* 18: 1109–1113. doi: http://dx.doi.org/10.1016/S0730-725X(00)00211-3.

Fujikawa A, Tsuchiya K, Honya K, Nitatori T (2006) Comparison of MRI sequences to detect ventriculitis. *AJR Am J Roentgenol* 187: 1048–1053. doi: http://dx.doi.org/10.2214/AJR.04.1923.

Gano D, Chau V, Poskitt KJ et al. (2013) Evolution of pattern of injury and quantitative MRI on days 1 and 3 in term newborns with hypoxic-ischemic encephalopathy. *Pediatr Res* 74: 82–87. doi: http://dx.doi.org/10.1038/pr.2013.69.

Gaschignard J, Levy C, Romain O et al. (2011) Neonatal Bacterial Meningitis: 444 Cases in 7 Years. *Pediatr Infect Dis J* 30: 212–217. doi: http://dx.doi.org/10.1097/INF.0b013e3181fab1e7.

Gaytant MA, Galama JM, Semmekrot BA et al. (2005) The incidence of congenital cytomegalovirus infections in the Netherlands. *J Med Virol* 76: 71–75. doi: http://dx.doi.org/10.1002/jmv.20325.

Ghei SK, Zan E, Nathan JE et al. (2014) MR imaging of hypoxic-ischemic injury in term neonates: Pearls and pitfalls. *Radiographics* 34: 1047–1061. doi: http://dx.doi.org/10.1148/rg.344130080.

Girard N, Raybaud C (2011) Neonates with seizures: What to consider, how to image. *Magn Reson Imaging Clin N Am* 19: 685–708 vii. doi: http://dx.doi.org/10.1016/j.mric.2011.08.003.

Grajkowska W, Kotulska K, Jurkiewicz E, Matyja E (2010) Brain lesions in tuberous sclerosis complex. Review. *Folia Neuropathol* 48: 139–149.

Grant PE, He J, Halpern EF et al. (2001) Frequency and clinical context of decreased apparent diffusion coefficient reversal in the human brain. *Radiology* 221: 43–50. doi: http://dx.doi.org/10.1148/radiol.2211001523.

Grant PE, Roche-Labarbe N, Surova A et al. (2009) Increased cerebral blood volume and oxygen consumption in neonatal brain injury. *J Cereb Blood Flow Metab* 29: 1704–1713. doi: http://dx.doi.org/10.1038/jcbfm.2009.90.

Greiner HM, Lynch ER, Fordyce S et al. (2012) Vigabatrin for childhood partial-onset epilepsies. *Pediatr Neurol* 46: 83–88. doi: http://dx.doi.org/10.1016/j.pediatrneurol.2011.11.020.

Griffiths PD, Gardner SA, Smith M, Rittey C, Powell T (1998) Hemimegalencephaly and focal megalencephaly in tuberous sclerosis complex. *AJNR Am J Neuroradiol* 19: 1935–1938.

Groenendaal F, Bianchi MC, Battini R et al. (2001) Proton magnetic resonance spectroscopy (1H-MRS) of the cerebrum in two young infants with Zellweger syndrome. *Neuropediatrics* 32: 23–27. doi: http://dx.doi.org/10.1055/s-2001-12218.

Gruetter R, Weisdorf SA, Rajanayagan V et al. (1998) Resolution improvements in in vivo 1H NMR spectra with increased magnetic field strength. *J Magn Reson* 135: 260–264. doi: http://dx.doi.org/10.1006/jmre.1998.1542.

Gunz AC, Choong K, Potter M, Miller E (2013) Magnetic resonance imaging findings and neurodevelopmental outcomes in neonates with urea-cycle defects. *Int Med Case Rep J* 6: 41–48. doi: http://dx.doi.org/10.2147/IMCRJ.S43513.

Ha JS, Kim TK, Eun BL et al. (2004) Maple syrup urine disease encephalopathy: A follow-up study in the acute stage using diffusion-weighted MRI. *Pediatr Radiol* 34: 163–166. doi: http://dx.doi.org/10.1007/s00247-003-1058-7.

Haacke EM, Mittal S, Wu Z, Neelavalli J, Cheng YC (2009) Susceptibility-weighted imaging: Technical aspects and clinical applications, Part 1. *AJNR Am J Neuroradiol* 30: 19–30. doi: http://dx.doi.org/10.3174/ajnr.A1400.

Han KT, Choi DS, Ryoo JW et al. (2007) Diffusion-weighted MR imaging of pyogenic intraventricular empyema. *Neuroradiology* 49: 813–818. doi: http://dx.doi.org/10.1007/s00234-007-0264-7.

Hanrahan JD, Sargentoni J, Azzopardi D et al. (1996) Cerebral metabolism within 18 hours of birth asphyxia: A proton magnetic resonance spectroscopy study. *Pediatr Res* 39: 584–590. doi: http://dx.doi.org/10.1203/00006450-199604000-00004.

Hoffmann C, Ben-Zeev B, Anikster Y et al. (2007) Magnetic resonance imaging and magnetic resonance spectroscopy in isolated sulfite oxidase deficiency. *J Child Neurol* 22: 1214–1221. doi: http://dx.doi.org/10.1177/0883073807306260.

Hopkins B, Sutton VR, Lewis RA, Van Den Veyver I, Clark G (2008) Neuroimaging aspects of Aicardi syndrome. *Am J Med Genet A* 146A: 2871–2878. doi: http://dx.doi.org/10.1002/ajmg.a.32537.

Hu J, Yu Y, Juhasz C et al. (2008) MR susceptibility weighted imaging (SWI) complements conventional contrast enhanced T1 weighted MRI in characterizing brain abnormalities of Sturge-Weber Syndrome. *J Magn Reson Imaging* 28: 300–317. doi: http://dx.doi.org/10.1002/jmri.21435.

Huisman TA, Phelps T, Bosemani T, Tekes A, Poretti A (2015) Parturitional injury of the head and neck. *J Neuroimaging* 25: 151–166. doi: http://dx.doi.org/10.1111/jon.12144.

Intrapiromkul J, Northington F, Huisman TA, Izbudak I, Meoded A, Tekes A (2013) Accuracy of head ultrasound for the detection of intracranial hemorrhage in preterm neonates: Comparison with brain MRI and susceptibility-weighted imaging. *J Neuroradiol* 40: 81–88. doi: http://dx.doi.org/10.1016/j.neurad.2012.03.006.

Izbudak I, Grant PE (2011) MR imaging of the term and preterm neonate with diffuse brain injury. *Magn Reson Imaging Clin N Am* 19: 709–731; vii. doi: http://dx.doi.org/10.1016/j.mric.2011.08.014.

Jacobs DS, Smith AS, Finelli DA, Lanzieri CF, Wiznitzer M (1993) Menkes kinky hair disease: Characteristic MR angiographic findings. *AJNR Am J Neuroradiol* 14: 1160–1163.

Jacobs S, Hunt R, Tarnow-Mordi W, Inder T, Davis P (2007) Cooling for newborns with hypoxic ischaemic encephalopathy. *Cochrane Database Syst Rev* CD003311. doi: http://dx.doi.org/10.1002/14651858.cd003311.pub2.

Jan W, Zimmerman RA, Wang ZJ, Berry GT, Kaplan PB, Kaye EM (2003) MR diffusion imaging and MR spectroscopy of maple syrup urine disease during acute metabolic decompensation. *Neuroradiology* 45: 393–399. doi: http://dx.doi.org/10.1007/s00234-003-0955-7.

Kalifa GL, Chiron C, Sellier N et al. (1987) Hemimegalencephaly: MR imaging in five children. *Radiology* 165: 29–33. doi: http://dx.doi.org/10.1148/radiology.165.1.3628788.

Kim SY, Goo HW, Lim KH, Kim ST, Kim KS (2006) Neonatal hypoglycaemic encephalopathy: Diffusion-weighted imaging and proton MR spectroscopy. *Pediatr Radiol* 36: 144–148. doi: http://dx.doi.org/10.1007/s00247-005-0020-2.

Kirton A, Armstrong-Wells J, Chang T et al. (2011) Symptomatic neonatal arterial ischemic stroke: The international pediatric stroke study. *Pediatrics* 128: e1402–e1410. doi: http://dx.doi.org/10.1542/peds.2011-1148.

Kitamura G, Kido D, Wycliffe N, Jacobson JP, Oyoyo U, Ashwal S (2011) Hypoxic-ischemic injury: Utility of susceptibility-weighted imaging. *Pediatr Neurol* 45: 220–224. doi: http://dx.doi.org/10.1016/j.pediatrneurol.2011.06.009.

Knaap MSVD, Valk J, Barkhof F, Knaap MSVD (2005) *Magnetic resonance of myelination and myelin disorders.* Berlin: New York, Springer. doi: http://dx.doi.org/10.1007/3-540-27660-2.

Knake S, Triantafyllou C, Wald LL et al. (2005) 3T phased array MRI improves the presurgical evaluation in focal epilepsies: A prospective study. *Neurology* 65: 1026–1031. doi: http://dx.doi.org/10.1212/01. wnl.0000179355.04481.3c.

Lee JH, Arcinue E, Ross BD (1994) Brief report: Organic osmolytes in the brain of an infant with hypernatremia. *N Engl J Med* 331: 439–442. doi: http://dx.doi.org/10.1056/NEJM199408183310704.

Lequin MH, Peeters EA, Holscher HC, De Krijger R, Govaert P (2004) Arterial infarction caused by carotid artery dissection in the neonate. *Eur J Paediatr Neurol* 8: 155–160. doi: http://dx.doi.org/10.1016/j. ejpn.2004.02.001.

Leventer RJ, Kornberg AJ, Phelan EM, Kean MJ (1997) Early magnetic resonance imaging findings in Menkes' disease. *J Child Neurol* 12: 222–224. doi: http://dx.doi.org/10.1177/088307389701200314.

Lin PY, Roche-Labarbe N, Dehaes M (2013a) Non-invasive optical measurement of cerebral metabolism and hemodynamics in infants. *J Vis Exp* e4379. doi: http://dx.doi.org/10.3791/4379.

Lin PY, Roche-Labarbe N, Dehaes M, Fenoglio A, Grant PE, Franceschini MA (2013b) Regional and hemispheric asymmetries of cerebral hemodynamic and oxygen metabolism in newborns. *Cereb Cortex* 23: 339–348. doi: http://dx.doi.org/10.1093/cercor/bhs023.

Low E, Boylan GB, Mathieson SR et al. (2012) Cooling and seizure burden in term neonates: An observational study. *Arch Dis Child Fetal Neonatal Ed* 97: F267–F272. doi: http://dx.doi.org/10.1136/ archdischild-2011-300716.

Lowe LH, Bailey Z (2011) State-of-the-art cranial sonography: Part 1, Modern techniques and image interpretation. *AJR Am J Roentgenol* 196: 1028–1033. doi: http://dx.doi.org/10.2214/AJR.10.6160.

Malamateniou C, Adams ME, Srinivasan L et al. (2009) The anatomic variations of the circle of Willis in preterm-at-term and term-born infants: An MR angiography study at 3T. *AJNR Am J Neuroradiol* 30: 1955–1962. doi: http://dx.doi.org/10.3174/ajnr.A1724.

Miller SP, Dilenge ME, Meagher-Villemure K, O'Gorman AM, Shevell MI (1998) Infantile epileptic encephalopathy (Ohtahara syndrome) and migrational disorder. *Pediatr Neurol* 19: 50–54. doi: http:// dx.doi.org/10.1016/S0887-8994(98)00009-5.

Nickerson JP, Richner B, Santy K et al. (2012) Neuroimaging of pediatric intracranial infection–Part 2: TORCH, viral, fungal, and parasitic infections. *J Neuroimaging* 22: e52–e63. doi: http://dx.doi. org/10.1111/j.1552-6569.2011.00699.x.

Nowinski WL, Puspitasaari F, Volkau I, Marchenko Y, Knopp MV (2013) Comparison of magnetic resonance angiography scans on 1.5, 3, and 7 Tesla units: A quantitative study of 3-dimensional cerebrovasculature. *J Neuroimaging* 23: 86–95. doi: http://dx.doi.org/10.1111/j.1552-6569.2011.00597.x.

Okada Y, Pratt K, Atwood C, Mascarenas A, Reineman R, Nurminen J, Paulson DN (2006) BabySQUID: A mobile, high-resolution multichannel magnetoencephalography system for neonatal brain assessment. Review Scientific Instrum 77(2): 24301–2430910.1063/1.2168672.

Okanishi T, Yamamoto H, Hosokawa T et al. (2015) Diffusion-weighted MRI for early diagnosis of neonatal herpes simplex encephalitis. *Brain Dev* 37: 423–31. doi: http://dx.doi.org/10.1016/j.braindev. 2014.07.006.

Papadelis C, Harini C, Ahtam B, Doshi C, Grant EP, Okada Y (2013) Current and Emerging Potential for Magnetoencephalography in Pediatric Epilepsy. *J Pediatr Epilepsy* 2: 1–13.

Patay Z (2011) MR imaging workup of inborn errors of metabolism of early postnatal onset. *Magn Reson Imaging Clin N Am* 19: 733–759; vii. doi: http://dx.doi.org/10.1016/j.mric.2011.09.001.

Pienaar R, Paldino MJ, Madan N et al. (2012) A quantitative method for correlating observations of decreased apparent diffusion coefficient with elevated cerebral blood perfusion in newborns presenting cerebral ischemic insults. *Neuroimage* 63: 1510–1518. doi: http://dx.doi.org/10.1016/j.neuroimage.2012.07.062.

Pierrat V, Haouari N, Liska A, Thomas D, Subtil D, Truffert P, Groupe D'etudes En Epidemiologie P (2005) Prevalence, causes, and outcome at 2 years of age of newborn encephalopathy: Population based study. *Arch Dis Child Fetal Neonatal Ed* 90: F257–F2561. doi: http://dx.doi.org/10.1136/adc.2003.047985.

Pollina J, Dias MS, Li V, Kachurek D, Arbesman M (2001) Cranial birth injuries in term newborn infants. *Pediatr Neurosurg* 35: 113–119. doi: http://dx.doi.org/10.1159/000050403.

Raets M, Dudink J, Raybaud C, Ramenghi L, Lequin M, Govaert P (2015) Brain vein disorders in newborn infants. *Dev Med Child Neurol* 57: 229–240. doi: http://dx.doi.org/10.1111/dmcn.12579.

Raju TN, Nelson KB, Ferriero D, Lynch JK, Participants N-NPSW (2007) Ischemic perinatal stroke: Summary of a workshop sponsored by the National Institute of Child Health and Human Development and the National Institute of Neurological Disorders and Stroke. *Pediatrics* 120: 609–616. doi: http://dx.doi.org/10.1542/peds.2007-0336.

Raybaud C, Widjaja E (2011) Development and dysgenesis of the cerebral cortex: Malformations of cortical development. *Neuroimaging Clin N Am* 21: 483–543, vii. doi: http://dx.doi.org/10.1016/j.nic.2011.05.014.

Roach ES, Gomez MR, Northrup H (1998) Tuberous sclerosis complex consensus conference: Revised clinical diagnostic criteria. *J Child Neurol* 13: 624–628. doi: http://dx.doi.org/10.1177/088307389801301206.

Roberts TP, Paulson DN, Hirschkoff E et al. (2014) Artemis 123: Development of a whole-head infant and young child MEG system. *Front Hum Neurosci* 8: 99. doi: http://dx.doi.org/10.3389/fnhum.2014.00099.

Sagar P, Grant PE (2006) Diffusion-weighted MR imaging: Pediatric clinical applications. *Neuroimaging Clin N Am* 16: 45–74, viii. doi: http://dx.doi.org/10.1016/j.nic.2005.11.003.

Sander TH, Preusser J, Mhaskar R, Kitching J, Trahms L, Knappe S (2012) Magnetoencephalography with a chip-scale atomic magnetometer. *Biomed Opt Express* 3: 981–990. doi: http://dx.doi.org/10.1364/BOE.3.000981.

Schneider JF, Hanquinet S, Severino M, Rossi A (2011) MR imaging of neonatal brain infections. *Magn Reson Imaging Clin N Am* 19: 761–775; vii–viii. doi: http://dx.doi.org/10.1016/j.mric.2011.08.013.

Shankaran S, Laptook AR, Ehrenkranz RA et al. (2005) Whole-body hypothermia for neonates with hypoxic-ischemic encephalopathy. *N Engl J Med* 353: 1574–1584. doi: http://dx.doi.org/10.1056/NEJMcps050929.

Smith JK, Mah JK, Castillo M (1996) Brain MR imaging findings in two patients with Alpers' syndrome. *Clin Imaging* 20: 235–237. doi: http://dx.doi.org/10.1016/0899-7071(95)00039-9.

Soares-Fernandes JP, Teixeira-Gomes R, Cruz R et al. (2008) Neonatal pyruvate dehydrogenase deficiency due to a R302H mutation in the PDHA1 gene: MRI findings. *Pediatr Radiol* 38: 559–562. doi: http://dx.doi.org/10.1007/s00247-007-0721-9.

Sofou K, Steneryd K, Wiklund LM, Tulinius M, Darin N (2013) MRI of the brain in childhood-onset mitochondrial disorders with central nervous system involvement. *Mitochondrion* 13: 364–371. doi: http://dx.doi.org/10.1016/j.mito.2013.04.008.

Stark JE, Seibert JJ (1994) Cerebral artery Doppler ultrasonography for prediction of outcome after perinatal asphyxia. *J Ultrasound Med* 13: 595–600.

Sudre G, Parkkonen L, Bock E, Baillet S, Wang W, Weber DJ (2011) rtMEG: A real-time software interface for magnetoencephalography. *Comput Intell Neurosci* 2011: 327953. doi: http://dx.doi.org/10.1155/2011/327953.

Sujansky E, Conradi S (1995) Sturge-Weber syndrome: Age of onset of seizures and glaucoma and the prognosis for affected children. *J Child Neurol* 10: 49–58. doi: http://dx.doi.org/10.1177/088307389501000113.

Takahashi S, Ishii K, Matsumoto K et al. (1993) Cranial MRI and MR angiography in Menkes' syndrome. *Neuroradiology* 35: 556–558. doi: http://dx.doi.org/10.1007/BF00588724.

Unay B, Kendirli T, Atac K, Gul D, Akin R, Gokcay E (2005) Caudothalamic groove cysts in Zellweger syndrome. *Clin Dysmorphol* 14: 165–167. doi: http://dx.doi.org/10.1097/00019605-200507000-00014.

Van Der Knaap MS, Jakobs C, Valk J (1996) Magnetic resonance imaging in lactic acidosis. *J Inherit Metab Dis* 19: 535–547. doi: http://dx.doi.org/10.1007/BF01799114.

Van Hove JL, Lohr NJ (2011) Metabolic and monogenic causes of seizures in neonates and young infants. *Mol Genet Metab* 104: 214–230. doi: http://dx.doi.org/10.1016/j.ymgme.2011.04.020.

Van Wezel-Meijler G, Leijser LM, De Bruine FT, Steggerda SJ, Van Der Grond J Walther FJ (2009) Magnetic resonance imaging of the brain in newborn infants: Practical aspects. *Early Hum Dev* 85: 85–92. doi: http://dx.doi.org/10.1016/j.earlhumdev.2008.11.009.

Vanhanen SL, Raininko R, Santavuori P (1994) Early differential diagnosis of infantile neuronal ceroid lipofuscinosis, Rett syndrome, and Krabbe disease by CT and MR. *AJNR Am J Neuroradiol* 15: 1443–1453.

Vanhanen SL, Raininko R, Santavuori P, Autti T, Haltia M (1995) MRI evaluation of the brain in infantile neuronal ceroid-lipofuscinosis. Part 1: Postmortem MRI with histopathologic correlation. *J Child Neurol* 10: 438–443. doi: http://dx.doi.org/10.1177/088307389501000603.

Vasudevan C, Levene M (2013) Epidemiology and aetiology of neonatal seizures. *Semin Fetal Neonatal Med* 18: 185–191. doi: http://dx.doi.org/10.1016/j.siny.2013.05.008.

Verrotti A, Carelli A, Coppola G (2014) Epilepsy in children with Menkes disease: A systematic review of literature. *J Child Neurol* 29: 1757–1764. doi: http://dx.doi.org/10.1177/0883073814541469.

Volpe JJ (2008) *Neurology of the Newborn*. Philadelphia: WB Saunders.

Weeke LC, Groenendaal F, Toet MC et al. (2015) The aetiology of neonatal seizures and the diagnostic contribution of neonatal cerebral magnetic resonance imaging. *Dev Med Child Neurol* 57: 248–256. doi: http://dx.doi.org/10.1111/dmcn.12629.

Weller S, Rosewich H, Gartner J (2008) Cerebral MRI as a valuable diagnostic tool in Zellweger spectrum patients. *J Inherit Metab Dis* 31: 270–280. doi: http://dx.doi.org/10.1007/s10545-008-0856-3.

Wheless JW, Carmant L, Bebin M et al. (2009) Magnetic resonance imaging abnormalities associated with vigabatrin in patients with epilepsy. *Epilepsia* 50: 195–205. doi: http://dx.doi.org/10.1111/j.1528-1167.2008.01896.x.

Wintermark P, Hansen A, Gregas MC et al. (2011) Brain perfusion in asphyxiated newborns treated with therapeutic hypothermia. *AJNR Am J Neuroradiol* 32: 2023–2029. doi: http://dx.doi.org/10.3174/ajnr.A2708.

Wolpert SM, Cohen A, Libenson MH (1994) Hemimegalencephaly: A longitudinal MR study. *AJNR Am J Neuroradiol* 15: 1479–1482.

Wusthoff CJ, Dlugos DJ, Gutierrez-Colina A et al. (2011a) Electrographic seizures during therapeutic hypothermia for neonatal hypoxic-ischemic encephalopathy. *J Child Neurol* 26: 724–728. doi: http://dx.doi.org/10.1177/0883073810390036.

Wusthoff CJ, Kessler SK, Vossough A et al. (2011b) Risk of later seizure after perinatal arterial ischemic stroke: A prospective cohort study. *Pediatrics* 127: e1550–e1557. doi: http://dx.doi.org/10.1542/peds.2010-1577.

Zand DJ, Simon EM, Pulitzer SB et al. (2003) In vivo pyruvate detected by MR spectroscopy in neonatal pyruvate dehydrogenase deficiency. *AJNR Am J Neuroradiol* 24: 1471–1474.

Zarifi MK, Astrakas LG, Poussaint TY, Plessis AD A, Zurakowski D, TZIKA AA (2002) Prediction of adverse outcome with cerebral lactate level and apparent diffusion coefficient in infants with perinatal asphyxia. *Radiology* 225: 859–70. doi: http://dx.doi.org/10.1148/radiol.2253011797.

7
NEONATAL EPILEPSIES AND EPILEPTIC ENCEPHALOPATHIES

Maria Roberta Cilio

Epileptic seizures have their highest incidence in the neonatal period. When considering seizures in neonates, one of the first issues of importance is recognizing that not all seizures have the same etiology. Early distinction and differentiation of acute seizures versus neonatal-onset epilepsies has significant therapeutic and prognostic implications. Acute seizures are often the only sign in the neonate of hypoxic-ischemic brain injury, an infection, hemorrhage of the central nervous system, or transient metabolic disturbance, and may require no pharmacological intervention, or only a very short course of treatment. Furthermore, searching for the cause of seizures may be limited to basic serum labs, a lumbar puncture, and/or head imaging (head ultrasound or magnetic resonance imaging [MRI]).

On the other hand, neonatal-onset epilepsies are rare, although often overlooked because their phenotype may be difficult to characterize. This is, in part, because of the fact that pediatricians or neonatologists frequently manage seizures in neonates without access to specialists with detailed knowledge of seizure semiology, epilepsy syndromes, and specific etiologies in this age group. Recognition is paramount, though, because these epilepsies may require targeted diagnostic evaluations, and prolonged treatment with antiepileptic drugs (AEDs). Furthermore, appropriate characterization of the epilepsy may lead to more rapid and focused diagnosis, and consideration of specific pharmacological therapy.

There are certain questions to answer when faced with a neonate having seizures. The neurological examination (i.e. normal versus abnormal between seizures) and the actual age at onset of seizures (i.e. first day versus first week versus within the first month of life) can help provide clues to the diagnosis. The specific semiology of the seizures and the ictal and interictal electroencepahalography (EEG) are also vital pieces of information.

Neonatal-onset epilepsies unrelated to prenatal, perinatal, or postnatal lesions present a major diagnostic and therapeutic challenge. However, genetic etiologies are being discovered for a growing proportion of these disorders, helping elucidate their molecular mechanisms (Nabbout and Dulac 2012). Neonatal-onset epilepsies have a broad spectrum phenotype: from relatively benign to much more severe. The association of epilepsy with the deterioration of cognitive functions forms a group of diseases known as 'epileptic encephalopathies', entities for which the EEG epileptiform abnormalities themselves are considered to have a major impact on brain development (Engel 2001, Berg et al. 2010).

This chapter will focus on the role of accurate definition of phenotype and seizure characterization at onset in achieving an early diagnosis and the possibility of targeted treatment in order to change the outcome, not only regarding seizures but also regarding neurological development.

The recent report of the International League against Epilepsy commission on classification and terminology (Berg et al. 2010) recognizes three neonatal electroclinical syndromes: benign familial neonatal epilepsy (BFNE), early myoclonic encephalopathy (EME), and Ohtahara syndrome. While BFNE is a self-limiting form of epilepsy in the newborn infant, associated in most cases with normal development, EME and Ohtahara syndrome are characterized by a severe disruption of cerebral functions and seizures often intractable. In the past few years, epileptic encephalopathies with onset in the neonatal period have been increasingly recognized including cyclin-dependent kinase-like 5 (CDKL5)-associated epileptic encephalopathy (Bahi-Buisson et al. 2008b), KCNQ2-encephalopathy (Weckhuysen et al. 2012, 2013), and epilepsy of infancy with migrating focal seizures (EIMFS) (Coppola et al. 1995, Cilio et al. 2008, Barcia et al. 2012). In addition, the use of video-EEG monitoring in the neonatal intensive care unit (NICU) has been implemented in many institutions, allowing for a better definition of the electroclinical phenotype of these severe forms of neonatal epilepsy.

Benign familial neonatal seizures

Benign familial neonatal seizures (BFNS) is an autosomal-dominant epilepsy syndrome of the newborn infant. Typically, seizures occur on day 2 or 3 of life, with the majority in the first week of life. Seizures are brief (1–2 minutes in duration), but can occur up to 30 times per day, sometimes evolving into status epilepticus. Family history reveals other members with seizures in the neonatal period. Newborn infants can continue to have seizures for several weeks or months before spontaneous remission, although seizures usually respond well to AEDs. There are a few reports of seizures lasting more than several months (Bjerre and Corelius 1968, Soldovieri et al. 2014).

The seizure semiology is characterized by initial asymmetric tonic posturing, often accompanied by autonomic features (apnea), sometimes with progression to unilateral or bilateral clonic jerks. Myoclonic seizures and epileptic spasms have not been reported. The ictal EEG is characterized by an electrodecremental pattern with superimposed muscle artifact during the tonic phase, and then rhythmic focal spike and wave discharges during the clonic phase (Fig. 7.1).

The interictal EEG may show some bilateral independent epileptiform abnormalities mainly over the central regions but is otherwise normal (personal observation). Poor prognostic patterns, such as burst suppression, have never been reported. Neonates with BFNS are neurologically normal in between seizures, and are able to breast- or bottle-feed without difficulty. All metabolic, infectious, hematologic studies, as well as brain imaging, are normal. The disorder is self-limited, as seizures stop spontaneously within the first year of life. However, up to 30% of patients in different series have febrile or afebrile seizures later

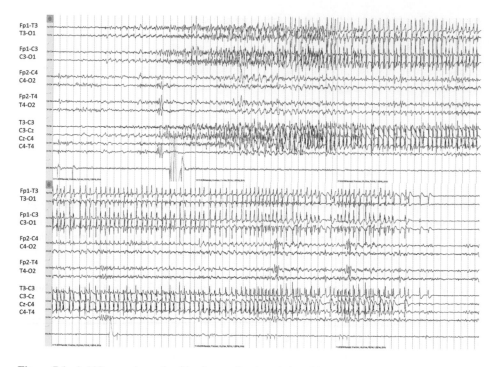

Figure 7.1. A 120-second epoch of ictal recording in a 4-day-old neonate with benign familial neonatal seizures showing a left focal seizure, which starts with a tonic phase of low amplitude fast activity, followed by rhythmic, high amplitude spikes over the left hemisphere. At the end of the ictal discharge, asymmetric postictal attenuation is seen over the right hemisphere. Gain, 7 μV/mm; high frequency filter, 70 Hz; paper speed, 15 mm/sec.

in life (Ronen et al. 1993, Grinton et al. 2015), while showing a normal psychomotor development.

The genes associated with BFNS are *KCNQ2* on chromosome 20q13.3 and *KCNQ3* on chromosome 8q24, and encode the voltage-gated potassium channel subunits KV 7.2 (Q2) and KV 7.3 (Q3), respectively (Biervert et al. 1998, Charlier et al. 1998, Singh et al. 1998). There are over 80 different mutations reported on *KCNQ2* and 6 mutations on *KCNQ3*. The Q2 and Q3 subunits of the potassium channel help mediate the M-current and play a key role in repolarizing action potentials by allowing the flow of potassium out of the cell. This process leads to hyperpolarization and decreased excitability. Reduction of the activity of these channels will cause increased neuronal excitability and the increased risk of seizures. (Soldovieri et al. 2007, Shah et al. 2008) Between 60% and 80% of families with BFNS will have a mutation or a deletion in either of these genes, the vast majority in *KCNQ2*. The majority of mutations are substitutions, insertions, or deletions; however, a few missense mutations have recently been identified (Soldovieri et al. 2014). In addition, the mutations are largely located in the long C-terminus region of Q2.

In the acute setting of the seizures, there is significant variability in medication usage – phenobarbital, valproate, phenytoin, levetiracetam, or combinations of these medications have all been reported (Soldovieri et al. 2014) – but there is lack of information regarding treatment response. The duration of therapy after cessation of seizures, and how prolonged pharmacological therapy may impact on the risk of seizure recurrence and epilepsy, is also unclear. Recently, it has been found that individuals with a greater number of seizures in the neonatal period were more likely to experience seizures later in life compared with individuals who experienced fewer neonatal seizures (Grinton et al. 2015).

KCNQ2 encephalopathy

More recently, the genetic screening for *KCNQ2/KCNQ3* mutations of patients with unexplained neonatal-onset epileptic encephalopathy led to the recognition of *de novo KCNQ2* mutations in patients with severe neonatal epileptic encephalopathy. This new entity has been named *KCNQ2* encephalopathy and is characterized by intractable seizures of neonatal onset and severe psychomotor impairment. Within the last two years, a number of studies with several dozen patients have been reported. However, most patients were diagnosed well after the neonatal period and their electroclinical phenotype could not be differentiated from EME or Ohtahara syndrome (Weckhuysen et al. 2012, 2013 Kato et al. 2013, Milh et al. 2013).

Several common features are seen in patients with *KCNQ2* encephalopathy when compared with BFNS. The onset of seizures is almost always in the first week of life. The seizure semiology also is very similar to BFNS – a prominent tonic component with or without associated clonic jerking of the face or limbs – and often associated with autonomic features such as apnea and desaturation. However, the seizure frequency in *KCNQ2* encephalopathy is quite high, with multiple seizures per day or even per hour, which tend to be therapy-resistant for weeks to months. In many cases, there is a tendency to seizure remission after the first years. All infants will have a severely abnormal interictal EEG pattern, either of burst suppression or of multifocal epileptiform activity.

A recent report on patients with *KCNQ2* encephalopathy diagnosed in the neonatal period and studied with continuous video-EEG recording allowed the description of a distinct electro-clinical phenotype as well as a dramatic response to oral carbamazepine (Numis et al. 2014). The ictal EEG is characterized by initial low-voltage fast activity over a single hemisphere followed by focal spike and wave complexes. While the seizures are quite short, the postictal phase is characterized by marked and prolonged diffuse voltage attenuation (Fig. 7.2).

While both age at onset and seizure semiology are similar to BFNS, the interictal EEG and clinical examination in infants with *KCNQ2* encephalopathy is very different and shows lack of physiological patterns and multifocal epileptiform abnormalities, intermixed with random, asynchronous attenuations (Fig. 7.3).

In addition, neonates with *KCNQ2* encephalopathy show severely abnormal neurological impairment already in the neonatal period, usually with lack of visual fixation or following, decreased spontaneous movements, and axial hypotonia. However, given the very

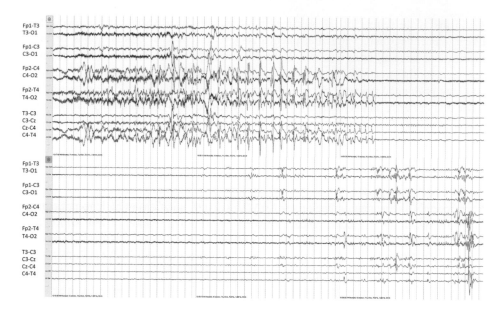

Figure 7.2. A 120-second epoch of ictal recording in a 6-week-old infant (ex-preterm born at 34 weeks, 40 weeks corrected age at the time of this recording) with *KCNQ2* encephalopathy showing a short focal seizure starting with focal low-voltage fast activity over the right hemisphere with superimposed muscle artifacts corresponding to the asymmetric tonic posturing phase, followed by focal rhythmic high amplitude spikes corresponding to the brief clonic phase. While the duration of the seizure is only about 40 seconds, there is a severe, diffuse, postictal attenuation lasting about 75 seconds with slow recovery of the background activity. Gain, 7 µV/mm; high frequency filter, 70 Hz; paper speed, 15 mm/sec.

frequent seizures and the resistance to AEDs, these patients are almost invariably treated with high doses of medications, including phenobarbital and benzodiazepines, very early after onset, which could, at least in part, contribute to the initial clinical neurological findings.

Many children with *KCNQ2* encephalopathy achieve seizure freedom after the first year of life; however, development remains, for the most part, profoundly impaired.

The fact that mutations in the same gene can give rise to either benign or severe epilepsies accompanied by neurological impairment demonstrates the importance of *KCNQ2* in brain development and suggests that the resulting potassium current may be differently affected in the two diseases. Explaining the mechanisms by which a mutation in the same gene can lead to both benign and severe epilepsies has been challenging. One study (Miceli et al. 2013) compared the impact of two mutations at the same position in *KCNQ2* found in children with BFNS (R213W mutation) and in children with neonatal epileptic encephalopathy (R213Q mutation), and showed that the R213Q caused a more pronounced functional defect, possibly reflected in the more severe phenotype. More recent data (Orhan et al. 2014) supported and extended this finding.

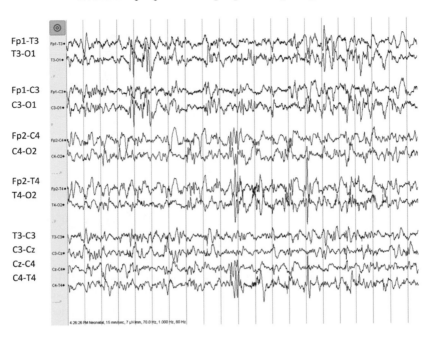

Figure 7.3. Interictal EEG in the same patient as Figure 7.2, characterized by multifocal spikes, sharp waves, and slow waves with short 1-second periods of asynchronous random attenuation. Gain, 7 µV/mm; high frequency filter, 70 Hz; paper speed, 15 mm/sec.

Finally, a more recent work by Miceli and collaborators showed that some of the mutations stabilized the activated state of the channel producing gain-of-function effects (Miceli et al. 2015).

Interestingly, sodium-channel blockers (carbamazepine and phenytoin) have been shown to be effective, resulting in a rapid dramatic reduction in seizure frequency and ultimately to seizure freedom (Numis et al. 2014, Pisano et al. 2015).

Ohtahara syndrome and early myoclonic encephalopathy
EME and Ohtahara syndrome share the important feature of burst suppression pattern on EEG associated with clinical signs of encephalopathy, although there has been much discussion concerning specific differences of the burst suppression pattern in each of these syndromes (Aicardi and Ohtahara 2005). Burst suppression consists of short periods of high voltage activity with mixed features but no age-appropriate activity alternating with periods of marked background attenuation (Fig. 7.4).

This pattern is typically unreactive and unaltered by exogenous or endogenous stimuli. Although neonates presenting with burst suppression may have different underlying etiologies, the pathophysiology of burst suppression is a fascinating question that has been addressed in research studies (Steriade et al. 1994). This study showed that suppression epochs are due to the absence of synaptic activity among cortical neurons. Interestingly, at

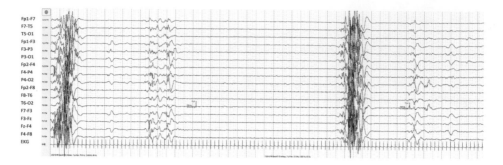

Figure 7.4. Burst suppression pattern in a 2-day-old infant with neonatal-onset epileptic encephalopathy. Short periods of high amplitude spikes, sharp waves, and slow waves are intermixed with prolonged periods of low voltage activity. Gain, 7 μV/mm; high frequency filter, 70 Hz; paper speed, 15 mm/sec.

variance with cortical neurons, only 60–70% of thalamic cells ceased firing and were completely silent during the suppressed periods of EEG activity. The remaining 30–40% of thalamic cells discharged rhythmic (1–4 Hz) spike bursts during periods of cortical silence.

EME is characterized by a burst suppression pattern associated with erratic, fragmentary myoclonus and the eventual development of focal seizures and infantile spasms. Onset of symptoms is almost always in the first days of life. The neurological status is always abnormal at onset (Aicardi and Ohtahara 2005): neonates are hypotonic and poorly responsive. The outcome of infants with EME is poor (Mizrahi and Milh 2012). There is a high incidence of death in the first few years of life. In the survivors, there is virtual absence of psychomotor development (Aicardi and Ohtahara 2005). While some authors indicated that the burst suppression pattern in EME is always present during both wakefulness and sleep (Schlumberger et al. 1992), others suggested that, in contrast with Ohtahara syndrome where burst suppression is invariably present in both states (Ohtahara and Yamatogi 2006), in EME burst suppression may be state-dependent and be only present during sleep.

In terms of causes, a metabolic etiology is highest on the differential, including glycine encephalopathy, propionic academia, D-glyceric acidemia, and methylmalonic aciduria (Dulac 2013). Numerous cases of pyridoxine dependency presenting as EME have been reported, supporting an early therapeutic trial with pyridoxine in this condition (Mills et al. 2010).

Ohtahara syndrome, first reported by Ohtahara in 1976 (Ohtahara et al. 1976, Ohtahara and Yamatogi 2006), is also characterized by onset within the first 3 months of life, most often in the neonatal period, persistent burst suppression pattern on EEG, and encephalopathy. The distinctive seizure type in this condition consists of tonic spasms, isolated or in cluster, symmetric or asymmetric. Partial seizures may also be present, while myoclonic seizures are very rare (Schlumberger et al. 1992). The suppression burst pattern, as described by Ohtahara et al. (Ohtahara et al. 1976, 1998, Ohtahara and Yamatogi 2003), is consistently observed in both wake and sleep states, and it is characterized by high-voltage bursts alternating with nearly isoelectric periods at an approximately regular rate. Bursts of 1 to 3 seconds comprise 150- to 350-microvolt high-voltage slow-waves intermixed with multifocal spikes. The duration of the suppression phase ranges from 2 to 5 seconds. Similar to EME, the prognosis of infants with Ohtahara syndrome is poor: developmental delay and evolution into West syndrome is common. Structural brain abnormalities, such as hemimegalencephaly and large focal cortical dysplasias, represent the most frequent etiology of Ohtahara syndrome, while metabolic disorders have been reported in only a few cases.

More recently, a main focus of investigation regarding pathophysiology of Ohtahara syndrome has been on genetic mutations. The first report of a genetic mutation associated with Ohtahara syndrome involved the *ARX* gene (Aristaless-related homeobox gene) (Kato et al. 2007). *ARX* encodes for a protein, a transcription factor, involved in the migration and development of cerebral interneurons. *De novo* mutations in the *STXBP1* (syntaxin binding protein 1) gene – also known as Munc18-1 – have also been found associated with Ohtahara syndrome (Saitsu et al. 2008), and this gene is now considered a major candidate in Ohtahara syndrome. STXBP1/Munc18-1 is a regulatory component of the soluble NSF attachment protein receptors (SNARE) complex that is placed in a late step of neuronal/ exocytic fusion (Shen et al. 2007). Synaptic vesicle fusion, like most intracellular membrane fusion, is mediated by the concerted action of the two SNARE protein families and plays a major role in the neurotransmitter release process. Recent studies shed light on the pathophysiology of Ohtahara syndrome that, in the setting of normal brain architecture, could be related to alterations of neurotransmission (Zhou et al. 2013).

There has been an ongoing discussion in the literature concerning the relationship between EME and Ohtahara syndrome and whether those may represent a continuum (Djukic et al. 2006) and the question is still open. It has been hypothesized that the presence of tonic seizure in Ohtahara syndrome versus absence of tonic seizures in EME may indicate the severity of brainstem dysfunction present at birth. According to this hypothesis, the brainstem dysfunction would be already present in neonates with Ohtahara syndrome, and would develop as a consequence of the disease in neonates with EME.

Epileptic encephalopathy associated with *CDKL5* mutations

Seen most frequently in females, with a 12:1 female-to-male ratio, the epileptic encephalopathy associated with *CDKL5* mutations can arise in the neonatal period, with the majority of patients having onset of seizures within the first 3 months of life.

Patients have severe psychomotor impairment. Hypotonia, gaze avoidance, and lack of development of language or fine motor skills are already evident early in the course of the disease. A significant proportion of children will have deceleration of head growth and hand stereotypies, similar to Rett syndrome. However, when compared to Rett syndrome, children with *CDKL5* have a much higher incidence of early-onset, treatment-resistant seizures.

Seizure onset is in the first few weeks of life, and almost always in the first 3 months. At onset, the interictal EEG can be normal. A three-stage electroclinical course was described by Bahi-Buisson and colleagues (2008b). Initially, affected individuals have frequent, albeit brief, seizures. Some of these children may reach seizure control after

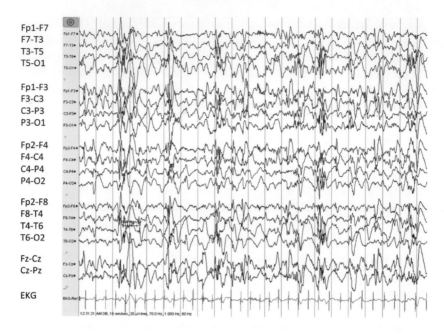

Figure 7.5. EEG of 2-year-old child with *CDKL5* associated epileptic encephalopathy. Interictal EEG recorded during sleep and showing diffuse slowing with intermixed frequent high amplitude generalized bursts of polyspikes, spikes, and waves. Gain, 20 µV/mm; high frequency filter, 70 Hz; paper speed, 15 mm/sec.

several weeks to months, with some even achieving a 'honeymoon period' of seizure freedom. Regardless of ultimate epilepsy course, all patients at this stage already exhibit hypotonia and poor eye contact. The second stage is characterized by a failure of developmental progression, and the appearance of epileptic spasms with or without hypsarrhythmia on EEG. Finally, in the third stage, children experience severe refractory epilepsy with multiple seizure types, including tonic, myoclonic, and spasms, occurring multiple times per day. By this point, the interictal EEG remains abnormal, with high-amplitude slow waves and bursts of spikes and polyspikes (Fig. 7.5).

A distinctive seizure type seen during the course of this epileptic encephalopathy is the hypermotor-tonic-spasms sequence (Klein et al. 2011), and the recognition of this quite specific sequence may lead the clinician to consider the diagnosis of a *CDKL5* encephalopathy. Identifying this disorder at presentation in the very first weeks of life can be challenging and most patients are still diagnosed only later in life. Nevertheless, the onset of brief tonic-spasms seizures in a girl with no interictal EEG abnormalities should suggest a *CDKL5* mutation (Fig. 7.6).

The *CDKL5* gene, also known as serine/threonine kinase 9 (STK9), is found at position 22 on the short arm of the X chromosome (Xp22). Many mutations have been found in the *CDKL5* gene, and as the clinical entity is more greatly recognized, some variability

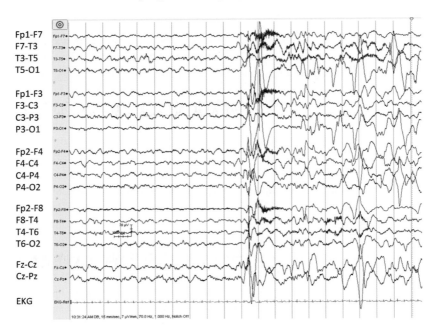

Figure 7.6. EEG recorded at 3 weeks of age in the same patient as Figure 7.5 showing the ictal pattern of a brief tonic seizure characterized by diffuse low amplitude fast activity preceded by a normal background. Gain, 7 μV/mm; high frequency filter, 70 Hz; paper speed, 15 mm/sec.

in phenotype does exist. In Bahi-Buisson's cohort (Bahi-Buisson et al. 2008b), there was trend toward clinical severity (earlier onset of epilepsy, intractable spasms, and worse psychomotor impairment) and mutations that impaired the catalytic domain, as opposed to truncating mutations that were downstream from the catalytic domain. Further research continues on pathogenicity and phenotypic variability as greater numbers of mutations are being found.

To date, no specific AEDs have been shown to have greater efficacy for seizure control in this particular epileptic encephalopathy. In addition, the medications chosen during the clinical course which includes infantile spasms are no different than other idiopathic or cryptogenic spasms, with most clinicians using adrenocorticotrophic hormone (ACTH) or another steroid derivative, and vigabatrin. Carbamazepine, valproate, and clobazam have also been trialed in order to control the tonic seizures with different results.

Epilepsy of infancy with migrating focal seizures
EIMFS is a newly recognized early-onset epilepsy syndrome (Engel 2001). First described in 1995, it is characterized by polymorphous, migrating, almost continuous, focal seizures associated with arrest of development, resulting in profound disability (Coppola et al. 1995). Most affected infants start to have seizures in the first few weeks of life and all start having seizures by six months of age (Cilio et al. 2008). Ictal discharges arise randomly

from various areas of both hemispheres and migrate from one region to another, conferring the main feature and name to this syndrome. The seizures are highly pharmacoresistant and overtreatment should be avoided. Conventional antiepileptic treatments, including pheno-barbital, phenytoin, carbamazepine, valproate, vigabatrin, benzodiazepines, lamotrigine, steroids, and ACTH, have proved ineffective. Vigabatrin and carbamazepine may worsen seizures. Various vitamins, including pyridoxine, biotin, and folinic acid, have been trialed without success. A ketogenic diet resulted in little or no improvement (Okuda et al. 2000, March et al. 2005). Potassium bromide and levetiracetam have been shown to control seizures to some extent (Okuda et al. 2000, Cilio et al. 2009. Unver et al. 2013, Caraballo et al. 2014). Only recently, *KCNT1 de novo* mutations have been identified in patients with EIMFS, confirming the genetic etiology of EIFMS and ascribing it to the large family of channelopathies (Barcia et al. 2012). *KCNT1* encodes a weakly voltage-dependent and intracellular sodium-activated potassium channel. *KCNT1* is a member of the Slo-type subfamily of potassium channel genes, also known as Slack (sequence like a calcium-activated potassium channel), and co-assembles with other Slo subunits (Kim et al. 2014). *KCNT1* is widely expressed in the nervous system and represents the largest known potas-sium channel subunit. Its activity contributes to the slow hyperpolarization that follows repetitive firing. Functional studies have shown that *KCNT1* mutations causing EIMFS are associated with a gain-of-function phenotype *in vitro*, leading to constitutive activation of the sodium-activated potassium channel (Barcia et al. 2012). While this could account for the increased excitability and seizure phenotype, the severity of developmental delay in children with EIMFS suggests an independent developmental role for this gene. Recent studies have established that, in addition to regulation ion flux, a number of channels have nonconducting functions that regulate biochemical activities independent of ion flux (Kac-zmarek 2006, Fleming and Kaczmarek 2009). This is likely to be the case for the *KCNT1* channel, which in its C-terminal domain interacts with a protein network including fragile X mental retardation protein (FMRP). It has been suggested that *KCNT1* mutations may alter the conformation of the C-terminal region of the protein, impairing not only the gating of the channel but also its ability to interact with developmentally relevant proteins such as FMRP, and accounting for the severe developmental delay (Barcia et al. 2012). Quinidine has been shown to reverse the increased conductance imparted by the pathological gain of function mutations *in vitro* and a case report has demonstrated efficacy in clinical practice (Bearden et al. 2014, Milligan et al. 2014). Seizure control has been suggested to improve neurodevelopmental outcomes (Bearden et al. 2014).

Conclusion

The gene discovery efforts of the past decade for severe epilepsies, particularly early onset epileptic encephalopathies, have shown that genetic mutations play a major role, and they must be considered in the differential diagnosis of seizures in neonates and infants. However, many unresolved questions remain. The electroclinical presentation in the neonatal period of neonatal-onset epilepsies is not yet well defined since many patients are diagnosed later in life, and clinical and EEG findings related to the neonatal period may be scarce. Addi-tionally, mutations in the same gene can be associated with both benign and severe epilepsies. In conclusion, the definition of the electroclinical phenotype remains important for a correct diagnosis, management, and prognosis. In the context of early diagnosis and targeted treatment, an accurate characterization of the neonatal phenotype is key to determine the best strategy to manage and treat neonatal-onset epilepsies, especially if the goal is not only seizures control but also a normal developmental outcome. The past 20 years have seen the development of prolonged video-EEG monitoring as a method for characterizing seizures in infants and children, providing the basis for a precise diagnosis of epilepsy type and syndrome and targeted therapy. We believe that similar care should be applied in neonates with seizures, since a number of them may benefit from an epileptological approach.

REFERENCES

Aicardi J, Ohtahara S (2005) Severe neonatal epilepsies with suppression-burst. In: Roger JB, Dravet M, Genton C, Tassinari P, CA. Wolf P, editors. *Epileptic Syndromes in Infancy, Childhood and Adolescence,* 2323–2328. Paris: John Libbey Eurotext.

Bahi-Buisson N, Kaminska A, Boddaert N et al. (2008a) The three stages of epilepsy in patients with CDKL5 mutations. *Epilepsia* 49 (6): 1027–1037. doi: http://dx.doi.org/10.1111/j.1528-1167.2007.01520.x.

Bahi-Buisson N, Nectoux J, Rosas-Vargas H et al. (2008b) Key clinical features to identify girls with CDKL5 mutations. *Brain* 131: 2647–2661. doi: http://dx.doi.org/10.1093/brain/awn197.

Barcia G, Fleming MR, Deligniere A et al. (2012) De novo gain-of-function KCNT1 channel mutations cause malignant migrating partial seizures of infancy. *Nature Genetics* 44: 1255–1259. doi: http://dx.doi.org/10.1038/ng.2441.

Bearden D, Strong A, Ehnot J, DiGiovine M, Dlugos D, Goldberg EM (2014) Targeted treatment of migrating partial seizures in infancy with quinidine. *Ann Neurol* 76: 457–461. doi: http://dx.doi.org/10.1002/ana.24229.

Berg AT, Berkovic SF, Brodies MJ et al. (2010) Revised terminology and concepts for organization of seizure and epilepsies: Report of the ILAE commission on classification and terminology, 2005–2009. *Epilepsia* 51: 676–685. doi: http://dx.doi.org/10.1111/j.1528-1167.2010.02522.x.

Biervert C, Schroeder BC, Kubisch C et al. (1998) A potassium channel mutation in neonatal human epilepsy. *Science* 279: 403–404. doi: http://dx.doi.org/10.1126/science.279.5349.403.

Bjerre I, Corelius E (1968) Benign neonatal familial convulsions. *Acta Paediat Scand* 57: 557–561. doi: http://dx.doi.org/10.1111/j.1651-2227.1968.tb06980.x.

Caraballo R, Pasteris MC, Fortini PS, Portuondo E (2014) Epilepsy of infancy with migrating focal seizures: Six patients treated with bromide. *Seizure* 23: 899–902. doi: http://dx.doi.org/10.1016/j.seizure.2014.06.016.

Charlier C, Singh NA, Ryan SG et al. (1998) A pore mutation in a novel KQT-like potassium channel gene in an idiopathic epilepsy family. *Nat Genet* 18: 53–55. doi: http://dx.doi.org/10.1038/ng0198-53.

Cilio MR, Bianchi R, Balestri M et al. (2009) Intravenous levetiracetam terminates refractory status epilepticus in two patients with migrating partial seizures in infancy. *Epilepsy Res* 86: 66–71. doi: http://dx.doi.org/10.1016/j.eplepsyres.2009.05.004.

Cilio MR, Dulac O, Guerrini R, Vigevano F (2008) Migrating partial seizures in infancy. In: Engel J et al., editors. *Epilepsy: A Comprehensive Textbook*, vol. 3, 2323–2328. Lippincott William & Wilkins, Philadelphia, PA, USA.

Coppola G, Plouin P, Chiron C, Robain O, Dulac O (1995) Migrating partial seizures in infancy – A malignant disorder with developmental arrest. *Epilepsia* 36: 1017–1024. doi: http://dx.doi.org/10.1111/j.1528-1157.1995.tb00961.x.

Djukic A, Lado FA, Shinnar S, Moshe SL (2006) Are early myoclonic encephalopathy (EME) and the Ohtahara syndrome (EIEE) independent of each other? *Epilepsy Research* 70: S68–S76. doi: http://dx.doi.org/10.1016/j.eplepsyres.2005.11.022.

Dulac O (2013) Epileptic encephalopathy with suppression-bursts and nonketotic hyperglycinemia. *Handbook of Clinical Neurology* 113: 1785–1797. doi: http://dx.doi.org/10.1016/B978-0-444-59565-2.00048-4.

Engel JJ (2001) A proposed diagnostic scheme for people with epileptic seizures and with epilepsy: Report of the ILAE task force on classification and terminology. *Epilepsia* 42: 796–803. doi: http://dx.doi.org/10.1046/j.1528-1157.2001.10401.x.

Fleming MR, Kaczmarek LK (2009) Use of optical biosensors to detect modulation of slack potassium channels by G protein-coupled receptors. *Journal of Receptors and Signal Transduction* 29: 173–181. doi: http://dx.doi.org/10.1080/10799890903056883.

Grinton BE, Heron SE, Pelekanos JT et al. (2015) Familial neonatal seizures in 36 families: Clinical and genetic features correlated with outcome. *Epilepsia* 56 (7): 1071–1080. doi: http://dx.doi.org/10.1111/epi.13020.

Kato M, Saitoh S, Kamei A et al. (2007) A longer polyalanine expansion mutation in the ARX gene causes early infantile epileptic encephalopathy with suppression-burst pattern (Ohtahara syndrome). *American Journal of Human Genetics* 81: 361–366. doi: http://dx.doi.org/10.1086/518903.

Kato M, Yamagata T, Kubota M et al. (2013) Clinical spectrum of early onset epileptic encephalopathies caused by KCNQ2 mutation. *Epilepsia* 54: 1282–1287. doi: http://dx.doi.org/10.1111/epi.12200.

Kaczmarek LK (2006) Non-conducting functions of voltage-gated ion channels. *Nat Rev Neurosci* 7: 761–771. doi: http://dx.doi.org/10.1038/nrn1988.

Kim GE, Kronengold J, Barcia G et al. (2014) Human slack potassium channel mutations increase positive cooperativity between individual channels. *Cell Reports* 9: 1661–1672. doi: http://dx.doi.org/10.1016/j.celrep.2014.11.015.

Klein KM, Yendle SC, Harvey AS et al. (2011) A distinctive seizure type in patients with CDKL5 mutations: Hypermotor-tonic-spasms sequence. *Neurology* 76: 1436–1438. doi: http://dx.doi.org/10.1212/WNL.0b013e3182166e58.

Marsch E, Melamed SE, Barron T, Clancy RR (2005) Migrating partial seizures in infancy: Expanding the phenotype of a rare seizure syndrome. *Epilepsia* 46: 568–572. doi: http://dx.doi.org/10.1111/j.0013-9580.2005.34104.x.

Miceli F, Soldovieri MV, Ambrosino P et al. (2013) Genotype-phenotype correlations in neonatal epilepsies caused by mutations in the voltage sensor of Kv7.2 potassium channel subunits. *Proc Natl Acad Sci USA* 110: 4386–4391. doi: http://dx.doi.org/10.1073/pnas.1216867110.

Miceli F, Soldovieri MV, Ambrosino P et al. (2015) Early-onset epileptic encephalopathy caused by gain-of-function mutations in the voltage sensor of Kv7.2 and Kv7.3 potassium channel subunits. *J Neurosci* 39: 3782–3793. doi: http://dx.doi.org/10.1523/JNEUROSCI.4423-14.2015.

Mills PB, Footitt EJ, Mills KA, et al. (2010) Genotypic and phenotypic spectrum of pyridoxine-dependent epilepsy (ALDH7A1 deficiency). *Brain* 133: 2148–2159.

Milh M, Boutry-Kryza N, Sutera-Sardo J et al. (2013) Similar early characteristics but variable neurological outcomes of patients with a de novo mutation of KCNQ2. *Orphanet J Rare Dis* 8: 80. doi: http://dx.doi.org/10.1186/1750-1172-8-80.

Milligan CJ, Li M, Gazina EV et al. (2014) KCNT1 gain of function in 2 epilepsy phenotypes is reversed by quinidine. *Ann Neurol* 75: 581–590. doi: http://dx.doi.org/10.1002/ana.24128.

Mizrahi E, Milh M (2012) Early severe neonatal and infantile epilepsies. In: Bureau M et al., editors. *Epileptic Syndromes in Infancy, Childhood and Adolescence*, 89–98. Paris: John Libbey Eurotext.

Nabbout R, Dulac O (2012) Genetics of early-onset epilepsy with encephalopathy. *Nat Rev Neurol* 8: 129–130. doi: http://dx.doi.org/10.1038/nrneurol.2012.12.

Numis AL, Angriman M, Sullivan JE et al. (2014) KCNQ2 encephalopathy: Delineation of the electroclinical phenotype and treatment response. *Neurology* 82: 368–370. doi: http://dx.doi.org/10.1212/WNL.0000000000000060.

Ohtahara S, Ishida S, Oka E, Yamatogi Y, Inoue H (1976) On the specific age dependent epileptic syndromes: The early-infantile epileptic encephalopathy with suppression bursts. *No To Hattatsu* 8: 270–280.

Ohtahara S, Ohtsuka Y, Erba G (1998) Early epileptic encephalopathy with suppression-burst. In: Engel J, Pedley TA, editors. *Epilepsy: A Comprehensive Textbook*, vol. 3, 2257–2261. Philadelphia: Lippincott-Raven.

Ohtahara S, Yamatogi Y (2006) Ohtahara syndrome: With special reference to its developmental aspects for differentiating from early myoclonic encephalopathy. *Epilepsy Research* 70: S58–S67. doi: http://dx.doi.org/10.1016/j.eplepsyres.2005.11.021.

Orhan G, Bock M, Schepers D et al. (2014) Dominant-negative effects of KCNQ2 mutations are associated with epileptic encephalopathy. *Ann Neurol* 75: 382–394. doi: http://dx.doi.org/10.1002/ana.24080.

Okuda K, Yasuhara A, Kamei A, Araki A, Kitamura N, Kobayashi Y (2000) Successful control with bromide of two patients with malignant migrating partial seizures in infancy. *Brain Dev* 22: 56–59. doi: http://dx.doi.org/10.1016/S0387-7604(99)00108-4.

Pisano T, Numis AL, Heavin SB et al. (2015) Early and effective treatment of KCNQ2 encephalopathy. *Epilepsia* 56: 685–691. doi: http://dx.doi.org/10.1111/epi.12984.

Ronen GM, Rosales TO, Connolly M, Anderson VE, Leppert M (1993) Seizure characteristics in chromosome 20 benign familial neonatal convulsions. *Neurology* 4: 1355–1360. doi: http://dx.doi.org/10.1212/WNL.43.7.1355.

Saitsu H, Kato M, Mizuguchi T et al. (2008) De novo mutations in the gene encoding STXBP1 (MUNC18-1) cause early infantile epileptic encephalopathy. *Nature Genetics* 40: 782–788. doi: http://dx.doi.org/10.1038/ng.150.

Schlumberger E, Dulac O, Plouin P (1992) Early infantile syndrome(s) with suppression-burst: Nosological considerations. In: Roger J et al., editors. *Epileptic Syndromes of Infancy, Childhood and Adolescence*, 35–42. London: John Libbey.

Shah MM, Migliore M, Valencia I, Cooper EC, Brown DA (2008) Functional significance of axonal Kv7 channels in hippocampal pyramidal neurons. *Proc Natl Acad Sci USA* 105: 7869–7874. doi: http://dx.doi.org/10.1073/pnas.0802805105.

Shen J, Tareste DC, Paumet F, Rothman JE, Melia TJ (2007) Selective activation of cognate SNAREpins by Sec1/Munc18 proteins. *Cell* 128: 183–195. doi: http://dx.doi.org/10.1016/j.cell.2006.12.016.

Singh NA, Charlier C, Stauffer D et al. (1998) A novel potassium channel gene, KCNQ2, is mutated in an inherited epilepsy of newborns. *Nat Genet* 18: 23–29. doi: http://dx.doi.org/10.1038/ng0198-25.

Soldovieri MV, Boutry-Kryza N, Milh M et al. (2014) Novel KCNQ2 and KCNQ3 mutations in a large cohort of families with benign neonatal epilepsy: First evidence for an altered channel regulation by syntaxin-1A. *Human Mutat* 35: 356–367. doi: http://dx.doi.org/10.1002/humu.22500.

Soldovieri MV, Cilio MR, Miceli F et al. (2007) Atypical gating of M-type potassium channels conferred by mutations in uncharged residues in the S4 region of KCNQ2 causing Benign Familial Neonatal Convulsions. *J Neurosci* 27: 4919–4928. doi: http://dx.doi.org/10.1523/JNEUROSCI.0580-07.2007.

Steriade M, Amzica F, Contreras D (1994) Cortical and thalamic cellular correlates of electroencephalographic burst-suppression. *Electroen Clin Neuro* 90: 1–16. doi: http://dx.doi.org/10.1016/0013-4694(94)90108-2.

Unver O, Incecik F, Dundar H, Komur M, Unver A, Okuyaz C (2013) Potassium bromide for treatment of malignant migrating partial seizures in infancy. *Pediatr Neurol* 49: 355–357. doi: http://dx.doi.org/10.1016/j.pediatrneurol.2013.05.016.

Weckhuysen S, Mandelstam S, Suls A et al. (2012) KCNQ2 encephalopathy: Emerging phenotype of a neonatal epileptic encephalopathy. *Ann Neurol* 71: 15–25. doi: http://dx.doi.org/10.1002/ana.22644.

Weckhuysen S, Ivanovic V, Hendrickx R et al. (2013) Extending the KCNQ2 encephalopathy spectrum: Clinical and neuroimaging findings in 17 patients. *Neurology* 81: 1697–1703. doi: http://dx.doi.org/10.1212/01.wnl.0000435296.72400.a1.

Yue C, Yaari Y (2006) Axo-somatic and apical dendritic Kv7/M channels differentially regulate the intrinsic excitability of adult rat CA1 pyramidal cells. *J Neurophysiol* 95: 3480–3495. doi: http://dx.doi.org/10.1152/jn.01333.2005.

Zhou P, Pang ZP, Yang X, et al. (2013) Syntaxin-1 N-peptide and H-abc-domain perform distinct essential functions in synaptic vesicle fusion. *Embo Journal* 32:159–171.

8
CLINICAL APPROACH TO A NEONATE WITH SEIZURES

Shripada Rao, Barry Lewis, Soumya Ghosh and Lakshmi Nagarajan

Neonatal seizures occur in 1.8–5 per 1000 live births, with majority occurring in the first few days of life (Jensen 2009, Ronen et al. 1999). Seizures occur more frequently in the neonatal period than at any other time of life. Although considered to be a manifestation of brain dysfunction, neonatal seizures themselves have been shown to adversely affect neurodevelopmental outcomes (Holmes 2009, Nagarajan et al. 2010, Glass et al. 2011, Shah et al. 2014). Hence it is important to (1) accurately diagnose the seizures, (2) identify the aetiology, (3) correct the underlying abnormality if possible, (4) treat the seizures with appropriate medications, (5) consider neuroprotective strategies and (6) provide appropriate supportive and follow-up care.

Accurate diagnosis

There is a wide variability in the estimates of incidence of neonatal seizures in published literature (Vasudevan and Levene 2013). This is because of different geographic populations, variable inclusion of term and preterm infants, inconsistent definitions of a seizure (clinical basis only, electrographically confirmed seizures only or both) and population-versus hospital-based studies. Another reason for the variable incidence is the fact that neonatal seizures are difficult to diagnose, classify and quantify.

Clinical examination alone has the potential to underdiagnose or over-report seizures (Murray et al. 2008, Malone et al. 2009, Nagarajan et al. 2011) and hence it is important not to rely solely on it. Neonatal seizures are now defined as those with epileptic brain activity (electrographic seizure) seen on electroencephalography (EEG), with or without clinical correlates (Ferriero 2009, Nagarajan et al. 2011, Wusthoff 2013). Electroclinical dissociation (ECD) is the detection of electrographic seizures without clinical correlates. It occurs frequently in neonates, when monitored with EEG. ECD is seen in term and preterm infants, in neonates undergoing therapeutic hypothermia and is common regardless of whether the child is getting a GABAergic drug or not, though thought to be more frequent in those who have received GABAnergic antiepileptic drugs (AEDs) (Boylan et al. 2013). The majority of the studies have included epileptic and non-epileptic phenomenon in the description of clinical features of neonatal seizures (Mizrahi and Kellaway 1987, Scher 2002, Volpe 2008). With increasing use of video-EEG (v-EEG) monitoring, the varied clinical correlates of electroclinical seizures are being better delineated. Most of the electroclinical seizures have multiple features. In a study of 61 epileptic seizures in neonates

(Nagarajan et al. 2012), oro-lingual features were reported most frequently at the onset, whereas ocular phenomena occurred most often during the seizure. Rhythmic clonic jerking is frequently epileptic in nature, and generalised myoclonic jerks are more likely to be epileptic than focal or multifocal myoclonus. Focal and multifocal tonic seizures may occur, and eye deviation and rhythmic jerking of eyes are likely to be epileptiform (Mizrahi and Kellaway 1987, Volpe 2008). Given the variable presenting features, an EEG is essential to diagnosing a neonatal seizure accurately, with or without clinical correlates. Hence, it is important to request a conventional multichannel v-EEG in any neonate who is at risk of seizures or who presents with clinical seizures. If facilities for v-EEG are not available on an emergency basis, limited-channel EEG with amplitude-integrated EEG (a-EEG) may be used as a screening tool in such situations.

Differentiating epileptic seizures from seizure like activities

When neonates demonstrate abnormal movements or behaviour, it is important to know whether they are seizures or paroxysmal non-epileptic phenomenon (Huntsman et al. 2008, Orivoli et al. 2015, Hart et al. 2015a). The following common movements need to be considered in the differential diagnosis of clinically suspected neonatal seizures (Table 8.1).

Jitteriness: Jitteriness is defined as rhythmic tremors of equal amplitude around a fixed axis. It is the most common involuntary movement in healthy neonates (Rosman et al. 1984), usually observed during the first 72 hours of life with improvement over 1–2 weeks. Conditions such as hypoglycaemia, hypocalcaemia, asphyxia and neonatal drug withdrawal syndrome (maternal marijuana or cocaine use) need to be considered while managing an infant with jitteriness (Parker et al. 1990). Maternal use of selective serotonin reuptake inhibitors is also associated with jitteriness (Zeskind and Stephens 2004, Olivier et al. 2013). Jitteriness can be brought on with stimuli and stopped with gentle passive flexion or restraint of the affected limb. It is not associated with ocular phenomena such as forced eye deviation or autonomic changes such as hypertension or apnoea (Huntsman et al. 2008). Treatment of jitteriness involves correcting the underlying cause, if identified. Special attention must be paid to mother-newborn infant bonding because jittery neonates tend to have decreased visual attention and are more difficult to console (Parker et al. 1990).

Benign neonatal sleep myoclonus: This is one of the most common neonatal seizure mimics (Malone et al. 2009, Maurer et al. 2010). Events are repetitive, generalised or multifocal rhythmic myoclonic jerks that occur only during sleep, in otherwise typical neonates, and disappear when awake. They mainly occur in the extremities and do not stop on holding the limbs. They will stop if you wake the infant. They are usually brief (<1 min), but occasionally can last longer than 30 minutes and mimic status epilepticus (Turanli et al. 2004). A v-EEG will show a normal background with no epileptiform activity in association with the myoclonic jerks. AEDs are not effective and may worsen the myoclonus. They usually resolve by 3 months of age without long-term sequelae (Maurer et al. 2010).

Motor automatisms: Repetitive stereotypical movements such as pedalling, cycling, boxing, swimming, drum-beating type of movements or myoclonic jerks may be observed in preterm infants and healthy newborn infants. They have also been reported during midazolam infusions. They are not associated with EEG changes and do not require AEDs (Zaw et al. 2001, Ishizaki et al. 2011). Oro-lingual and ocular phenomenon may be epileptic (Nagarajan et al. 2012).

Dystonic and tonic movements: Generalised stiffening, dystonia and rigidity may be misdiagnosed as tonic seizures, and can be a result of hypoxic-ischaemic encephalopathy (HIE), affecting the basal ganglia and thalami, meningitis, maternal drug use, acute bilirubin encephalopathy, neuromuscular or neuro-metabolic disorders (Hart et al. 2015b). Paroxysmal tonic up-gaze and paroxysmal tonic down-gaze may occasionally be seen in the normal and neurologically impaired neonates (Hans and Sanger 2004). A more frequent seizure mimic is the Sutcliffe-Sandiper syndrome: the association of gastroesophageal reflux with dystonic movements and posturing, often related to feeding (Cross 2013).

Hyperekplexia: Also called startle disease, it is a rare neurological disorder with an excessive startle response which may be associated with generalised rigidity and nocturnal myoclonus. Occurrence of the startle response, by nose tapping, with lack of habituation, is thought to be characteristic of this disorder. Hyperekplexia may be sporadic or of genetic origin – with autosomal dominantly inherited mutations in the alpha-1 subunit of the glycine receptor gene being seen in the majority. Clonazepam is useful for the exaggerated startle reflex, but does not appear to influence the hypertonicity or the reported association of sudden infant death syndrome (Zhou et al. 2002, Orivoli et al. 2015).

Paroxysmal extreme pain disorder: It was previously called the familial rectal pain syndrome. It may present in infants with flushing, stiffening or tonic phenomenon and bradycardia. It is an autosomal dominant disorder due to a sodium channel mutation – mostly SCN9A (Fertleman et al. 2007).

Repetitive eye phenomenon: This can be quite challenging. Eye deviation, rhythmic jerking and eye flickering can be epileptic (Volpe 2008, Nagarajan et al. 2012), whereas disconjugate eye movements are frequently not epileptiform. Opsoclonus may rarely occur in the neonatal period; autoimmune phenomenon needs to be considered with inclusion of investigation for neuroblastoma (Hero 2013).

EEG

The definitive diagnosis of neonatal seizures is based on their detection on EEG (Boylan et al. 2013, Mccoy et al. 2013). While a standard v-EEG of approximately 60 minutes' duration may capture neonatal seizures (Nagarajan et al. 2010), continuous long-term v-EEG is considered to be the criterion standard for the diagnosis, classification, quantification and prognostication of neonatal seizures and to monitor response to medication (Shellhaas 2015).

The American Clinical Neurophysiology Society's guideline recommends that neonates at high risk for seizures be monitored with v-EEG for 24 hours (Shellhaas et al. 2011). Difficulties in implementing this guideline include the need for appropriate equipment, special training for the application and expertise for the interpretation of the recording and high cost (Glass 2014). A recent international survey of 210 neonatal intensive care unit

TABLE 8.1
Non-epileptic movements that can mimic neonatal seizures

	Clinical features	EEG
Jitteriness/tremor	Irregular, stimulus sensitive; disappear when the limb is held firmly	Normal
Benign neonatal sleep myoclonus	Repetitive, focal or multifocal rhythmic myoclonic jerks that occur during sleep in otherwise healthy normal neonates; disappear when the neonate is awake	Normal
Motor automatisms	Repetitive stereotypical movements such as pedalling, cycling, boxing, swimming, drum-beating type of movements or myoclonic jerks	Normal
Dystonic and tonic movements	Generalised stiffening of all four limbs	Abnormal but no seizure correlates
Sandiper syndrome	Associated with gastro-oesophageal reflux	Normal
Hyperekplexia	Excessive startle response	Normal
Paroxysmal extreme pain disorder	Flushing, stiffening or tonic phenomenon and bradycardia	Normal
Opsoclonus	Chaotic rapid multidirectional eye movements; consider neuroblastoma	Normal
Cardiac arrhythmias	Long QT syndrome, WPW syndrome, etc	Hypoxic slowing during prolonged episodes

WPW, Wolf-Parkinson-White syndrome

(NICU) staff found that v-EEG was available only during daytime on weekdays in majority of the NICUs (Boylan et al. 2010).

In view of the resource issues with v-EEG, a-EEG has gained widespread acceptance in recent times as an alternate modality for bedside monitoring of neonatal seizures. The a-EEG is commonly used to assess the degree of encephalopathy in term infants undergoing therapeutic hypothermia after HIE (Hallberg et al. 2010). The evolution of a-EEG over 48–72 hours is also a useful adjunct in prognosticating long-term neurodevelopmental outcomes in HIE (Cseko et al. 2013). However, the ability of limited channel a-EEG to correctly diagnose electrographic seizures is debatable (Toet et al. 2002, Shah et al. 2008, Lawrence et al. 2009, Evans et al. 2010). In view of the variable sensitivity and specificity, a-EEG alone is not recommended for seizure detection in neonates (Shellhaas et al. 2011, Rakshasbhuvankar et al., 2015).

In current clinical practice, a judicious combination of v-EEG and a-EEG is often used for the diagnosis and management of neonates with seizures.

Aetiology of neonatal seizures
An underlying aetiology can be identified in nearly 90% of neonates with seizures with appropriate investigations (Weeke et al. 2015a). Neonatal seizures are a manifestation of brain impairment due to wide variety of causes, with HIE, intracranial haemorrhages and perinatal ischaemic strokes (PAIS) being some of the most common aetiologies. Transient

TABLE 8.2
Aetiological classification of neonatal seizures

Aetiology	Aetiology and time of onset of neonatal seizures[1]	Incidence[2]
Hypoxic-ischaemic encephalopathy	4–48 hours	37.1–57.5%
Metabolic or electrolyte disorders	Glucose ↓: day 2 Calcium ↓ / Magnesium ↓: day 2–3 or week 2–6, Sodium ↑or ↓: any time, Bilirubin ↑: day 3	3–19%
Intracranial haemorrhage	Subdural:<12 hours Subarachnoid:<5 days, often day 2	4.8–17%
Ischaemic infarction or sinovenous thrombosis	12–76 hours	7–18%
Intracranial infections	Meningitis: any time, often 1st week; encephalitis: <3 days HIV and HSV: 1st week neurotropic virus: any time	3–20%
Congenital malformations of the CNS	Any time	3.2–11.3%
Inborn errors of metabolism	Any time	1–11.3%
Idiopathic	Any time	0.5–14%
Intoxications	Intoxication by local anaesthesia: <6 hours; withdrawal: <3 days	0.5%

[1]Adapted from Loman et al. (2014). [2]Adapted from Loman et al. (2014), Tekgul et al. (2006), Mastrangelo et al. (2005) and Ronen et al. (1999)

metabolic disturbances and inherited metabolic disorders, central nervous system (CNS) infections (viral, bacterial), cerebral venous sinus thrombosis, brain malformation disorders and genetic epilepsies (benign and the epileptic encephalopathy) constitute most of other causative disorders of neonatal seizures (Loman et al. 2014). In low-income countries incidence of neonatal seizures is higher, and infectious causes may be responsible for >50% of neonatal seizures (Idro et al. 2008).

Investigation and treatment of the underlying abnormality
INVESTIGATION OF A NEONATE WITH SEIZURES
History: Detailed history could provide clues to the following causes of neonatal seizures (Tables 8.2 and 8.3).
    a. Drugs used by mothers such as SSRIs, alcohol, opiates and cocaine. In a large observational study of 997 infants (987 mothers on antidepressants) Källén et al. reported that nine neonates developed seizures. Infants of mothers who were on tricyclic antidepressants were at higher risk compared to those on Selective Serotonin Re-uptake Inhibitors (SSRI) (5/395 vs. 4/559) (Kallen 2004). However, it

is reassuring to know that multiple systematic reviews have reported that neonatal seizures are very rare occurrences with maternal use of SSRI and Selective Nor-epineprhine Re-uptake Inhibitors (SNRI) (Moses-Kolko et al. 2005, Sie et al. 2011). Neonates born to mothers on chronic medications or substance abuse with opioids can develop severe withdrawal symptoms including seizures in the first week of life (Dahan et al. 2011, Grim et al. 2013).

b. History of excessive fetal movements during pregnancy. Aberrant foetal movements may indicate seizures. Occasionally, seizures could be identified on foetal ultrasounds (Patane and Ghidini 2001, Sheizaf et al. 2007).

c. History of maternal illness. History of maternal illness during pregnancy such as pre-eclampsia, chorioamnionitis and prolonged rupture of membranes need to be elicited. In addition, detailed labour and birth history including duration of labour, presence of fetal distress, need for resuscitation at birth, Apgar scores and cord blood gases are important (Jensen, 2009, Yildiz et al. 2012). It is also essential to elicit history of maternal herpes infection during pregnancy (Pinninti and Kimberlin 2014).

d. Parental description of events. It is important to elicit history of the type of events, duration, involvement of one or both sides and associated symptoms such as apnoea, colour change. It is worth enquiring if parents have taken a video of the events on their smart phones.

e. Family history of seizure disorders. Benign familial neonatal seizures and other genetic epilepsies, neurocutaneous syndromes, brain malformations and certain metabolic disorders can run in families.

f. Preterm. Preterm infants are more susceptible to seizures because of the risk of intra-ventricular haemorrhage and meningitis.

CLINICAL EXAMINATION

A thorough examination of the nervous system as well as other systems is important. A relatively well neonate with focal seizures may suggest perinatal stroke (Kirton et al. 2011, van der Aa et al. 2014). A well neonate with multifocal seizures may have electrolyte abnormalities such as hypocalcacmia. Neonates with perinatal asphyxia and CNS infections

TABLE 8.3
Clinical history in neonatal seizures

Maternal diseases	Preeclampsia, herpes, chorioamnionitis, antepartum haemorrhage, excessive fatal movements
Maternal medications	Antidepressants, opioid analgesics, benzodiazepines, alcohol
History of perinatal asphyxia	Fetal heart rate monitoring, growth retardation, difficult labour, Apgar scores, delivery room resuscitation details, type of delivery, cord blood gases
Parental description of the observed seizures	Ask if they have taken a video of the episode; encourage them to do so

are usually unwell and may have associated multiorgan dysfunction. The presence of jaundice, petechiae, purpura and anaemia in a sick infant may be suggestive of meningitis. Inborn errors of metabolism (IEMs) need to be kept in mind; the EEG, neuroimaging or clinical features may provide a clue. Dysmorphic features may point to underlying syndromic disorders. It is important to look for the presence of microcephaly, macrocephaly, neuro-cutaneous signs, hepatosplenomegaly, ophthalmologic examinations and bruit over the fontanels (vein of Galen malformation).

Investigations: Initial investigation should focus on identifying conditions that are treatable and if untreated can lead to brain damage. The most important are hypoglycaemia, bacterial meningitis, herpes meningitis and some IEM (Table 8.4). Hence blood glucose, full blood count, C-reactive protein (CRP), blood culture, lumbar puncture with cerebrospinal fluid (CSF) examination for microscopy, culture and herpes simplex DNA using polymerase chain reaction (PCR), throat and rectal swabs for herpes simplex virus (HSV) and plasma ammonia should be performed on a priority basis.

Other important treatable causes of seizures are hypocalcaemia, hypomagnesaemia, hyponatremia and hypokalaemia, which can be easily diagnosed by monitoring plasma levels. Occasionally, subdural and epidural haemorrhages can give rise to seizures. They can be diagnosed with bedside cranial ultrasound. Emergency evacuation of the blood can prevent brain damage secondary to compression effect (Noguchi et al. 2010).

Once these investigations are completed, the next line of investigations will need to focus on conditions where curative therapy may not be available, but a definitive diagnosis will facilitate provision of supportive treatment and prognostication (Table 8.5).

IMAGING STUDIES

Cranial ultrasound: The most commonly performed imaging study in the NICUs is head ultrasound (Table 8.6). It is a good initial imaging modality for conditions such as intraventricular haemorrhage, intraparenchymal haemorrhage, structural abnormalities of the brain, gross ischemic stroke, arteriovenous malformations, hydrocephalus, basal ganglia changes in HIE and others (Daneman et al. 2006). Ultrasound may also be useful in suspected IEM (Leijser et al. 2007).

TABLE 8.4

Emergency investigations to identify potentially treatable conditions, where delay can be harmful

Condition	Investigations
Metabolic	Blood glucose, plasma sodium, potassium, calcium, magnesium, blood gas, lactate, ammonia, liver function tests, renal function tests
Infections	Full blood count, CRP, blood culture, CSF microscopy and culture, throat and rectal swabs for HSV, Blood PCR for HSV, urine microscopy and culture
Intracranial haemorrhage	Cranial ultrasound

TABLE 8.5
Investigations to make a diagnosis, in order to facilitate prognostication and supportive treatment (curative therapy may not available)

Condition	Investigations
Disorders of amino acid metabolism	Plasma, CSF and urine amino acids
Disorders of organic acid metabolism	Urine organic acids, plasma acyl carnitines
Mitochondrial and respiratory chain disorders	Blood and CSF lactate and pyruvate, muscle and/
Peroxisome disorders	or liver enzymology, specific gene testing
Pyridoxine-responsive seizures (antiquitin deficiency)	Very long chain fatty acids
	Response to pyridoxine under EEG monitoring, urine, plasma and/or CSF aminoadipate semi aldehyde or piperideine-6-carboxylate
Pyridoxal phosphate-responsive seizures (PNPO deficiency) (Mills et al. 2014)	Response to pyridoxal phosphate, CSF amino acids and biogenic amines, urine vanillactate
Infections	CSF, blood, throat swab, rectal swab PCR for enterovirus, para-echo virus and other viruses
Chromosome disorders, neonatal epileptic encephalopathies	Chromosome analysis, microarray, whole-exome sequencing, epilepsy gene panels
Idiopathic and refractory seizures	Liver biopsy, muscle biopsy, skin biopsy for DNA storage and analysis
Brain malformation disorders, some metabolic encephalopathies	MRI, CT scan, cranial ultrasound

CSF, cerebrospinal fluid; PCR, polymerase chain reaction; PNPO, pyridoxamine 5'-phosphate oxidase.

Magnetic resonance imaging of the brain

Magnetic resonance imaging (MRI) is the imaging modality of choice and has the ability to help diagnose the cause of seizures as well as in prognostication (Leth et al. 1997, Cheong et al. 2012, Van Laerhoven et al. 2013, Osmond et al. 2014, Weeke et al. 2015a). In a prospective study, Osmond et al. (2014) followed term infants with seizures until 18–24 months of age and found that the probability of developing neurodevelopmental impairment or recurrence of seizures was extremely low in the absence of major cerebral lesions on MRI.

MRI is very useful in diagnosing PAIS and to prognosticate in infants with PAIS (Lequin et al. 2009, Gunny and Lin 2012, van der Aa et al. 2013).

MRI and magnetic resonance spectroscopy are beneficial in diagnosing a variety of IEM such as non-ketotic hyperglycenemia, mitochondrial disorders maple syrup urine disease, etc (Khong et al. 2003, Mourmans et al. 2006, Kilicarslan et al. 2012, Rossi and Biancheri 2013, Sato et al. 2014).

MRI is useful in assessing the extent of brain damage in neonates with hypoglycaemic seizures: Patterns of injury may be transient, age dependent and more varied than the traditional descriptions of diffuse cortical and subcortical white matter damage involving the parietal and occipital lobes (Barkovich et al. 1998, Burns et al. 2008).

In infections of the CNS, MRI helps in identifying ventriculitis, encephalitis, subdural collection, ventriculomegaly and intracranial abscess (Jaremko et al. 2011).

TABLE 8.6
Conditions where neuroimaging is useful

Intraventricular haemorrhage, subdural haemorrhage, subarachnoid haemorrhage, parenchymal
  haemorrhage.

Perinatal arterial stroke

Certain metabolic disorders

Hypoxic ischemic encephalopathy, hypoglycaemic encephalopathy

Hydrocephalus

Infections: encephalitis, cerebral abscess

Cerebral malformations: lissencephaly, pachygyria, absent corpus callosum

Hamartomas, tumours, cortical dysplasias

Computed tomography

In the past decade, there has been a decrease in the use of computed tomography (CT)
because of risks of high dose of radiation. In addition, the image contrast is inferior to MRI
(apart from recognition of calcification). Hence CT is reserved for emergency situations
where MRI is not available or when the critical condition of the neonate requires rapid
scanning (Tekgul et al. 2006).

Treatment of neonatal seizures

The main principles of management are antiseizure medication, supportive management and treatment of the underlying aetiology. Supportive management might neces-
sitate the administration of IV fluids, mechanical ventilation and correction of
hypotension, if required. Conditions such as meningitis, hypoglycaemia, hypocalcaemia, hypomagnesemia, electrolyte imbalances and HSV encephalitis should be treated
aggressively. Specific treatment options for neonatal seizures are discussed in detail
in chapter 9.

Neuroprotection of neonates with hypoxic-ischemic encephalopathy

Therapeutic cooling has been shown to decrease the risk of long-term adverse outcomes in
neonates with HIE and is widely undertaken in infants with moderate to severe encephalopathy (Jacobs et al. 2013, Srinivasakumar et al. 2013, Gardiner et al. 2014).

Providing appropriate supportive and follow-up care

Neurocritical care for a neonate with seizures involves multiple disciplines: neurology,
neonatology, radiology, haematology, biochemistry, microbiology and many more.
Neonates with seizures need to be followed up and assessed appropriately and early
interventional strategies should be instigated proactively. Genetic and prenatal counselling for the future may be necessary for some parents. Besides medical care the
family needs supportive care: emotional, psychosocial and financial, both in the short
and long term.

Conclusion

The management of neonatal seizures is challenging. They are difficult to diagnose and treat and are associated with adverse outcomes. Neonatal seizures need to be differentiated from non-epileptic motor phenomena, as over-diagnosis may result in inappropriate treatment and unnecessary parental anxiety. Clinicians need to be aware that the majority of neonatal seizures have no clinical correlates – they are electrographic-only (subclinical) seizures. The gold standard investigation to diagnose seizures is continuous v-EEG preferably for about 24 hours; however, resource limitations are a hindrance to its universal applicability. Standard one-hour v-EEG recordings and a-EEG may be useful as screening tools to identify infants who need continuous v-EEG. Neonatal seizures are associated with a variety of aetiologies, with HIE being the most common. Initial investigations and management should focus on potentially treatable conditions, where delay in treatment can lead to worse outcomes. MRI, ultrasound and CT scan can complement each other as imaging modalities in neonatal seizures. Phenobarbitone, phenytoin, midazolam, lignocaine, and more recently levetiracetam are commonly used anticonvulsants in the neonatal period, but evidence to support their efficacy and safety is limited. Therapeutic cooling is an accepted neuroprotective strategy in moderate to severe HIE. Supportive care and long-term follow-up in infants with neonatal seizures is essential.

REFERENCES

Barkovich AJ, Ali FA, Rowley HA, Bass N (1998) Imaging patterns of neonatal hypoglycemia. *AJNR Am J Neuroradiol* 19: 523–528.

Boylan G, Burgoyne L, Moore C, O'Flaherty B, Rennie J (2010) An international survey of EEG use in the neonatal intensive care unit. *Acta Paediatr* 99: 1150–1155. doi: http://dx.doi.org/10.1111/j.1651-2227.2010.01809.x.

Boylan GB, Stevenson NJ, Vanhatalo S (2013) Monitoring neonatal seizures. *Semin Fetal Neonatal Med* 18: 202–208. doi: http://dx.doi.org/10.1016/j.siny.2013.04.004.

Burns CM, Rutherford MA, Boardman JP, Cowan FM (2008) Patterns of cerebral injury and neurodevelopmental outcomes after symptomatic neonatal hypoglycemia. *Pediatrics* 122: 65–74. doi: http://dx.doi.org/10.1542/peds.2007-2822.

Cheong JL, Coleman L, Hunt, R. W., Lee, K. J., Doyle, L. W., Inder, T.E., Jacobs, S. E., & Infant Cooling Evaluation C (2012). Prognostic utility of magnetic resonance imaging in neonatal hypoxic-ischemic encephalopathy: Substudy of a randomized trial. *Arch Pediatr Adolesc Med* 166: 634–640. doi: http://dx.doi.org/10.1001/archpediatrics.2012.284.

Cross JH (2013) Differential diagnosis of epileptic seizures in infancy including the neonatal period. *Semin Fetal Neonatal Med* 18: 192–195. doi: http://dx.doi.org/10.1016/j.siny.2013.04.003.

Cseko AJ, Bango M, Lakatos P, Kardasi J, Pusztai L, Szabo M (2013) Accuracy of amplitude-integrated electroencephalography in the prediction of neurodevelopmental outcome in asphyxiated infants receiving hypothermia treatment. *Acta Paediatr* 102: 707–711. doi: http://dx.doi.org/10.1111/apa.12226.

Dahan S, Elefant E, Girard I, Azcona B, Champion V, Mitanchez D (2011) Neonatal seizures, buprenorphine abstinence syndrome, and substitutive treatment with morphine. *Arch Pediatr* 18: 287–290. doi: http://dx.doi.org/10.1016/j.arcped.2010.12.003.

Daneman A, Epelman M, Blaser S, Jarrin JR (2006) Imaging of the brain in full-term neonates: Does sonography still play a role? *Pediatr Radiol* 36: 636–646. doi: http://dx.doi.org/10.1007/s00247-006-0201-7.

Evans E, Koh S, Lerner J, Sankar R, Garg M (2010) Accuracy of amplitude integrated EEG in a neonatal cohort. *Arch Dis Child Fetal Neonatal Ed* 95: F169–F173. doi: http://dx.doi.org/10.1136/adc.2009.165969.

Ferriero DM (2009) Controversies and advances in neonatal neurology: Introduction. Introduction. *Pediatr Neurol* 40: 145–146. doi: http://dx.doi.org/10.1016/j.pediatrneurol.2008.09.015.

Fertleman CR, Ferrie CD, Aicardi J, Bednarek NA et al. (2007) Paroxysmal extreme pain disorder (previously familial rectal pain syndrome). *Neurology* 69: 586–595. doi: http://dx.doi.org/10.1212/01.wnl.0000268065.16865.5f.

Gardiner J, Wagh D, Mcmichael J, Hakeem M, Rao S (2014) Outcomes of hypoxic ischaemic encephalopathy treated with therapeutic hypothermia using cool gel packs – experience from Western Australia. *Eur J Paediatr Neurol,* 18: 391–398. doi: http://dx.doi.org/10.1016/j.ejpn.2014.02.003.

Glass HC (2014) Neonatal seizures: Advances in mechanisms and management. *Clin Perinatol* 41: 177–190. doi: http://dx.doi.org/10.1016/j.clp.2013.10.004.

Glass HC, Nash KB, Bonifacio SL et al. (2011) Seizures and magnetic resonance imaging-detected brain injury in newborns cooled for hypoxic-ischemic encephalopathy. *J Pediatr* 159: 731e1–735e1.

Grim K, Harrison TE, Wilder RT (2013) Management of neonatal abstinence syndrome from opioids. *Clin Perinatol* 40: 509–524. doi: http://dx.doi.org/10.1016/j.clp.2013.05.004.

Gunny RS, Lin D (2012) Imaging of perinatal stroke. *Magn Reson Imaging Clin N Am* 20: 1–33. doi: http://dx.doi.org/10.1016/j.mric.2011.10.001.

Hallberg B, Grossmann K, Bartocci M, Blennow M (2010) The prognostic value of early aEEG in asphyxiated infants undergoing systemic hypothermia treatment. *Acta Paediatr* 99: 531–536. doi: http://dx.doi.org/10.1111/j.1651-2227.2009.01653.x.

Hans JS, Sanger T (2004) Neonatal movement disorders. *Neo Reviews* 5: e321–e326.

Hart AR, Pilling EL, Alix JJ (2015a) Neonatal seizures-part 1: Not everything that jerks, stiffens and shakes is a fit. *Arch Dis Child Educ Pract Ed* 100: 170–175. doi: http://dx.doi.org/10.1136/archdischild-2014-306385.

Hero B, Schleiermacher G (2013) Update on pediatric opsoclonus myoclonus. *Neuropediatrics* 44 (6): 324–329. doi: http://dx.doi.org/10.1055/s-0033-1358604.

Holmes GL (2009) The long-term effects of neonatal seizures. *Clin Perinatol* 36: 901–914 vii-viii. doi: http://dx.doi.org/10.1016/j.clp.2009.07.012.

Huntsman RJ, Lowry NJ, Sankaran K (2008) Nonepileptic motor phenomena in the neonate. *Paediatr Child Health* 13: 680–684.

Idro R, Gwer S, Kahindi M et al. (2008) The incidence, aetiology and outcome of acute seizures in children admitted to a rural Kenyan district hospital. *BMC Pediatr* 8: 5. doi: http://dx.doi.org/10.1186/1471-2431-8-5.

Ishizaki Y, Watabe S, Mimaki N, Arakaki Y, Ohtsuka Y (2011) Paroxysmal automatic movements mimicking neonatal seizures induced by midazolam. *No To Hattatsu* 43: 291–294.

Jacobs SE, Berg M, Hunt R, Tarnow-Mordi WO, Inder TE, Davis PG (2013) Cooling for newborns with hypoxic ischaemic encephalopathy. *Cochrane Database Syst Rev* 1: CD003311. doi: http://dx.doi.org/10.1002/14651858.cd003311.pub3.

Jaremko JL, Moon AS, Kumbla S (2011) Patterns of complications of neonatal and infant meningitis on MRI by organism: A 10 year review. *Eur J Radiol* 80: 821–827. doi: http://dx.doi.org/10.1016/j.ejrad.2010.10.017.

Jensen FE (2009) Neonatal seizures: An update on mechanisms and management. *Clin Perinatol* 36: 881–900, vii. doi: http://dx.doi.org/10.1016/j.clp.2009.08.001.

Kallen B (2004) Neonate characteristics after maternal use of antidepressants in late pregnancy. *Arch Pediatr Adolesc Med* 158: 312–316. doi: http://dx.doi.org/10.1001/archpedi.158.4.312.

Khong PL, Lam BC, Chung BH, Wong KY, Ooi GC (2003) Diffusion-weighted MR imaging in neonatal nonketotic hyperglycinemia. *AJNR Am J Neuroradiol* 24: 1181–1183.

Kilicarslan R, Alkan A, Demirkol D, Toprak H, Sharifov R (2012) Maple syrup urine disease: Diffusion-weighted MRI findings during acute metabolic encephalopathic crisis. *Jpn J Radiol* 30: 522–525. doi: http://dx.doi.org/10.1007/s11604-012-0079-2.

Kirton A, Armstrong-Wells J, Chang T et al. (2011) Symptomatic neonatal arterial ischemic stroke: The international pediatric stroke study. *Pediatrics* 128: e1402–e1410. doi: http://dx.doi.org/10.1542/peds.2011-1148.

Lawrence R, Mathur A, Nguyen The Tich S, Zempel J, Inder T (2009) A pilot study of continuous limited-channel aEEG in term infants with encephalopathy. *J Pediatr* 154: 835e1–841e1.

Leijser LM, De Vries LS, Rutherford MA et al. (2007) Cranial ultrasound in metabolic disorders presenting in the neonatal period: Characteristic features and comparison with MR imaging. *AJNR Am J Neuroradiol* 28: 1223–1231. doi: http://dx.doi.org/10.3174/ajnr.A0553.

Lequin MH, Dudink J, Tong KA, Obenaus A (2009) Magnetic resonance imaging in neonatal stroke. *Semin Fetal Neonatal Med* 14: 299–310. doi: http://dx.doi.org/10.1016/j.siny.2009.07.005.

Leth H, Toft PB, Herning M, Peitersen B, Lou HC (1997) Neonatal seizures associated with cerebral lesions shown by magnetic resonance imaging. *Arch Dis Child Fetal Neonatal Ed* 77: F105–F110. doi: http://dx.doi.org/10.1136/fn.77.2.F105.

Loman AM, Ter Horst HJ, Lambrechtsen FA, Lunsing RJ (2014) Neonatal seizures: Aetiology by means of a standardized work-up. *Eur J Paediatr Neurol* 18: 360–367. doi: http://dx.doi.org/10.1016/j.ejpn.2014.01.014.

Malone A, Ryan CA, Fitzgerald A, Burgoyne L, Connolly S, Boylan GB (2009) Interobserver agreement in neonatal seizure identification. *Epilepsia* 50: 2097–2101. doi: http://dx.doi.org/10.1111/j.1528-1167.2009.02132.x.

Mastrangelo M, Van Lierde A, Bray M, Pastorino G, Marini A, Mosca F (2005) Epileptic seizures, epilepsy and epileptic syndromes in newborns: A nosological approach to 94 new cases by the 2001 proposed diagnostic scheme for people with epileptic seizures and with epilepsy. *Seizure* 14: 304–311. doi: http://dx.doi.org/10.1016/j.seizure.2005.04.001.

Maurer VO, Rizzi M, Bianchetti MG, Ramelli GP (2010) Benign neonatal sleep myoclonus: A review of the literature. *Pediatrics* 125: e919–e924. doi: http://dx.doi.org/10.1542/peds.2009-1839.

Mills PB, Camuzeaux SS, Footitt EJ et al. (2014) Epilepsy due to PNPO mutations: Genotype, environment and treatment affect presentation and outcome. *Brain* 137: 1350–1360. doi: http://dx.doi.org/10.1093/brain/awu051.

Mizrahi EM, Kellaway P (1987) Characterization and classification of neonatal seizures. *Neurology* 37: 1837–1844. doi: http://dx.doi.org/10.1212/WNL.37.12.1837.

Moses-Kolko EL, Bogen D, Perel J et al. (2005) Neonatal signs after late in utero exposure to serotonin reuptake inhibitors: Literature review and implications for clinical applications. *JAMA* 293: 2372–2383. doi: http://dx.doi.org/10.1001/jama.293.19.2372.

Mourmans J, Majoie CB, Barth PG, Duran M, Akkerman EM, Poll-The BT (2006) Sequential MR imaging changes in nonketotic hyperglycinemia. *AJNR Am J Neuroradiol* 27: 208–211.

Murray DM, Boylan GB, Ali I, Ryan CA, Murphy BP, Connolly S (2008) Defining the gap between electrographic seizure burden, clinical expression and staff recognition of neonatal seizures. *Arch Dis Child Fetal Neonatal Ed* 93: F187–F191. doi: http://dx.doi.org/10.1136/adc.2005.086314.

Nagarajan L, Ghosh S, Palumbo L (2011) Ictal electroencephalograms in neonatal seizures: Characteristics and associations. *Pediatr Neurol* 45: 11–16. doi: http://dx.doi.org/10.1016/j.pediatrneurol.2011.01.009.

Nagarajan L, Palumbo L, Ghosh S (2010) Neurodevelopmental outcomes in neonates with seizures: A numerical score of background encephalography to help prognosticate. *J Child Neurol* 25: 961–968. doi: http://dx.doi.org/10.1177/0883073809355825.

Nagarajan L, Palumbo L, Ghosh S (2012) Classification of clinical semiology in epileptic seizures in neonates. *Eur J Paediatr Neurol* 16: 118–125. doi: http://dx.doi.org/10.1016/j.ejpn.2011.11.005.

Noguchi M, Inamasu J, Kawai F et al. (2010) Ultrasound-guided needle aspiration of epidural hematoma in a neonate after vacuum-assisted delivery. *Childs Nerv Syst* 26: 713–716. doi: http://dx.doi.org/10.1007/s00381-009-1072-7.

Olivier JD, Akerud H, Kaihola H et al. (2013) The effects of maternal depression and maternal selective serotonin reuptake inhibitor exposure on offspring. *Front Cell Neurosci* 7: 73. doi: http://dx.doi.org/10.3389/fncel.2013.00073.

Orivoli S, Facini C, Pisani F (2015) Paroxysmal nonepileptic motor phenomena in newborn. *Brain Dev* 37(9): 833–839. doi: http://dx.doi.org/10.1016/j.braindev.2015.01.002.

Osmond E, Billetop A, Jary S, Likeman M, Thoresen M, Luyt K (2014) Neonatal seizures: Magnetic resonance imaging adds value in the diagnosis and prediction of neurodisability. *Acta Paediatr* doi: http://dx.doi.org/10.1111/apa.12583.

Parker S, Zuckerman B, Bauchner H, Frank D, Vinci R, Cabral H (1990) Jitteriness in full-term neonates: Prevalence and correlates. *Pediatrics* 85: 17–23.

Patane L, Ghidini A (2001) Fetal seizures: Case report and literature review. *J Matern Fetal Med* 10: 287–289. doi: http://dx.doi.org/10.1080/jmf.10.4.287.289.

Pinninti SG, Kimberlin DW (2014) Management of neonatal herpes simplex virus infection and exposure. *Arch Dis Child Fetal Neonatal Ed* 99: F240–F244. doi: http://dx.doi.org/10.1136/archdischild-2013-303762.

Rakshasbhuvankar A, Paul S, Nagarajan L, Ghosh S, Rao S (2015) Amplitude-integrated EEG for detection of neonatal seizures: a systematic review. *Seizure* 33: 90–98.

Ronen GM, Penney S, Andrews W (1999) The epidemiology of clinical neonatal seizures in Newfoundland: A population-based study. *J Pediatr* 134: 71–75. doi: http://dx.doi.org/10.1016/S0022-3476(99)70374-4.

Rosman NP, Donnelly JH, Braun MA (1984) The jittery newborn and infant: A review. *J Dev Behav Pediatr* 5: 263–273. doi: http://dx.doi.org/10.1097/00004703-198410000-00008.

Rossi A, Biancheri R (2013) Magnetic resonance spectroscopy in metabolic disorders. *Neuroimaging Clin N Am* 23: 425–448. doi: http://dx.doi.org/10.1016/j.nic.2012.12.013.

Sato T, Muroya K, Hanakawa J, Asakura Y et al. (2014) Neonatal case of classic maple syrup urine disease: usefulness of (1) H-MRS in early diagnosis. *Pediatr Int* 56: 112–115. doi: http://dx.doi.org/10.1111/ped.12211.

Scher MS (2002) Controversies regarding neonatal seizure recognition. *Epileptic Disord* 4: 139–158.

Shah DK, Mackay MT, Lavery S et al. (2008) Accuracy of bedside electroencephalographic monitoring in comparison with simultaneous continuous conventional electroencephalography for seizure detection in term infants. *Pediatrics* 121: 1146–1154. doi: http://dx.doi.org/10.1542/peds.2007-1839.

Shah DK, Wusthoff CJ, Clarke P et al. (2014) Electrographic seizures are associated with brain injury in newborns undergoing therapeutic hypothermia. *Arch Dis Child Fetal Neonatal Ed* 99: F219–F224. doi: http://dx.doi.org/10.1136/archdischild-2013-305206.

Sheizaf B, Mazor M, Landau D, Burstein E, Bashiri A, Hershkovitz R (2007) Early sonographic prenatal diagnosis of seizures. *Ultrasound Obstet Gynecol* 30: 1007–1009. doi: http://dx.doi.org/10.1002/uog.5153.

Shellhaas RA (2015) Continuous long-term electroencephalography: The gold standard for neonatal seizure diagnosis. *Semin Fetal Neonatal Med* 20: 149–153. doi: http://dx.doi.org/10.1016/j.siny.2015.01.005.

Shellhaas RA, Chang T, Tsuchida T et al. (2011) The American clinical neurophysiology society's guideline on continuous electroencephalography monitoring in neonates. *J Clin Neurophysiol* 28: 611–617. doi: http://dx.doi.org/10.1097/WNP.0b013e31823e96d7.

Sie SD, Wennink JM, Van Driel JJ et al. (2011) Maternal use of SSRIs, SNRIs and NaSSAs: Practical recommendations during pregnancy and lactation. *Arch Dis Child Fetal Neonatal Ed* 97(6): F472–476.

Srinivasakumar P, Zempel J, Wallendorf M, Lawrence R, Inder T, Mathur A (2013) Therapeutic hypothermia in neonatal hypoxic ischemic encephalopathy: Electrographic seizures and magnetic resonance imaging evidence of injury. *J Pediatr* 163: 465–470. doi: http://dx.doi.org/10.1016/j.jpeds.2013.01.041.

Tekgul H, Gauvreau K, Soul J et al. (2006) The current etiologic profile and neurodevelopmental outcome of seizures in term newborn infants. *Pediatrics* 117: 1270–1280. doi: http://dx.doi.org/10.1542/peds.2005-1178.

Toet MC, Van Der Meij W, De Vries LS, Uiterwaal CS, Van Huffelen KC (2002) Comparison between simultaneously recorded amplitude integrated electroencephalogram (cerebral function monitor) and standard electroencephalogram in neonates. *Pediatrics* 109: 772–779. doi: http://dx.doi.org/10.1542/peds.109.5.772.

Turanli G, Senbil N, Altunbasak S, Topcu M (2004) Benign neonatal sleep myoclonus mimicking status epilepticus. *J Child Neurol* 19: 62–63. doi: http://dx.doi.org/10.1177/08830738040190010708.

Van Der Aa N, Benders M, Groenendaal F, De Vries L (2014) Neonatal stroke: A review of the current evidence on epidemiology, pathogenesis, diagnostics and therapeutic options. *Acta Paediatr* 103: 356–364. doi: http://dx.doi.org/10.1111/apa.12555.

Van Der Aa NE, Northington FJ, Stone BS et al. (2013) Quantification of white matter injury following neonatal stroke with serial DTI. *Pediatr Res* 73: 756–762. doi: http://dx.doi.org/10.1038/pr.2013.45.

Van Laerhoven H, De Haan TR, Offringa M, Post B, Van Der Lee JH (2013) Prognostic tests in term neonates with hypoxic-ischemic encephalopathy: A systematic review. *Pediatrics* 131: 88–98. doi: http://dx.doi.org/10.1542/peds.2012-1297.

Vasudevan C, Levene M (2013) Epidemiology and aetiology of neonatal seizures. *Semin Fetal Neonatal Med* 18: 185–191. doi: http://dx.doi.org/10.1016/j.siny.2013.05.008.

Volpe, J. J. (2008) *Neurology of the newborn* (5th ed.). Philadelphia: Saunders/Elsevier.

Weeke LC, Groenendaal F, Toet MC et al. (2015a) The aetiology of neonatal seizures and the diagnostic contribution of neonatal cerebral magnetic resonance imaging. *Dev Med Child Neurol* 57: 248–256. doi: http://dx.doi.org/10.1111/dmcn.12629.

Wusthoff CJ (2013) Diagnosing neonatal seizures and status epilepticus. *J Clin Neurophysiol* 30: 115–121. doi: http://dx.doi.org/10.1097/WNP.0b013e3182872932.

Yildiz EP, Tatli B, Ekici B et al. (2012) Evaluation of etiologic and prognostic factors in neonatal convulsions. *Pediatr Neurol* 47: 186–192. doi: http://dx.doi.org/10.1016/j.pediatrneurol.2012.05.015.

Zaw W, Knoppert DC, Da Silva O (2001) Flumazenil's reversal of myoclonic-like movements associated with midazolam in term newborns. *Pharmacotherapy* 21: 642–646. doi: http://dx.doi.org/10.1592/phco.21.6.642.34545.

Zeskind PS, Stephens LE (2004) Maternal selective serotonin reuptake inhibitor use during pregnancy and newborn neurobehavior. *Pediatrics* 113: 368–375. doi: http://dx.doi.org/10.1542/peds.113.2.368.

Zhou L, Chillag KL, Nigro MA (2002) Hyperekplexia: A treatable neurogenetic disease. *Brain Dev* 24: 669–674. doi: http://dx.doi.org/10.1016/S0387-7604(02)00095-5.

9
TREATMENT OF NEONATAL SEIZURES

Lakshmi Nagarajan

There are many controversies in the diagnosis and management of neonatal seizures (Scher 2002, Sankar and Painter 2005, Wirrell 2005, Kaminska et al. 2007, McCoy and Hahn 2013, van Rooij et al. 2013b, Thoresen and Sabir 2015). Neonatal seizures (NS) occur frequently, with wide variance in estimates of incidence (Silverstein and Jensen 2007, Uria-Avellanal et al. 2013). The true incidence is difficult to determine as only some electroencepahalography (EEG) confirmed seizures (ECSz) in the neonatal period have clinical features (Bye and Flanagan 1995, Nagarajan et al. 2012) and majority of the neonatal seizures are electrographical (ESz) only (Volpe 1989, Scher et al. 2003, Sankar and Rho 2007, Nagarajan et al. 2011a). Adding to the complexity however there are many seizure mimics that do not have any EEG correlates (Mizrahi 1987, Clancy 2006, Murray et al. 2008) and have been considered and treated as neonatal seizures.

Neonatal seizures are manifestations of significant neurological dysfunction and have a wide spectrum of aetiologies (Tekgul et al. 2006, Scher 2009), with hypoxic-ischaemic encephalopathy (HIE) being the most common. Identification and treatment of the underlying or contributory disorder are obviously important. Are seizures themselves harmful and do they independently contribute to worse outcomes? Current thinking is weighted towards considering that both ESz and ECSz, and even brief EEG rhythmic discharges (BERDs) add to the adverse outcomes associated with neonatal seizures (Boylan et al. 1999, Sankar and Rho 2007, Glass et al. 2009, 2011, Nagarajan et al. 2011b, Shah et al. 2014, Pappas et al. 2015).

Therapeutic options to treat neonatal seizures are limited and the frequently used antiepileptic drugs (AEDs) for neonatal seizures are not very effective (Volpe 2008, Pressler and Mangum 2013, Slaughter et al. 2013, van Rooij et al. 2013a, Shetty 2015). Concerns exist regarding the safety and adverse effects (short- and long-term) of the AEDs, including the effects on brain development and neurodevelopmental outcomes (Bittigau et al. 2002, Pennell et al. 2012, Maitre et al. 2013, Velez-Ruiz and Meador 2015). In this chapter the most frequently used AEDs, the most promising AEDs and the second- and third-line drugs, as well as emerging treatment options, combinations and concepts will be discussed.

Pharmacological treatment of seizures
A 2004 Cochrane review on pharmacological treatment of seizures found only two randomised control trials (RCTs) and concluded that there was little evidence to support the

choice of any AED for neonatal seizures (Booth and Evans 2004). The first RCT by Painter et al. in 1999 showed that both phenobarbital and phenytoin (PHT) were similarly effective and controlled seizures in less than 50% of infants (Painter et al. 1999). The second RCT by Boylan et al. in 2004 randomised infants who failed to respond to phenobarbital to receive either lidocaine or midazolam (MDZ) as second-line agents. There was a trend for lidocaine to be more effective in reducing the seizure burden (Boylan et al. 2004). Recent systematic reviews (Slaughter et al. 2013, Hellstrom-Westas et al. 2015) again found only the same two RCTs and concluded that there is limited evidence regarding the best pharmacological treatment option in neonatal seizures. In the absence of evidence from RCTs, various anticonvulsants including phenobarbital, PHT, MDZ, lignocaine, clonazepam, valproate, levetiracetam, topiramate (TPM), vigabatrin, zonisamide and oxcarbazepine have been used by clinicians (Silverstein and Ferriero 2008, Slaughter et al. 2013). Neuroprotective strategies and new treatment options and combinations are emerging (Pressler and Mangum 2013).

First-line antiepileptic drugs
PHENOBARBITONE

Since its introduction in 1912, phenobarbital has been recognised as a first-line agent for the treatment of seizures, in the neonatal as well as other age groups. Phenobarbital has emerged as the most frequently used AED for neonatal seizures and remains the drug of first choice (Vento et al. 2010, van Rooij et al. 2013a). Phenobarbital acts by prolonging the opening of post-synaptic cell membrane chloride ion channels within $GABA_A$ receptors, thus hyperpolarising the neuronal cell membrane (Vajda and Eadie 2014).

In Painter's randomised cross-over trial (Painter et al. 1999), seizures were controlled in 43% of infants treated with phenobarbital compared with 45% in the PHT-treated group. Painter and colleagues found that addition of the second drug, when the first was not effective, did not significantly improve seizure outcome. In a non-randomised study (Castro Conde et al. 2005) of amplitude-integrated EEG (a-EEG) confirmed seizures, seizures persisted in 53% of 45 infants who received phenobarbital or PHT. In a small randomised study (Boylan et al. 2004) 11 of 22 neonates were reported to respond to a phenobarbital dose of up to 40 mg/kg as a first-line AED. In an open label randomised control trial of phenobarbital versus PHT treatment of neonatal seizures, phenobarbital was reported to be more efficacious, irrespective of aetiology in term and near-term infants (Pathak et al. 2013).

Phenobarbital is thought to have a reasonably good safety profile; however there are concerns that it may increase neuronal apoptosis and adversely affect neurodevelopmental outcomes (Bittigau et al. 2002, Loring and Meador 2004, Tomson et al. 2011, Hernandez-Diaz et al. 2012, Pennell et al. 2012). Early treatment with phenobarbital in children with febrile seizures has been associated with adverse cognitive effects (Farwell et al. 1990, Sulzbacher et al. 1999). Prophylactic phenobarbital in preterm infants, in neonates with HIE, or even antenatal use has not been shown to improve neurodevelopmental outcomes

(Whitelaw and Odd 2007). The possible effects of phenobarbital on the developing brain continue to remain a significant concern.

Suggested dosage guidelines for phenobarbital and other AEDs are shown in Table 9.1. Rapid sequential loading (to 40 mg/kg) may improve seizure response (van Rooij et al. 2013b).

TABLE 9.1
Suggested doses of antiepileptic drugs used for neonatal seizures

Drug name	Loading dose	Maintenance dose
Phenobarbitone	20 mg/kg IV Repeat doses 10–20 mg/kg, total up to 40 mg/kg	3–5 mg/kg/day, may be given once daily (enteral or parenteral); monitor levels
Phenytoin	20 mg/kg IV Over 30–60 minutes	5–8 mg/kg/day in 2 divided doses (enteral or parenteral); monitor levels
Levetiracetam	20–40 mg/kg IV, repeat up to 20 mg/kg	20–40 mg/kg/day in 2–3 divided doses (enteral or parenteral)
Midazolam	0.05–0.2 mg/kg IV	IV 0.05–0.75 mg//kg/h (max 1 mg/kg/h); start weaning 24 hours after seizure freedom Caution with use in <28 weeks.
Clonazepam	0.01–0.1 mg/kg IV	0.03–0.5 mg/kg/24 h in 3–4 doses (enteral or parenteral)
Lorazepam	0.05–0.1 mg/kg IV	None; loading dose may be repeated if necessary
Diazepam	0.1–0.5 mg/kg IV	
Lidocaine	Normothermia	Normothermia
<2.5 kg	2 mg/kg/ IV	IV 6 mg/kg/h for 4 h, then 3 mg/kg/h for 12 h, 1.5 mg/kg/h for 12 h
>2.5 kg	2 mg/kg/ IV	IV 7 mg/kg/h for 4 h, then 3.5 mg/kg/h for 12 h, 1.75 mg/kg/h for 12 h
Lidocaine	Therapeutic hypothermia	Therapeutic hypothermia
<2.5 kg	2 mg/kg IV	IV 6 mg/kg/h for 3.5 h, then 3 mg/kg/h for 12 h, 1.5 mg/kg/h for 12 h
>2.5 kg	2 mg/kg/ IV	IV 7 mg/kg/h for 3.5 h, then 3.5 mg/kg/h for 12 h, 1.75 mg/kg/h for 12 h
Topiramate	5 mg/kg/day Enteral	5 mg/kg/day enteral
Valproate	20–25 mg/kg Oral 20–30 mg/kg Rectal 10–25 mg/kg IV	10–30 mg/kg/day in 2 divided doses (enteral or parenteral); monitor levels; monitor ammonia level and liver function
Carbamazepine	5–20 mg/kg Enteral	5–8 mg/kg given 8–12 hourly (enteral); monitor levels
Paraldehyde	0.3 ml/kg rectally	

PHENOBARBITAL IN COMBINATION WITH OTHER INTERVENTIONS

Therapeutic hypothermia

HIE remains one the most frequent causes of neonatal seizures. Therapeutic hypothermia has been shown to be beneficial for infants with HIE in many trials (Gano et al. 2014). Though seizure rates may not have changed significantly with the use of cooling, the reduction in seizure burden, alteration of temporal evolution of seizures and increase in electro-clinical dissociation (ECD) have been well demonstrated (Lynch et al. 2012, Srinivasakumar et al. 2013, Boylan et al. 2015). Clinicians should be cognisant of the possible effects of therapeutic hypothermia on the pharmacodynamic and pharmacokinetic properties of AEDs used for neonatal seizures (Pokorna et al. 2015).

It has been suggested that phenobarbital, by itself or with bumetanide (BTN), may augment the therapeutic effect of hypothermia in animal models (Barks et al. 2010, Liu et al. 2012), but only a few studies in neonates have explored this. No clinically relevant effect of moderate hypothermia was identified on phenobarbital pharmacokinetics in a study exploring the pharmacokinetics and clinical efficacy of phenobarbital in asphyxiated neonates (van den Broek et al. 2012). The authors also suggest that the combination may have a neuroprotective effect, as evidenced by reduction in the number of infants who showed a worsening (continuous normal voltage to discontinuous normal voltage) of the a-EEG background. Therapeutic hypothermia did not influence the clearance of phenobarbital in a retrospective study of 39 infants (Shellhaas et al. 2013). In cooled infants who received prophylactic phenobarbital, a retrospective analysis showed fewer clinical seizures; however no reduction in the neurodevelopmental impairment was observed (Meyn et al. 2010). In a study of 68 infants (Sarkar et al. 2012), phenobarbital treatment before cooling did not improve the composite outcome of neonatal death or the presence of an abnormal post-hypothermia brain magnetic resonance imaging; however, long-term outcomes were not reported.

Modulators of cation-chloride co-transporters

Bumetanide is a loop diuretic, previously used in neonates, with rapid onset and short duration of action as well as a relatively good safety profile (Pressler and Mangum 2013). In the immature brain there is overexpression of the sodium potassium chloride co-transporter (CCC) isoform 1 (NKCC1) and low expression of the potassium CCC (KCC2). This results in high intra-neuronal chloride concentrations, causing GABA receptor activation to have a paradoxical excitatory or depolarising effect (instead of the hyper-polarising action seen in the mature brain). BTN inhibits NKCC1 and reduces intra-neuronal chloride and hence the depolarising effect of GABA. BTN has been reported to supress seizures in some animal models of epilepsy. Studies in a rat model of neonatal seizures showed that BTN in combination with phenobarbital was effective in reducing seizures, without any increases in neuronal apoptosis, and this, along with other studies, provided support for clinical trials of BTN in neonates at risk of HIE and neonatal seizures (Cleary et al. 2013). However BTN in some animal and *in vitro* models has been found to enhance or have no effect on paroxysmal activity, lack target specificity and have different effects on interictal spikes as opposed to ictal epileptic rhythms (Vanhatalo et al. 2009).

A recent trial of BTN for neonatal seizures refractory to phenobarbital (NEMO trial) was stopped early because of the lack of efficacy and increased incidence of adverse effects such as hearing impairment, dehydration, hypotension and electrolyte imbalance (Pressler et al. 2015). The decision to stop the trial may have been overcautious (Thoresen and Sabir 2015). There have been efforts to find other drugs that target CCCs and may be effective for treatment of neonatal seizures (Puskarjov et al. 2014). Modulation of CCCs, with or without phenobarbital and/or hypothermia, remains a promising and novel therapeutic option to be explored further.

Novel therapies

Melatonin, erythropoietin and anti-inflammatory compounds are reported to have anticonvulsant and neuroprotective effects, which may be additive when administered with phenobarbital and other neuroprotective strategies in animal models. Their role in clinical management of neonatal seizures is being explored (Johnston et al. 2011, Forcelli et al. 2013, Hagberg et al. 2015, Wu and Gonzalez 2015).

The role of phenobarbital in the treatment of neonatal seizures in future is yet to be determined, in the light of its efficacy, the adverse effects on neurodevelopmental outcomes and potential neuroprotective effects, especially in conjunction with other strategies. For the present phenobarbital remains the most frequently used AED for neonatal seizures worldwide.

PHENYTOIN

Phenytoin is another first-line AED for neonatal seizures. Painter et al. (1999) reported that PHT and phenobarbital were equally but incompletely effective as AEDs in neonates (Painter et al. 1999). When either drug was given alone, the seizures were controlled in fewer than half of the neonates. A few other studies have compared phenobarbital versus PHT for neonatal seizures (Castro Conde et al. 2005, Pathak et al. 2013, van Rooij et al. 2013b). PHT is thought to limit repetitive firing of action potentials by its effects on the voltage-dependant sodium channel (Vajda and Eadie 2014). As sodium and potassium channels co-localise at the neuronal membrane it may also modulate the potassium channel and be useful in epileptic encephalopathies and benign familial neonatal epilepsies associated with sodium and potassium channel mutations (Bellini et al. 1993, Boerma et al. 2015, Howell et al. 2015, Pisano et al. 2015).

PHT has been one of the mainstays of AED management of seizures and epilepsy. It has both enteral and parenteral preparations. Intravenous PHT cannot be mixed with other drugs, has to be administered slowly and may cause tissue irritation and discolouration. PHT infusions have been associated with hypotension, cardiac arrhythmias and collapse. Difficulties in administration of intravenous PHT and the availability of other treatment options have resulted in some waning of use of PHT for neonatal seizures. Loading and maintenance doses for PHT are shown in Table 9.1.

Second- and third-line antiepileptic drugs

LEVETIRACETAM

Levetiracetam (LEV) is a relatively new wide spectrum AED, with a good efficacy and safety profile in children and adults and is thought to be the most promising AED for neonatal seizures. It has a unique structure (pyrrolidine derivative) and a novel mode of action. It is thought to influence excitability by binding to the synaptic vesicle gly-coprotein 2A receptor (SV2A) on neuronal cells and reduces presynaptic neurotransmitter release. This receptor appears to be involved in the generation of focal and generalised seizures (Kaminski et al. 2008, Crepeau and Treiman 2010). The precise mechanisms of action of LEV are still being elucidated (Beaulieu 2013). Several observational studies in term and preterm infants a with small sample size (*n*=6–38) have suggested that it is useful for seizures with efficacies ranging from 35% to 100% (Furwentsches et al. 2010, Abend et al. 2011, Ramantani et al. 2011, Khan et al. 2013, Rakshasbhu-vankar et al. 2013, Dilena et al. 2015). Small numbers, variable neonatal seizure characteristics (ECSz, ESz, both, clinically diagnosed Sz), varying clinical profiles and aetiologies may account for the differences in efficacy. In a prospective feasibility study of 38 neonates with EEG-identified seizures, LEV was reported to result in seizure freedom in 30 at the end of the first week (Ramantani et al. 2011). The medication was well tolerated in all the studies, with no serious clinical or laboratory side effects. The availability in liquid and intravenous forms, the safety and tolerance to rapid infusion of loading doses (Wheless et al. 2009), no requirement to monitor levels, twice daily dosage schedule for maintenance, the renal excretion, minimal protein binding, lack of significant interactions with most other drugs and lack of evidence regarding neurode-generative effects make LEV an attractive and easy-to-use drug in neonates (Kim et al. 2007, Mruk et al. 2015). LEV is also thought to result in better long-term neurodevel-opmental outcomes compared with phenobarbital administration in the neonate (Maitre et al. 2013).

LEV is rapidly becoming the most popular new AED for adjunctive treatment of neonatal seizures, despite not having official regulatory approval for use for neonatal seizures in many parts of the world (Silverstein and Ferriero 2008, Mruk et al. 2015). RCTs to compare LEV versus phenobarbital, PHT or another drug as first or second-line AED are needed to determine the place of this drug in the hierarchical treatment of neonatal seizures (Loiacono et al. 2014). An international phase IIB randomised control trial (NEOLEV2) of LEV versus phenobarbital in term neonates with seizures is under way.

A study (Sharpe et al. 2012) to determine pharmacokinetics, safety and efficacy in neonatal seizures showed clearance of LEV in neonates was higher than expected on the basis of immature renal function in term infants and increased significantly during the first week of life. The authors suggest that a higher loading dose and more frequent dosing of LEV are needed in term infants to maintain serum concentrations in the range seen in children and adults. A systematic review of pharmacokinetics of AEDs in neonates (Tulloch et al. 2012) found limited pharmacokinetic data for the use of LEV in neonates and suggested similar loading and maintenance doses for infants and young children. The optimal dosage schedule is still not clear. Table 9.1 provides some guidelines.

BENZODIAZEPINES

Clonazepam, diazepam, lorazepam and MDZ have been used as boluses or infusions in many centres as first-, second- or third-line drugs (Deshmukh et al. 1986, Bye and Flanagan 1995, Castro Conde et al. 2005, Lundqvist et al. 2013). Benzodiazepines bind to the $GABA_A$ receptor and increase the frequency with which chloride channels open, increasing inhibitory neurotransmission. They may have some effects on sodium and calcium channels (Vajda and Eadie 2014).

Midazolam is probably the most frequently used and studied benzodiazepine, though clonazepam and diazepam have been used previously for neonatal seizures. MDZ has been used as second- and third-line AED for neonatal seizures. The dosages have varied with infusions at 100–1000 micrograms/kg/hour (Sheth et al. 1996, Boylan et al. 2004, van Leuven et al. 2004, Shany et al. 2007). Levels of MDZ in plasma were not reported to correlate to response (van Leuven et al. 2004). The reported efficacies in these studies have ranged from 0% to 100%. Small numbers, heterogeneous patient cohorts, variability in other AEDs and non-randomised nature of most studies probably account for the wide variability in response and limitations of the studies. Even though MDZ is reasonably well tolerated, respiratory depression may occur, and cardiac depression and seizure exacerbation may occasionally be a problem (Gelissen et al. 1996, Montenegro et al. 2001). Suggested dosage, schedules for the benzodiazepines are shown in Table 9.1.

LIDOCAINE

Lidocaine is infrequently used and generally considered third line; however in some centres and countries it is considered second line (Vento et al. 2010, Lundqvist et al. 2013). Lidocaine is a sodium channel blocker and this is probably how it influences seizures and neuronal excitability (Diao et al. 2013, Borowicz and Banach 2014). The efficacy of lidocaine for neonatal seizures was shown to be 60%–92% when administered after phenobarbital. Cardiovascular side effects have been reported after lidocaine and may occur more frequently if used in infants with congenital heart disease, hypokalaemia and concurrent use of PHT (Weeke et al. 2015). Cardiac toxicity in adult studies (antiarrhythmic drug) has been associated mostly when the plasma levels are >9 mg/ml (Malingre et al. 2006). More recent studies and protocols suggest that cardiac side effects occur much less frequently than previously thought (Hellstrom-Westas et al. 1988, Boylan et al. 2004, van Rooij et al. 2004, Malingre et al. 2006, Shany et al. 2007, van den Broek et al. 2011, Lundqvist et al. 2013, van den Broek et al. 2013, Weeke et al. 2015). Nevertheless it would be prudent to have continuous cardiac monitoring in neonates on lidocaine infusions and to discontinue if a cardiac arrhythmia occurs (van Rooij et al. 2004). Lidocaine does not appear to modify the background EEG pattern (van den Broek et al. 2011). If neonatal seizures are responsive to intravenous lidocaine, oral mexiletene may be considered in the longer term (Nakazawa et al. 2013). Dosage schedules (Malingre et al. 2006, Shany et al. 2007, Lundqvist et al. 2013) for lidocaine are outlined in Table 9.1. In neonates with HIE receiving therapeutic hypothermia, modification of the regime should be considered as hypothermia reduces lidocaine clearance by 24% (van den Broek et al. 2013).

Lidocaine is probably underutilised in neonatal seizures; in view of its efficacy and safety profile with current protocols it should be considered in future trials of AEDs for neonatal seizures.

Other drugs and therapies
TOPIRAMATE
TPM has multiple mechanisms of action that include inhibition of glutamate receptors and GABA$_A$R activated ion channels and blockade of voltage-activated sodium and calcium channels as well as inhibition of carbonic anhydrase. Considering the developmental profile of neonatal neuronal excitatory and inhibitory systems, TPM would be a good drug to consider for neonatal seizures and has been used 'off label' (Silverstein and Ferriero 2008, Pressler and Mangum 2013, Vesoulis and Mathur 2014). Filippi et al. (2009) used a dosage of 5 mg/kg/day and showed no significant difference in pharmacokinetic parameters between neonates treated with deep and mild hypothermia. This is an arbitrary dose and though it resulted in appropriate levels for a short period of time, additional studies are required over a longer period of time in different populations. Metabolic acidosis, irritability and feeding problems are some of the adverse effects reported with TPM. The lack of availability of a parenteral solution or even liquid preparation makes it difficult to use in a sick neonate. TPM appears not to induce neuronal cell death and may have neuroprotective and antiepileptogenic effects in developing animal models (Koh et al. 2004, Kim et al. 2007). Despite the possible adverse events (neurological and metabolic), TPM is an option worth exploring further for neonatal seizures.

VALPROATE
Valproate is thought to act through increased GABA-mediated inhibition, sodium channel blockade and modulation of N-methyl-D-aspartate (NMDA) receptors. It has been shown to have neuroprotective effects in animal models (Suda et al. 2013). Small case series suggest it is effective in neonatal seizures at doses of 20–30 mg/kg given through nasogastric tube or rectally (Steinberg et al. 1986, Gal et al. 1988). The availability of liquid and parenteral preparations makes it an easy-to-use option; however hyperammonaemia that may associated with valproate therapy is of concern, especially when metabolic disorders may be the cause of neonatal seizures. The optimal doses and the place of valproate in the armamentarium to treat neonatal seizures are yet to be determined.

CARBAMAZEPINE AND OXCARBAZEPINE
Carbamazepine (CBZ) is thought to prevent repetitive firing of action potentials in depolarised neurons by its action on voltage-dependant sodium channels (Vajda and Eadie 2014). In small groups of neonates, the therapeutic effects of loading doses of 5–20 mg/kg

day and maintenance doses of 5–8 mg/kg given 8–12 hourly have been studied (Singh et al. 1996, Tulloch et al. 2012). The ideal reference range for CBZ in neonatal seizures is unknown. It may play a role in neonatal seizures due to chanellopathies (Pisano et al. 2015). The low activity of isoenzyme CYP3A4 at birth (needed to metabolize CBZ to the active CBZ epoxide), the immaturity of the epoxide hydrolase enzymes, the reduced renal elimination and the lack of an intravenous preparation limit the use of CBZ in neonatal seizures. Oxcarbazepine appears to have a similar mechanism of action. Oxcarbazepine has less drug-to-drug interaction, is less sedating and may be better tolerated. It is also being used 'off label' in neonatal seizures, probably more frequently than CBZ (Slaughter et al. 2013).

Vigabatrin

Vigabatrin is a selective enzyme activated irreversible inhibitor of GABA transaminases and acts by increasing GABA in the brain. A dosage schedule of 125 mg twice daily has been reported (Tulloch et al. 2012). It has been known to be useful in spasms and seizures in neonatal epileptic encephalopathies and tuberous sclerosis complex (Vigevano et al. 2013, Overwater et al. 2015). Treatment with vigabatrin, directed at the metabolic defect in neurotransmitter disorders, is reported to have been disappointing (Pearl et al. 2006). Vigabatrin use is associated with a risk of visual impairment and loss (van Rooij et al. 2013b) and therefore vigabatrin should be used with caution, if at all, in neonatal seizures.

Lamotrigine

Lamotrigine is an AED that inhibits excitatory activity through the voltage-dependant sodium channel (stabilising neuronal membrane potential) and by inhibiting glutamate and aspartate release. It has a good safety profile that makes it attractive for neonatal seizures (Barr et al. 1999, van Rooij et al. 2013a, 2013b). However, the need to introduce it slowly often limits its use in the neonate with frequent seizures.

Zonisamide

Zonisamide is a broad-spectrum AED effective for multiple seizure types. Its actions are thought to include effects on the voltage-sensitive Na^+ channels, the voltage-dependant T-type calcium current and modulation of GABAnergic inhibition. Zonisamide has been reported to be used in neonatal seizures, especially in the early epileptic encephalopathies (Ohno et al. 2000, Kato et al. 2013, Slaughter et al. 2013).

Paraldehyde

Paraldehyde has been reported to have been used as second-line drug in one study, at 0.3 ml/kg rectally or 1–3 ml/kg/hour intravenously with equivocal efficacy (Slaughter et al. 2013). In neonatal seizures, if used, it is primarily administered rectally, as there are concerns regarding adverse effects such as pulmonary oedema, pulmonary haemorrhage and hypotension with intravenous doses (Tulloch et al. 2012). The mode of action of paraldehyde is unclear.

THIOPENTONE

Thiopentone has been reported to be quick acting and efficacious at 10 mg/kg intravenously in one study in nine infants with phenobarbital-resistant seizures. Hypotension needing intervention occurred in the majority (Bonati et al. 1990).

XENON

Xenon is a general anaesthetic agent; it is an NMDA glutamate receptor antagonist. Preliminary studies suggest Xenon may have antiseizure as well as neuroprotective effects (Azzopardi et al. 2013). It is a potential new therapy for neonatal seizures, especially in combination with hypothermia.

METABOLIC DISORDERS AND VITAMIN RESPONSIVE SEIZURES

Although treatable metabolic causes of neonatal seizures are uncommon, a prompt diagnosis is important in order to initiate treatment and prevent irreversible neurological injury. Abnormalities in glucose, sodium, calcium and magnesium levels should be looked for and treated. They may exacerbate seizures even if they are not the primary cause. The early diagnosis of inborn errors of metabolism (IEMs) is crucial, considering that many have effective treatments (e.g. dietary supplementation or restriction) with favourable long-term outcomes (Ficicioglu and Bearden 2011, Campistol and Plecko 2015).

Antiquitin (alpha-aminoadipic semialdehyde dehydrogenase) deficiency is the main cause of pyridoxine-dependant epilepsy (PDE). Responsiveness to pyridoxine may also be seen in neonatal seizures associated with conditions such as neonatal/infantile hypophosphotasia, familial hyperphosphotasia, nutritional vitamin B6 deficiency, pyridoxamine 5'-phosphate oxidase (PNPO) deficiency and other yet to be identified causes (Stockler et al. 2011). Seizures in infants who are pyridoxine-dependant must be treated using pharmacologic doses of pyridoxine (vitamin B6), and life-long therapy is required. To interrupt seizures an intravenous dose of 100 mg is often administered initially and followed by 15–30 mg/kg/day of pyridoxine. As respiratory arrest has been reported with parenteral pyridoxine, it should be given with adequate monitoring and respiratory support facility. Consideration should be given to a lysine-restricted diet to address the potential toxicity of accumulated toxic compounds in PDE and fortification with arginine (van Karnebeek and Jaggumantri 2015).

Pyridoxal phosphate-dependant seizures result from a deficiency of PNPO: exome sequencing can detect *PNPO* mutations. Patients with PNPO deficiency may respond to pyridoxal phosphate at initial doses ranging from 18 mg to 55 mg followed by maintenance of 6–26 mg/kg/day in several divided doses. Infants with PNPO deficiency may not respond to pyridoxine, though changing from pyridoxine to pyridoxal phosphate may worsen seizures occasionally (Mills et al. 2014).

Folinic acid responsive seizures are treated with supplements of folinic acid (5-formyltetrahydrofolate) at 5 mg/kg/day. They are thought to be identical to PDE associated with antiquitin mutations, though there are reports of folinic acid responsiveness in other conditions (Tso et al. 2014).

Supplementation with selected drugs may be considered in specific IEM, for example with creatine in creatine deficiency syndromes, serine and glycine in defects of serine biogenesis, sodium benzoate in non-ketotic hyperglycinaemia and biotin in biotinidase deficiency (Ficicioglu and Bearden 2011, Campistol and Plecko 2015).

KETOGENIC DIET

A ketogenic diet may be considered for refractory seizures. While well established for children, there is scant information in the neonatal population (Cobo et al. 2015). Ketogenic diet is also the treatment of choice for neonates with Glut 1 deficiency and may be useful in non-ketotic hyperglycinemia (Cusmai et al. 2012, Pong et al. 2012).

Genes and epilepsy

With the advent of next generation sequencing there are rapid advances in genetic causes of epilepsy of early onset (Mastrangelo 2015). This is expected to result in the development of unique targeted therapies, such as the use of quinidine in KCNT1 gain in function mutations that may be seen in epilepsy of infancy with migrating focal seizures or memantine in a GRIN 2A mutation with early onset epilepsy (Milligan et al. 2014, Pierson et al. 2014).

Duration of therapy

The optimal duration of AED therapy for neonatal seizures is unknown (Bartha et al. 2007, Bassan et al. 2008, Guillet and Kwon 2008, Blume et al. 2009, Wickstrom et al. 2013). The rationale for continuation of AEDs after seizure cessation in the newborn period is to prevent or decrease the occurrence of further seizures. However, it is imperative to assess the risk of further seizures versus the potential long-term neurodevelopmental sequelae from commonly used AEDS. The neurological status of the infant, EEG, neuroimaging and underlying aetiology need to be considered in this decision regarding duration of therapy. In genetic and metabolic disorders duration of targeted therapy may be necessary lifelong. In most neonates stopping AEDs after 72 hours of seizure freedom and restarting if necessary seems a reasonable strategy (WHO Guidelines 2011). Further research is essential to develop evidence-based guidelines regarding optimal duration and choice of AED in neonatal seizures.

Challenges for the future

Seizures are reported to occur much more frequently in preterm infants compared with term infants on EEG monitoring. Do these seizures warrant treatment and should they be treated differently? Should the management of neonatal seizures with AEDs be tailored to the aetiology?

Any treatment effect is difficult to evaluate as the majority of neonatal seizures will resolve within days (at least in the short term), independent of therapeutic intervention. This may result in unwarranted efficacy being attributed to the last AED used (Lynch et al. 2012). International guidelines for AED trials in neonatal seizures are required.

Randomised controlled trials for AEDs and other seizure interventions need to be thoughtfully designed to address the age-specific challenges in the neonatal period, provide guidelines for the duration of therapy, as well as evaluate the potential effect on long-term neurodevelopmental outcome.

REFERENCES

Abend N, Gutierrez-Colina AM, Monk HM, Dlugos DJ, Clancy RR (2011) Levetiracetam for treatment of neonatal seizures. *J Child Neurol* 26: 465–470. doi: http://dx.doi.org/10.1177/0883073810384263.

Azzopardi D, Robertson NJ, Kapetanakis A et al. (2013) Anticonvulsant effect of xenon on neonatal asphyxial seizures. *Arch Dis Child Fetal Neonatal Ed* 98: F437–F439. doi: http://dx.doi.org/10.1136/archdischild-2013-303786.

Barks JD, Liu YQ, Shangguan Y, Silverstein FS (2010) Phenobarbital augments hypothermic neuroprotection. *Pediatr Res* 67: 532–537. doi: http://dx.doi.org/10.1203/PDR.0b013e3181d4ff4d.

Barr PA, Buettiker VE, Antony JH (1999) Efficacy of lamotrigine in refractory neonatal seizures. *Pediatr Neurol* 20: 161–163. doi: http://dx.doi.org/10.1016/S0887-8994(98)00125-8.

Bartha AI, Shen J, Katz KH et al. (2007) Neonatal seizures: Multicenter variability in current treatment practices. *Pediatr Neurol* 37: 85–90. doi: http://dx.doi.org/10.1016/j.pediatrneurol.2007.04.003.

Bassan H, Bental Y, Shany E et al. (2008) Neonatal seizures: Dilemmas in workup and management. *Pediatr Neurol* 38: 415–421. doi: http://dx.doi.org/10.1016/j.pediatrneurol.2008.03.003.

Beaulieu MJ (2013) Levetiracetam. *Neonatal Netw* 32: 285–288. doi: http://dx.doi.org/10.1891/0730-0832.32.4.285.

Bellini G, Miceli F, Soldovieri MV et al. (1993) KCNQ3-Related Disorders. In: Pagon RA, Adam MP, Ardinger HH, Wallace SE, Amemiya A, Bean LJH, Bird TD, Dolan CR, Fong CT, Smith RJH, Stephens K, editors. *GeneReviews(R)*. Seattle: University of Washington, Seattle. All rights reserved.

Bittigau P, Sifringer M, Genz K et al. (2002) Antiepileptic drugs and apoptotic neurodegeneration in the developing brain. *Proceedings of the National Academy of Sciences of the United States of America* 99: 15089–15094. doi: http://dx.doi.org/10.1073/pnas.222550499.

Blume HK, Garrison MM, Christakis DA (2009) Neonatal seizures: Treatment and treatment variability in 31 United States pediatric hospitals. *J Child Neurol* 24: 148–154. doi: http://dx.doi.org/10.1177/0883073808321056.

Boerma RS, Braun KP, Van De Broek MP et al. (2016) Remarkable phenytoin sensitivity in 4 children with SCN8A-related epilepsy: A molecular neuropharmacological approach. *Neurotherapeutics* 13(1): 192–7. doi: 10.1007/s13311-015-0372-8.

Bonati M, Marraro G, Celardo A et al. (1990) Thiopental efficacy in phenobarbital-resistant neonatal seizures. *Dev Pharmacol Ther* 15: 16–20.

Booth D, Evans DJ (2004) Anticonvulsants for neonates with seizures. *Cochrane Database Syst Rev.* 18(4): CD004218.

Borowicz KK, Banach M (2014) Antiarrhythmic drugs and epilepsy. *Pharmacol Rep* 66: 545–551. doi: http://dx.doi.org/10.1016/j.pharep.2014.03.009.

Boylan GB, Kharoshankaya L, Wusthoff CJ (2015) Seizures and hypothermia: Importance of electroencephalographic monitoring and considerations for treatment. *Semin Fetal Neonatal Med* 20: 103–108. doi: http://dx.doi.org/10.1016/j.siny.2015.01.001.

Boylan GB, Pressler RM, Rennie JM et al. (1999) Outcome of electroclinical, electrographic, and clinical seizures in the newborn infant. *Dev Med Child Neurol* 41: 819–825. doi: http://dx.doi.org/10.1111/j.1469-8749.1999.tb00548.x.

Boylan GB, Rennie JM, Chorley G et al. (2004) Second-line anticonvulsant treatment of neonatal seizures: A video-EEG monitoring study. *Neurology* 62: 486–488. doi: http://dx.doi.org/10.1212/01.WNL.0000106944.59990.E6.

Brito S, Thompson K, Campistol J, Colomer J, Hardy SA, He L, Fernández-Marmiesse A, Palacios L, Jou C, Jiménez-Mallebrera C, Armstrong J, Montero R, Artuch R, Tischner C, Wenz T, McFarland R, Taylor RW (2015) Corrigendum: Long-term survival in a child with severe encephalopathy, multiple respiratory chain deficiency and GFM1 mutations. *Front Genet* 6: 254. doi: 10.3389/fgene.2015.00254. eCollection 2015.

Bye A, Flanagan D (1995) Electroencephalograms, clinical observations and the monitoring of neonatal seizures. *J Paediatr Child Health* 31: 503–507. doi: http://dx.doi.org/10.1111/j.1440-1754.1995.tb00872.x.

Campistol J, Plecko B (2015) Treatable newborn and infant seizures due to inborn errors of metabolism. *Epileptic Disord* 17(3): 229–42. doi: http://dx.doi.org/10.1684/epd.2015.0754.

Castro Conde JR, Hernandez Borges AA, Domenech Martinez E, Gonzalez Campo C, Perera Soler R (2005) Midazolam in neonatal seizures with no response to phenobarbital. *Neurology* 64: 876–879. doi: http://dx.doi.org/10.1212/01.WNL.0000152891.58694.71.

Clancy RR (2006) Prolonged electroencephalogram monitoring for seizures and their treatment. *Clin Perinatology* 33: 649–665, vi. doi: http://dx.doi.org/10.1016/j.clp.2006.06.004.

Cleary RT, Sun H, Huynh T et al. (2013) Bumetanide enhances phenobarbital efficacy in a rat model of hypoxic neonatal seizures. *PLoS One* 8: e57148. doi: http://dx.doi.org/10.1371/journal.pone.0057148.

Cobo NH, Sankar R, Murata KK, Sewak SL, Kezele MA, Matsumoto JH (2015) The ketogenic diet as broad-spectrum treatment for super-refractory pediatric status epilepticus: Challenges in implementation in the pediatric and neonatal intensive care units. *J Child Neurol* 30: 259–266. doi: http://dx.doi.org/10.1177/0883073813516192.

Crepeau AZ, Treiman DM (2010) Levetiracetam: A comprehensive review. *Expert Rev Neurother* 10: 159–171. doi: http://dx.doi.org/10.1586/ern.10.3.

Cusmai R, Martinelli D, Moavero R et al. (2012) Ketogenic diet in early myoclonic encephalopathy due to non ketotic hyperglycinemia. *Eur J Paediatr Neurol* 16: 509–513. doi: http://dx.doi.org/10.1016/j.ejpn.2011.12.015.

Deshmukh A, Wittert W, Schnitzler E, Mangurten HH (1986) Lorazepam in the treatment of refractory neonatal seizures. A pilot study. *Am J Dis Child* 140: 1042–1044. doi: http://dx.doi.org/10.1001/archpedi.1986.02140240088032.

Diao L, Hellier JL, Uskert-Newsom J, Williams PA, Staley KJ, Yee, AS (2013) Diphenytoin, riluzole and lidocaine: Three sodium channel blockers, with different mechanisms of action, decrease hippocampal epileptiform activity. *Neuropharmacology* 73: 48–55. doi: http://dx.doi.org/10.1016/j.neuropharm.2013.04.057.

Dilena R, Striano P, Traverso M et al. (2015) Dramatic effect of levetiracetam in early-onset epileptic encephalopathy due to STXBP1 mutation. *Brain Dev.* 38(1): 128–31. doi: 10.1016/j.braindev.2015.07.002. Epub 2015 Jul 23.

Farwell JR, Lee YJ, Hirtz DG, Sulzbacher SI, Ellenberg JH, Nelson KB (1990) Phenobarbital for febrile seizures–effects on intelligence and on seizure recurrence. *N Engl J Med* 322: 364–369. doi: http://dx.doi.org/10.1056/NEJM199002083220604.

Ficicioglu C, Bearden D (2011) Isolated neonatal seizures: When to suspect inborn errors of metabolism. *Pediatr Neurol* 45: 283–291. doi: http://dx.doi.org/10.1016/j.pediatrneurol.2011.07.006.

Filippi L, La Marca G, Fiorini P et al. (2009) Topiramate concentrations in neonates treated with prolonged whole body hypothermia for hypoxic ischemic encephalopathy. *Epilepsia* 50: 2355–2361. doi: http://dx.doi.org/10.1111/j.1528-1167.2009.02302.x.

Forcelli PA, Soper C, Duckles A, Gale K, Kondratyev A (2013) Melatonin potentiates the anticonvulsant action of phenobarbital in neonatal rats. *Epilepsy Res* 107: 217–223. doi: http://dx.doi.org/10.1016/j.eplepsyres.2013.09.013.

Furwentsches A, Bussmann C, Ramantani G et al. (2010). Levetiracetam in the treatment of neonatal seizures: A pilot study. *Seizure* 19: 185–189. doi: http://dx.doi.org/10.1016/j.seizure.2010.01.003.

Gal P, Oles KS, Gilman JT, Weaver R (1988) Valproic acid efficacy, toxicity, and pharmacokinetics in neonates with intractable seizures. *Neurology* 38: 467–471. doi: http://dx.doi.org/10.1212/WNL.38.3.467.

Gano D, Orbach SA, Bonifacio SL, Glass HC (2014) Neonatal seizures and therapeutic hypothermia for hypoxic-ischemic encephalopathy. *Mol Cell Epilepsy* 1(3): pii: e88.

Gelissen HP, Epema AH, Henning RH, Krijnen HJ, Hennis PJ, Den Hertog A (1996) Inotropic effects of propofol, thiopental, midazolam, etomidate, and ketamine on isolated human atrial muscle. *Anesthesiology* 84: 397–403.

Glass HC, Bonifacio SL, Sullivan J et al. (2009) Magnetic resonance imaging and ultrasound injury in preterm infants with seizures. *J Child Neurol* 24: 1105–1111. doi: http://dx.doi.org/10.1177/0883073809338328.

Glass HC, Hong KJ, Rogers EE et al. (2011) Risk factors for epilepsy in children with neonatal encephalopathy. *Pediatr Res* 70: 535–540. doi: http://dx.doi.org/10.1203/PDR.0b013e31822f24c7.

Guillet R, Kwon JM (2008) Prophylactic phenobarbital administration after resolution of neonatal seizures: Survey of current practice. *Pediatrics* 122: 731–735. doi: http://dx.doi.org/10.1542/peds.2007-3278.

Hagberg H, Mallard C, Ferriero DM et al. (2015) The role of inflammation in perinatal brain injury. *Nat Rev Neurol* 11: 192–208. doi: http://dx.doi.org/10.1038/nrneurol.2015.13.

Hellstrom-Westas L, Boylan G, Agren J (2015) Systematic review of neonatal seizure management strategies provides guidance on anti-epileptic treatment. *Acta Paediatr* 104: 123–129. doi: http://dx.doi.org/10.1111/apa.12812.

Hellstrom-Westas L, Westgren U, Rosen I, Svenningsen NW (1988) Lidocaine for treatment of severe seizures in newborn infants. I. Clinical effects and cerebral electrical activity monitoring. *Acta Paediatr Scand* 77: 79–84. doi: http://dx.doi.org/10.1111/j.1651-2227.1988.tb10602.x/

Hernandez-Diaz S, Smith CR, Shen A et al. (2012) Comparative safety of antiepileptic drugs during pregnancy. *Neurology* 78: 1692–1699. doi: http://dx.doi.org/10.1212/WNL.0b013e3182574f39.

Howell KB, Mcmahon JM, Carvill GL et al. (2015) SCN2A encephalopathy: A major cause of epilepsy of infancy with migrating focal seizures. *Neurology* 85(11): 958–66. doi: 10.1212/WNL.0000000000001926. Epub 2015 Aug 19.

Johnston MV, Fatemi A, Wilson MA, Northington F (2011) Treatment advances in neonatal neuroprotection and neurointensive care. *Lancet Neurol* 10: 372–382. doi: http://dx.doi.org/10.1016/S1474-4422(11)70016-3.

Kaminska A, Mourdie J, Barnerias C, Bahi-Buisson N, Plouin P, Huon C (2007) Management of neonatal seizures. *Arch Pediatr* 14: 1137–1151. doi: http://dx.doi.org/10.1016/j.arcped.2007.05.004.

Kaminski RM, Matagne A, Leclercq K et al. (2008) SV2A protein is a broad-spectrum anticonvulsant target: Functional correlation between protein binding and seizure protection in models of both partial and generalized epilepsy. *Neuropharmacology* 54: 715–720. doi: http://dx.doi.org/10.1016/j.neuropharm.2007.11.021.

Kato M, Yamagata T, Kubota M et al. (2013) Clinical spectrum of early onset epileptic encephalopathies caused by KCNQ2 mutation. *Epilepsia* 54: 1282–1287. doi: http://dx.doi.org/10.1111/epi.12200.

Khan O, Cipriani C, Wright C, Crisp E, Kirmani B (2013) Role of intravenous levetiracetam for acute seizure management in preterm neonates. *Pediatr Neurol* 49: 340–343. doi: http://dx.doi.org/10.1016/j.pediatrneurol.2013.05.008.

Kim J, Kondratyev A, Gale K (2007) Antiepileptic drug-induced neuronal cell death in the immature brain: Effects of carbamazepine, topiramate, and levetiracetam as monotherapy versus polytherapy. *J Pharmacol Exp Ther* 323: 165–173. doi: http://dx.doi.org/10.1124/jpet.107.126250.

Koh S, Tibayan FD, Simpson JN, Jensen FE (2004) NBQX or topiramate treatment after perinatal hypoxia-induced seizures prevents later increases in seizure-induced neuronal injury. *Epilepsia* 45: 569–575. doi: http://dx.doi.org/10.1111/j.0013-9580.2004.69103.x.

Liu Y, Shangguan Y, Barks JD, Silverstein, FS (2012) Bumetanide augments the neuroprotective efficacy of phenobarbital plus hypothermia in a neonatal hypoxia-ischemia model. *Pediatr Res* 71: 559–565. doi: http://dx.doi.org/10.1038/pr.2012.7.

Loiacono G, Masci M, Zaccara G, Verrotti A (2014) The treatment of neonatal seizures: Focus on Levetiracetam. *J Matern Fetal Neonatal Med* 29(1): 69–74. doi: 10.3109/14767058.2014.986651. Epub 2014 Dec 5.

Loring DW, Meador KJ (2004) Cognitive side effects of antiepileptic drugs in children. *Neurology* 62: 872–877. doi: http://dx.doi.org/10.1212/01.WNL.0000115653.82763.07.

Lundqvist M, Agren J, Hellstrom-Westas L, Flink R, Wickstrom R (2013) Efficacy and safety of lidocaine for treatment of neonatal seizures. *Acta Paediatr* 102: 863–867. doi: http://dx.doi.org/10.1111/apa.12311.

Lynch NE, Stevenson NJ, Livingstone V, Murphy BP, Rennie JM, Boylan GB (2012) The temporal evolution of electrographic seizure burden in neonatal hypoxic ischemic encephalopathy. *Epilepsia* 53: 549–557. doi: http://dx.doi.org/10.1111/j.1528-1167.2011.03401.x.

Maitre NL, Smolinsky C, Slaughter JC, Stark AR (2013) Adverse neurodevelopmental outcomes after exposure to phenobarbital and levetiracetam for the treatment of neonatal seizures. *J Perinatol* 33: 841–846. doi: http://dx.doi.org/10.1038/jp.2013.116.

Malingre MM, Van Rooij LG, Rademaker CM et al. (2006) Development of an optimal lidocaine infusion strategy for neonatal seizures. *Eur J Pediatr* 165: 598–604. doi: http://dx.doi.org/10.1007/s00431-006-0136-x.

Mastrangelo M (2015) Novel genes of early-onset epileptic encephalopathies: From genotype to phenotypes. *Pediatr Neurol* 53: 119–129. doi: http://dx.doi.org/10.1016/j.pediatrneurol.2015.04.001.

McCoy B, Hahn CD (2013) Continuous EEG monitoring in the neonatal intensive care unit. *J Clin Neurophysiol* 30: 106–114. doi: http://dx.doi.org/10.1097/WNP.0b013e3182872919.

Meyn DF Jr., Ness J, Ambalavanan N, Carlo WA (2010) Prophylactic phenobarbital and whole-body cooling for neonatal hypoxic-ischemic encephalopathy. *J Pediatr* 157: 334–336. doi: http://dx.doi.org/10.1016/j.jpeds.2010.04.005.

Milligan CJ, Li M, Gazina EV et al. (2014) KCNT1 gain of function in 2 epilepsy phenotypes is reversed by quinidine. *Ann Neurol* 75: 581–590. doi: http://dx.doi.org/10.1002/ana.24128.

Mills PB, Camuzeaux SS, Footitt EJ, Mills KA, Gissen P, Fisher L et al. (2014) Epilepsy due to PNPO mutations: genotype, environment and treatment affect presentation and outcome. *Brain* 137(Pt 5): 1350–60. doi: 10.1093/brain/awu051. Epub 2014 Mar 18.

Mizrahi EM (1987) Neonatal seizures: Problems in diagnosis and classification. *Epilepsia* 28 (Suppl 1): S46–S55. doi: http://dx.doi.org/10.1111/j.1528-1157.1987.tb05757.x.

Montenegro MA, Guerreiro MM, Caldas JP, Moura-Ribeiro MV, Guerreiro CA (2001) Epileptic manifestations induced by midazolam in the neonatal period. *Arq Neuropsiquiatr* 59: 242–243. doi: http://dx.doi.org/10.1590/S0004-282X2001000200018.

Mruk AL, Garlitz KL, Leung NR (2015) Levetiracetam in neonatal seizures: A review. *J Pediatr Pharmacol Ther* 20: 76–89.

Murray DM, Boylan GB, Ali I, Ryan CA, Murphy BP, Connolly S (2008) Defining the gap between electrographic seizure burden, clinical expression and staff recognition of neonatal seizures. *Arch Dis Child Fetal Neonatal Ed* 93: F187–F191. doi: http://dx.doi.org/10.1136/adc.2005.086314.

Nagarajan L, Ghosh S, Palumbo L (2011a) Ictal electroencephalograms in neonatal seizures: Characteristics and associations. *Pediatr Neurol* 45: 11–16. doi: http://dx.doi.org/10.1016/j.pediatrneurol.2011.01.009.

Nagarajan L, Palumbo L, Ghosh S (2011b) Brief electroencephalography rhythmic discharges (BERDs) in the neonate with seizures: Their significance and prognostic implications. *J Child Neurol* 26: 1529–1533. doi: http://dx.doi.org/10.1177/0883073811409750.

Nagarajan L, Palumbo L, Ghosh S (2012) Classification of clinical semiology in epileptic seizures in neonates. *Eur J Paediatr Neurol* 16: 118–125. doi: http://dx.doi.org/10.1016/j.ejpn.2011.11.005.

Nakazawa M, Okumura A, Niijima S et al. (2013) Oral mexiletine for lidocaine-responsive neonatal epilepsy. *Brain Dev* 35: 667–669. doi: http://dx.doi.org/10.1016/j.braindev.2012.10.011.

Ohno M, Shimotsuji Y, Abe J, Shimada M, Tamiya H (2000) Zonisamide treatment of early infantile epileptic encephalopathy. *Pediatr Neurol* 23: 341–344. doi: http://dx.doi.org/10.1016/S0887-8994(00)00197-1.

Overwater IE, Bindels-De Heus K, Rietman AB et al. (2015) Epilepsy in children with tuberous sclerosis complex: Chance of remission and response to antiepileptic drugs. *Epilepsia* 56: 1239–1245. doi: http://dx.doi.org/10.1111/epi.13050.

Painter MJ, Scher MS, Stein AD et al. (1999) Phenobarbital compared with phenytoin for the treatment of neonatal seizures. *N Engl J Med* 341: 485–489. doi: http://dx.doi.org/10.1056/NEJM199908123410704.

Pappas A, Shankaran S, Mcdonald SA et al. (2015) Cognitive outcomes after neonatal encephalopathy. *Pediatrics* 135: e624–e634. doi: http://dx.doi.org/10.1542/peds.2014-1566.

Pathak G, Upadhyay A, Pathak U, Chawla D, Goel SP (2013) Phenobarbitone versus phenytoin for treatment of neonatal seizures: An open-label randomized controlled trial. *Indian Pediatr* 50: 753–757. doi: http://dx.doi.org/10.1007/s13312-013-0218-6.

Pearl PL, Hartka TR, Taylor J (2006) Diagnosis and treatment of neurotransmitter disorders. *Curr Treat Options Neurol* 8: 441–450. doi: http://dx.doi.org/10.1007/s11940-006-0033-7.

Pennell PB, Klein AM, Browning N et al. (2012) Differential effects of antiepileptic drugs on neonatal outcomes. *Epilepsy Behav* 24: 449–456. doi: http://dx.doi.org/10.1016/j.yebeh.2012.05.010.

Pierson TM, Yuan H, Marsh ED et al. (2014) Mutation and early-onset epileptic encephalopathy: Personalized therapy with memantine. *Ann Clin Transl Neurol* 1: 190–198. doi: http://dx.doi.org/10.1002/acn3.39.

Pisano T, Numis AL, Heavin SB et al. (2015) Early and effective treatment of KCNQ2 encephalopathy. *Epilepsia* 56: 685–691. doi: http://dx.doi.org/10.1111/epi.12984.

Plecko B, Paul K, Mills P, Clayton P, Paschke E, Maier O, Hasselmann O, Schmiedel G, Kanz S, Connolly M, Wolf N, Struys E, Stockler S, Abela L, Hofer D (2014) Pyridoxine responsiveness in novel mutations of the PNPO gene. *Neurology* 82(16): 1425–33. doi: 10.1212/WNL.0000000000000344. Epub 2014 Mar 21.

Pokorna P, Wildschut ED, Vobruba V, Van Den Anker J, Tibboel D (2015) The impact of hypothermia on the pharmacokinetics of drugs used in neonates and young infants. *Curr Pharm Des* 21(39): 5705–24.

Pong AW, Geary BR, Engelstad KM, Natarajan A, Yang H, De Vivo DC (2012) Glucose transporter type I deficiency syndrome: Epilepsy phenotypes and outcomes. *Epilepsia* 53: 1503–1510. doi: http://dx.doi.org/10.1111/j.1528-1167.2012.03592.x.

Pressler RM, Boylan GB, Marlow N et al. (2015) Bumetanide for the treatment of seizures in newborn babies with hypoxic ischaemic encephalopathy (NEMO): An open-label, dose finding, and feasibility phase 1/2 trial. *Lancet Neurol* 14: 469–477. doi: http://dx.doi.org/10.1016/S1474-4422(14)70303-5.

Pressler RM, Mangum B (2013) Newly emerging therapies for neonatal seizures. *Semin Fetal Neonatal Med* 18: 216–223. doi: http://dx.doi.org/10.1016/j.siny.2013.04.005.

Puskarjov M, Kahle KT, Ruusuvuori E, Kaila K (2014) Pharmacotherapeutic targeting of cation-chloride cotransporters in neonatal seizures. *Epilepsia* 55: 806–818. doi: http://dx.doi.org/10.1111/epi.12620.

Rakshasbhuvankar A, RaoS, Kohan R, Simmer K, Nagarajan L (2013) Intravenous levetiracetam for treatment of neonatal seizures. *J Clin Neurosci* 20: 1165–1167. doi: http://dx.doi.org/10.1016/j.jocn.2012.08.014.

Ramantani G, Ikonomidou C, Walter B, Rating D, Dinger J (2011) Levetiracetam: Safety and efficacy in neonatal seizures. *Eur J Paediatr Neurol* 15: 1–7. doi: http://dx.doi.org/10.1016/j.ejpn.2010.10.003.

Sankar R, Painter MJ (2005) Neonatal seizures: After all these years we still love what doesn't work. *Neurology* 64: 776–777. doi: http://dx.doi.org/10.1212/01.WNL.0000157320.78071.6D.

Sankar R, Rho JM (2007) Do seizures affect the developing brain? Lessons from the laboratory. *J Child Neurol* 22: 21S–29S. doi: http://dx.doi.org/10.1177/0883073807303072.

Sarkar S, Barks JD, Bapuraj JR et al. (2012) Does phenobarbital improve the effectiveness of therapeutic hypothermia in infants with hypoxic-ischemic encephalopathy? *J Perinatol* 32: 15–20. doi: http://dx.doi.org/10.1038/jp.2011.41.

Scher MS (2002) Controversies regarding neonatal seizure recognition. *Epileptic Disord* 4: 139–158.

Scher MS, Alvin J, Gaus L, Minnigh B, Painter MJ (2003) Uncoupling of EEG-clinical neonatal seizures after antiepileptic drug use. *Pediatr Neurol* 28: 277–280. doi: http://dx.doi.org/10.1016/S0887-8994(02)00621-5.

Scher MS, Loparo KA. (2009). Neonatal EEG/sleep state analyses: A complex phenotype of developmental neural plasticity. *Dev Neurosci* 31(4): 259–75. doi: 10.1159/000216537. Epub 2009 Jan 2.

Shah DK, Wusthoff CJ, Clarke P et al. (2014) Electrographic seizures are associated with brain injury in newborns undergoing therapeutic hypothermia. *Arch Dis Child Fetal Neonatal Ed* 99: F219–F224. doi: http://dx.doi.org/10.1136/archdischild-2013-305206.

Shany E, Benzaqen O, Watemberg N (2007) Comparison of continuous drip of midazolam or lidocaine in the treatment of intractable neonatal seizures. *J Child Neurol* 22: 255–259. doi: http://dx.doi.org/10.1177/0883073807299858.

Sharpe CM, Capparelli EV, Mower A, Farrell MJ, Soldin SJ, Haas RH (2012) A seven-day study of the pharmacokinetics of intravenous levetiracetam in neonates: Marked changes in pharmacokinetics occur during the first week of life. *Pediatr Res* 72: 43–49. doi: http://dx.doi.org/10.1038/pr.2012.51.

Shellhaas RA, Ng CM, Dillon CH, Barks JD, Bhatt-Mehta V (2013) Population pharmacokinetics of phenobarbital in infants with neonatal encephalopathy treated with therapeutic hypothermia. *Pediatr Crit Care Med* 14: 194–202. doi: http://dx.doi.org/10.1097/PCC.0b013e31825bbbc2.

Sheth RD, Buckley DJ, Gutierrez AR, Gingold M, Bodensteiner JB, Penney S (1996) Midazolam in the treatment of refractory neonatal seizures. *Clin Neuropharmacol* 19: 165–170.

Shetty J (2015) Neonatal seizures in hypoxic-ischaemic encephalopathy – risks and benefits of anticonvulsant therapy. *Dev Med Child Neurol* 57 (Suppl. 3): 40–43. doi: http://dx.doi.org/10.1111/dmcn.12724.

Silverstein FS, Ferriero DM (2008) Off-label use of antiepileptic drugs for the treatment of neonatal seizures. *Pediatr Neurol* 39: 77–79. doi: http://dx.doi.org/10.1016/j.pediatrneurol.2008.04.008.

Silverstein FS, Jensen FE (2007) Neonatal seizures. *Ann Neurol* 62: 112–120. doi: http://dx.doi.org/10.1002/ana.21167

Singh B, Singh P, Al Hifzi I, Khan M, Majeed-Saidan M (1996) Treatment of neonatal seizures with carbamazepine. *J Child Neurol* 11: 378–382. doi: http://dx.doi.org/10.1177/088307389601100506.

Slaughter LA, Patel AD, Slaughter JL (2013) Pharmacological treatment of neonatal seizures: A systematic review. *J Child Neurol* 28: 351–364. doi: http://dx.doi.org/10.1177/0883073812470734.

Srinivasakumar P, Zempel J, Wallendorf M, Lawrence R, Inder T, Mathur A (2013) Therapeutic hypothermia in neonatal hypoxic ischemic encephalopathy: electrographic seizures and magnetic resonance imaging evidence of injury. *J Pediatr* 163(2): 465–70. doi: 10.1016/j.jpeds.2013.01.041. Epub 2013 Feb 26.

Steinberg A, Shalev RS, Amir N (1986) Valproic acid in neonatal status convulsivus. *Brain Dev* 8: 278–279. doi: http://dx.doi.org/10.1016/S0387-7604(86)80082-1.

Stockler S, Plecko B, Gospe SM et al. (2011) Pyridoxine dependent epilepsy and antiquitin deficiency: Clinical and molecular characteristics and recommendations for diagnosis, treatment and follow-up. *Mol Genet Metab* 104: 48–60. doi: http://dx.doi.org/10.1016/j.ymgme.2011.05.014.

Suda S, Katsura K, Kanamaru T, Saito M, Katayama Y (2013) Valproic acid attenuates ischemia-reperfusion injury in the rat brain through inhibition of oxidative stress and inflammation. *Eur J Pharmacol* 707: 26–31. doi: http://dx.doi.org/10.1016/j.ejphar.2013.03.020.

Sulzbacher S, Farwell JR, Temkin N, Lu AS, Hirtz DG (1999) Late cognitive effects of early treatment with phenobarbital. *Clin Pediatr (Phila)* 38: 387–394. doi: http://dx.doi.org/10.1177/000992289903800702.

Tekgul H, Gauvreau K, Soul J et al. (2006) The current etiologic profile and neurodevelopmental outcome of seizures in term newborn infants. *Pediatrics* 117: 1270–1280. doi: http://dx.doi.org/10.1542/peds.2005-1178.

Thoresen M, Sabir H (2015) Epilepsy: Neonatal seizures still lack safe and effective treatment. *Nat Rev Neurol* 11: 311–312. doi: http://dx.doi.org/10.1038/nrneurol.2015.74.

Tomson T, Battino D, Bonizzoni E et al. (2011) Dose-dependent risk of malformations with antiepileptic drugs: An analysis of data from the EURAP epilepsy and pregnancy registry. *Lancet Neurol* 10: 609–617. doi: http://dx.doi.org/10.1016/S1474-4422(11)70107-7.

Tso WW, Kwong AK, Fung CW, Wong VC (2014) Folinic acid responsive epilepsy in Ohtahara syndrome caused by STXBP1 mutation. *Pediatr Neurol* 50: 177–180. doi: http://dx.doi.org/10.1016/j.pediatrneurol.2013.10.006.

Tulloch JK, Carr RR, Ensom MH (2012) A systematic review of the pharmacokinetics of antiepileptic drugs in neonates with refractory seizures. *J Pediatr Pharmacol Ther* 17: 31–44.

Uria-Avellanal C, Marlow N, Rennie JM (2013) Outcome following neonatal seizures. *Semin Fetal Neonatal Med* 18: 224–232. doi: http://dx.doi.org/10.1016/j.siny.2013.01.002.

Vajda FJ, Eadie MJ (2014) The clinical pharmacology of traditional antiepileptic drugs. *Epileptic Disord* 16: 395–408.

Van Den Broek MP, Groenendaal F, Toet MC et al. (2012) Pharmacokinetics and clinical efficacy of phenobarbital in asphyxiated newborns treated with hypothermia: A thermopharmacological approach. *Clin Pharmacokinet* 51: 671–679. doi: http://dx.doi.org/10.1007/s40262-012-0004-y.

Van Den Broek MP, Huitema AD, Van Hasselt JG et al. (2011) Lidocaine (lignocaine) dosing regimen based upon a population pharmacokinetic model for preterm and term neonates with seizures. *Clin Pharmacokinet* 50: 461–469. doi: http://dx.doi.org/10.2165/11589160-000000000-00000.

Van Den Broek MP, Rademaker CM, Van Straaten HL et al. (2013) Anticonvulsant treatment of asphyxiated newborns under hypothermia with lidocaine: Efficacy, safety and dosing. *Arch Dis Child Fetal Neonatal Ed* 98: F341–F345. doi: http://dx.doi.org/10.1136/archdischild-2012-302678.

Van Karnebeek CD, Jaggumantri S (2015) Current treatment and management of pyridoxine-dependent epilepsy. *Curr Treat Options Neurol* 17: 335. doi: http://dx.doi.org/10.1007/s11940-014-0335-0.

Van Leuven K, Groenendaal F, Toet MC et al. (2004) Midazolam and amplitude-integrated EEG in asphyxiated full-term neonates. *Acta Paediatr* 93: 1221–1227. doi: http://dx.doi.org/10.1111/j.1651-2227.2004.tb02753.x.

Van Rooij LG, Hellstrom-Westas L, De Vries LS (2013a) Treatment of neonatal seizures. *Semin Fetal Neonatal Med* 18: 209–215. doi: http://dx.doi.org/10.1016/j.siny.2013.01.001.

Van Rooij LG, Toet MC, Rademaker KM, Groenendaal F, De Vries LS (2004) Cardiac arrhythmias in neonates receiving lidocaine as anticonvulsive treatment. *Eur J Pediatr* 163: 637–641. doi: http://dx.doi.org/10.1007/s00431-004-1513-y.

Van Rooij LG, Van Den Broek MP, Rademaker CM, De Vries LS (2013b) Clinical management of seizures in newborns: Diagnosis and treatment. *Paediatr Drugs* 15: 9–18. doi: http://dx.doi.org/10.1007/s40272-012-0005-1.

Vanhatalo S, Hellstrom-Westas L, De Vries LS (2009) Bumetanide for neonatal seizures: Based on evidence or enthusiasm? *Epilepsia* 50: 1292–1293. doi: http://dx.doi.org/10.1111/j.1528-1167.2008.01894.x.

Velez-Ruiz NJ, Meador KJ (2015) Neurodevelopmental effects of fetal antiepileptic drug exposure. *Drug Saf* 38: 271–278. doi: http://dx.doi.org/10.1007/s40264-015-0269-9.

Vento M, De Vries LS, Alberola A et al. (2010) Approach to seizures in the neonatal period: a European perspective. *Acta Paediatr* 99: 497–501. doi: http://dx.doi.org/10.1111/j.1651-2227.2009.01659.x.

Vesoulis ZA, Mathur AM (2014) Advances in management of neonatal seizures. *Indian J Pediatr* 81: 592–598. doi: http://dx.doi.org/10.1007/s12098-014-1457-9.

Vigevano F, Arzimanoglou A, Plouin P, Specchio N (2013) Therapeutic approach to epileptic encephalopathies. *Epilepsia* 54 (Suppl. 8): 45–50. doi: http://dx.doi.org/10.1111/epi.12423.

Volpe JJ (1989) Neonatal seizures: Current concepts and revised classification. *Pediatrics* 84: 422–428.

Volpe JJ (2008) Neurology of the newborn. In: Volpe JJ, editor. *Neonatal Seizures* 203–244. 5th ed. Philadelphia, PA: WB Saunders Elsevier.

Weeke LC, Schalkwijk S, Toet MC, Van Rooij LG, De Vries LS, Van Den Broek MP (2015) Lidocaine-Associated cardiac events in newborns with seizures: Incidence, symptoms and contributing factors. *Neonatology* 108: 130–136. doi: http://dx.doi.org/10.1159/000430767.

Wheless JW, Clarke D Hovinga CA et al. (2009) Rapid infusion of a loading dose of intravenous levetiracetam with minimal dilution: A safety study. *J Child Neurol* 24: 946–951. doi: http://dx.doi.org/10.1177/0883073808331351.

Whitelaw A, Odd D (2007) Postnatal phenobarbital for the prevention of intraventricular hemorrhage in preterm infants. *Cochrane Database Syst Rev* Cd001691. doi: http://dx.doi.org/10.1002/14651858.cd001691.pub2.

Wickstrom R, Hallberg B, Bartocci M (2013) Differing attitudes toward phenobarbital use in the neonatal period among neonatologists and child neurologists in Sweden. *Eur J Paediatr Neurol* 17: 55–63. doi: http://dx.doi.org/10.1016/j.ejpn.2012.09.001.

Wirrell EC (2005) Neonatal seizures: To treat or not to treat? *Semin Pediatr Neurol* 12: 97–105. doi: http://dxdoi.org/10.1016/j.spen.2005.03.004.

World Health Organization Guidelines (2011) Approved by the Guidelines Review Committee. *Guidelines on Neonatal Seizures*. Geneva: World Health Organization Copyright (c) World Health Organization 2011.

Wu YW, Gonzalez FF (2015) Erythropoietin: A novel therapy for hypoxic-ischaemic encephalopathy? *Dev Med Child Neurol* 57 (Suppl. 3): 34–39. doi: http://dx.doi.org/10.1111/dmcn.12730.

10
PREDICTORS OF NEURODEVELOPMENTAL OUTCOME IN INFANTS WITH NEONATAL SEIZURES

Lakshmi Nagarajan, Andrea Poretti, Thierry A G M Huisman and Soumya Ghosh

Seizures occur frequently in the neonatal period and may be due to a variety of causes (Volpe 2008, Uria-Avellanal et al. 2013). They are the most common manifestation of serious injury or impairment of the immature brain. There have been significant advances in diagnosis (electroclinical and electrographic seizures), investigation and treatment of infants with neonatal seizures (NS). However, 25–70% of infants with neonatal seizures (often with encephalopathy) have adverse neurodevelopmental outcomes – impairment of cognition, language, learning, motor function, behaviour, growth and epilepsy (Sankar and Painter 2005, Sankar and Rho 2007, Nagarajan et al. 2010, Uria-Avellanal et al. 2013, Pappas et al. 2015). Mortality is also increased in infants with neonatal seizures with reported rates of 7–20% (Garcias Da Silva et al. 2004, Tekgul et al. 2006, Pisani et al. 2007, 2008, Volpe 2008, Nagarajan et al. 2010a, 2010b). Mortality and morbidity are higher in the preterm compared to term infants, being highest in extreme (<28 weeks) preterm birth (Volpe 2008).

The ability to accurately predict outcome early in the neonatal period will help to determine the best care options and enable early treatment and neuroprotective strategies. The electroencephalography (EEG) background and the aetiology of the underlying disorder are the best predictors of outcome (Volpe 2008). In this chapter, we shall discuss the role of EEG, clinical findings, aetiology, neuroimaging, evoked potentials and laboratory biomarkers as prognostic factors of neurodevelopmental outcome in infants with neonatal seizures.

EEG background as predictor of outcome
The background on a neonatal EEG remains one of the most useful predictors of outcome, irrespective of the aetiology, in both term and preterm infants with seizures (Watanabe et al. 1980, Tharp et al. 1981, Lombroso 1983, Holmes and Lombroso 1993, Volpe 2008, Nagarajan et al. 2010a, Zhang et al. 2013). Interpretation of a neonatal EEG must be undertaken by neurologists with expertise in this field. The maturational patterns at different gestational ages vary and it may be challenging to differentiate between normal and abnormal background (Boylan et al. 2010).

The continuity, the amplitude, the variability and reactivity, the synchronicity, the symmetry, interburst intervals, sleep cycling, the interictal epileptiform activity and the maturational patterns are taken into consideration to assess the background on a neonatal EEG (Watanabe et al. 1980, Tharp et al. 1981, Lombroso and Matsumiya 1985, Shewmon 1990, Lombroso and Holmes 1993, Laroia et al. 1998, Nagarajan et al. 2010). Burst suppression patterns, discontinuous EEG activity and persistent very low amplitude usually indicate a severely abnormal background. The background is often classified as (1) normal, (2) mildly abnormal, (3) moderately abnormal or (4) severely abnormal based on visual assessment of these features. Figures 10.1a and 10.1b show normal to near-normal backgrounds in term and preterm infants, while Figures 10.2 to 10.5 show epochs of EEG with abnormal backgrounds of varying severity. Numerous studies have demonstrated the value of the conventional video EEG (v-EEG) in outcome prediction (see Chapter 4). The background on amplitude-integrated EEG (a-EEG) has also been shown to be useful in prognostication (Zhang et al. 2013, Shah and Wusthoff 2015).

Most studies suggest that a normal or mildly abnormal background is associated with normal outcomes in approximately 90% of infants with neonatal seizures, whereas the incidence of adverse outcomes is ~50% in those with moderately abnormal and in ~90% in those with severely abnormal backgrounds (Lombroso 1983, Lombroso and Holmes 1993; Boylan et al. 1999, Menache et al. 2002, Volpe 2008, Nagarajan et al. 2010, 2010a, 2012, Uria-Avellanal et al. 2013). Changes in the EEG background (improvement, persistence or worsening of abnormalities) with time are also of prognostic significance (Watanabe et al. 1980, Tharp et al. 1981). Electroclinical syndromes with EEGs (showing burst suppression patterns), suggesting epileptic encephalopathies such as Ohtahara syndrome and early myoclonic encephalopathy, are indicators of poor prognosis (Beal et al. 2012). Therapeutic hypothermia may influence the background and studies are required to explore the potential pitfalls in using pre-cooling era criteria for determination of the degree of abnormality on an EEG in a cooled infant (Thoresen et al. 2010, Cseko et al. 2013, Boylan et al. 2015, Merchant and Azzopardi 2015). The advent of background EEG scores, novel EEG parameters, automated background analysis, seizure detection algorithms, a-EEG and conventional multiple-channel v-EEG for standard as well as prolonged studies further add to the role of the EEG as a powerful predictor of outcome and perhaps an investigational tool that will help improve outcomes (Volpe 2008, Nagarajan et al. 2010, Boylan 2011, Shellhaas et al. 2011).

Electroclinical and electrographic features of neonatal seizures

The literature regarding neonatal seizures is sometimes difficult to interpret as studies with clinically identified seizures generally underestimate the electrographic seizure burden (Murray et al. 2008). The occurrence of clinical seizures has been shown to be associated with adverse outcomes in some studies (Glass et al. 2009), with increasing severity resulting in worse outcomes. EEG confirmation of clinical seizures increases the rate of unfavourable outcome (van Rooij et al. 2010, West et al. 2011).

Infants who present with frequent recurrent seizures or those with status epilepticus have been associated with a high incidence of poor outcome (Legido et al. 1991, McBride

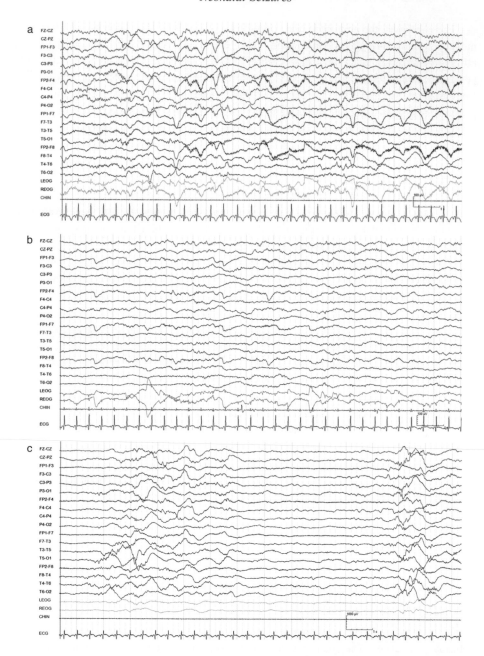

Figure 10.1a. Normal. EEG in the wake (panel a), active sleep (panel b) and quiet sleep (panel c) states in normal early term infants. Note the muscle and eye movement artefacts in the wake trace, eye movements in active sleep and trace alternant pattern in quiet sleep. The EEGs are shown in a double banana montage with top two channels (in black) showing midline derivations, the next four (in blue) left parasagittal, followed by four right parasagittal (in maroon), then four left temporal (in blue) and four right temporal (in maroon). The last four traces show electro-oculography, electromyography and electrocardiography. Calibration bars in right lower part of each panel.

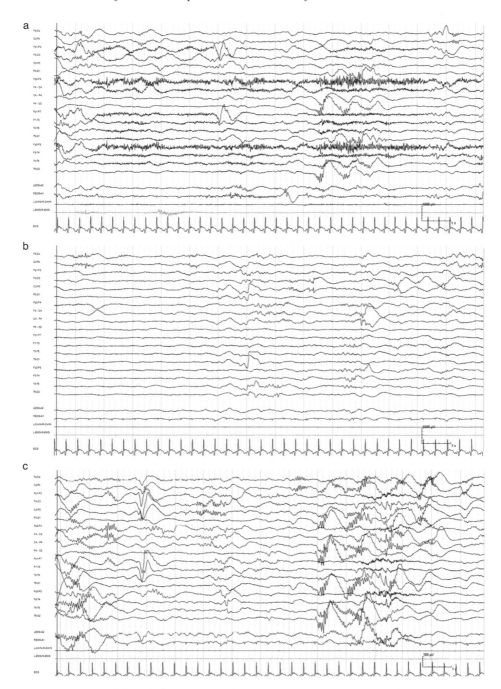

Figure 10.1b. Preterm EEG (near normal). EEG of a preterm infant (born at 27 weeks, age 21 days) showing (a) near normal wake, (b) active sleep and (c) quiet sleep states. Note the prominent delta brushes in panel c. Montage and calibration bars as in Figure 10.1a.

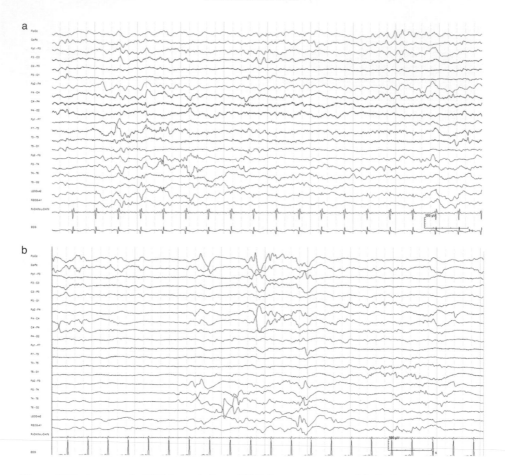

Figure 10.2. Asymmetric EEG due to infarcts. EEG shows asymmetry of the background and sharps in two infants with cerebral infarcts. The background in panel b is more abnormal than in panel a (note the difference in asynchrony, amplitude and asymmetry). Montage and calibration bars as in Figure 10.1.

et al. 2000, Pisani et al. 2007, Volpe 2008, van Rooij et al. 2010). Whether seizures respond to treatment and the number of antiepileptic drugs (AEDs) used appear to correlate with EEG background activity and outcome (Toet et al. 2005, Ronen et al. 2007, van der Heide et al. 2012, Shah et al. 2014). In the neonate, focal clonic seizures are frequently associated with a perinatal arterial ischaemic stroke (PAIS). The presence of clonic features during an electroclinical seizure has been shown to be associated with a better prognosis in some studies, but not in all (Mizrahi and Kellaway 1987, Brunquell et al. 2002, Pisani et al. 2008, Garfinkle and Shevell 2011, Nagarajan et al. 2012). Clinically diagnosed tonic seizures are thought to be associated with a poor prognosis; however, the associations between seizure types and prognosis is not consistent (Tekgul et al. 2006, Volpe 2008).

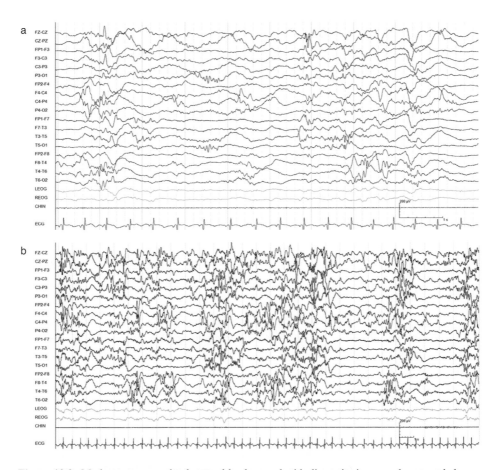

Figure 10.3. Moderate to severely abnormal background with discontinuity, asynchrony and sharps. EEG epoch shows a moderate to severely abnormal background with excessive discontinuity through portions of the recording, asynchrony and sharps. Panel a is a 10s epoch and panel b is a 30s epoch from the same EEG. Montage and calibration bars as in Figure 10.1.

Electroclinical dissociation (ECD) describes seizures on EEG without any associated clinical features. ECD occurs frequently in neonates with seizures (more frequently in the preterm than term). There appears to be no difference in prognosis between infants with and without ECD (Nagarajan et al. 2010), although the background was found to be more impaired in those with ECD. The data in different studies suggest that electrographic and electroclinical seizures are important in the evaluation of seizure burden, for clinical research and in therapeutic interventional protocols (Hellstrom-Westas et al. 1995, Silverstein et al. 2008, West et al. 2011, Shah et al. 2012, Uria-Avellanal et al. 2013).

An electrographic seizure in a neonate is conventionally defined as one in which a rhythmic EEG discharge lasts 10 seconds or longer, and could have variable morphology, frequency and field (Lombroso and Holmes 1993, Volpe 2008, Nagarajan et al. 2010). Certain

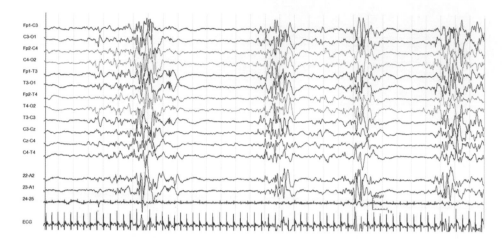

Figure 10.4. Burst suppression in hypoxic-ischaemic encephalopathy (HIE) shows a severely abnormal background with burst suppression in an infant with HIE born at 41 weeks. Montage and calibration bars as in Figure 10.1.

electrographic seizure patterns may have prognostic significance. The prognostic value of EEG features such as multiple seizure foci, ictal fractions and bihemispheric involvement is not clear (Ortibus et al. 1996, Bye et al. 1997, Pisani et al. 2008, Volpe 2008, Nagarajan et al. 2011a). Low amplitude and low frequency of the seizure discharge have been associated with poor prognosis (Nagarajan et al. 2011a). The ictal alpha seizure pattern is associated with a poor outcome (Volpe 2008). Some features such as ictal fast activity on EEG are not helpful prognostic factors of outcome in neonatal seizures (Nagarajan et al. 2011b). Brief rhythmic discharges, of less than 10 seconds' duration (not fulfilling the conventional criterion of seizure), may also contribute to the epileptic burden and hence to neurodevelopmental outcomes (Shewmon 1990, Oliveira et al. 2000, Nagarajan et al. 2010, 2011c).

Aetiology

The aetiology underlying the impairment in brain function that causes neonatal seizures (and encephalopathy) is an important determinant of outcome. Neonatal seizures may be due to a variety of causes – some transient, some permanent.

Hypoxic-ischaemic encephalopathy (HIE) is the most common cause of neonatal seizures and the most studied. The more severe the HIE, the worse the outcome. Hypothermia is neuroprotective and improves outcome in infants with HIE. Brain malformations, meningitis/encephalitis and (IEM) are generally associated with a high incidence of mortality and morbidity (Huang et al. 2012, Uria-Avellanal et al. 2013).

Preterm infants with encephalopathy have a less favourable outcome than term neonates and the outcome is worst for the extremely (<28 weeks) preterm (Uria-Avellanal et al. 2013, Shankaran 2014).

Children with symptomatic cerebral venous sinus thrombosis have an increased incidence of mortality and neurodevelopmental sequelae whereas those with PAIS fare better

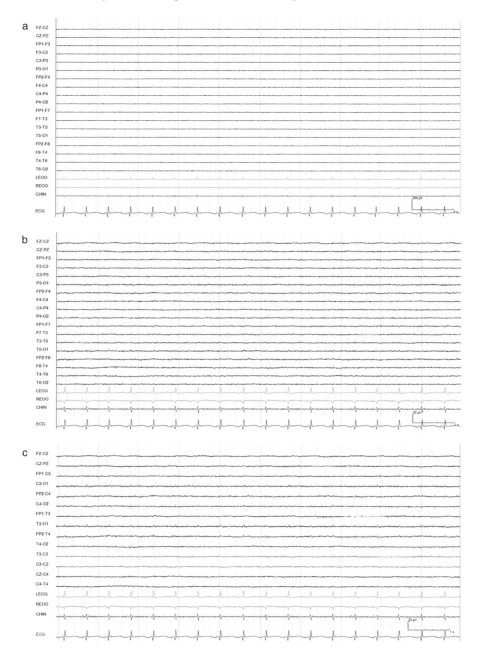

Figure 10.5. EEG epoch showing electro-cerebral inactivity (indicating severe background abnormality), at different gains and montages. Panels a and b show the same epoch on a bipolar double banana montage at sensitivity of 7μV/mm (panel a) and 2μV/mm (panel b). Panel c shows the epoch on a montage with long interelectrode distances at a sensitivity of 2μV/mm. A montage with long interelectrode distances is important to confirm an isoelectric EEG. Montage and calibration bars as in Figure 10.1.

(Berfelo et al. 2010, Kersbergen et al. 2011, Rutherford et al. 2012). Infants with intraventricular haemorrhages and seizures have a poor prognosis. When primary subarachnoid haemorrhage in a term infant is the cause of seizures, the prognosis is good (Uria-Avellanal et al. 2013).

Infants with neuroglucopenia resulting in seizures often have neuroimaging abnormalities and up to 50% have neurodevelopmental disorders (Koivisto et al. 1972, Menni et al. 2001, Uria-Avellanal et al. 2013). The occurrence and impact of many transient and mild metabolic disturbances (such as electrolyte and glucose abnormalities) have been minimised because of improved neonatal intensive care. Early diagnosis and treatment of infants with neonatal seizures due to pyridoxine-dependant epilepsy and or pyridoxal 5 phosphate responsive epilepsy is important (Stockler et al. 2011, Mills et al. 2014). These disorders (due to pyridoxamine 5'-phosphate oxidase (PNPO) deficiency, *antiquitin* deficiency and other conditions) are associated with long-term cognitive deficits, and early treatment may result in normal outcomes in some (Guerin et al. 2014).

Epileptic syndromes are rare in neonates. Infants with benign familial neonatal convulsions have a good prognosis for neurodevelopmental outcome, while the early infantile epileptic encephalopathies uniformly appear to have a poor prognosis (Beal et al. 2012, Mastrangelo and Leuzzi 2012, Zara et al. 2013).

Neuroimaging

Head ultrasonography is a valuable first-line imaging modality to study the neonate presenting with the acute onset of seizures, and may help in the diagnosis of several underlying causes including HIE, intraventricular haemorrhages and arterial ischemic stroke. The main advantage of head ultrasonography is that it can be performed at the bedside, does not use ionizing radiation, is widely available and does not require sedation. Magnetic resonance imaging (MRI) including conventional anatomical sequences and advanced sequences such as diffusion weighted imaging, diffusion tensor imaging, susceptibility weighted imaging, and ^{1}H-magnetic resonance spectroscopy is currently the 'standard of care'. Multisequence MRI provides more sensitive and specific information and consequently facilitates diagnosis, helps guiding treatment and may predict outcome. A strong correlation between neuroimaging findings and functional/cognitive outcome in neonates with seizures has been shown by several studies (Tekgul et al. 2006, Painter et al. 2012, Osmond et al. 2014). Painter et al. correlated the severity of neuroimaging findings and outcome in 48 neonates with seizures and found that newborn infants with normal neuroimaging studies were more likely to have a better outcome than those with diffuse and severe imaging abnormalities (Painter et al. 2012). A strong relationship between neuroimaging abnormalities and subsequent outcome has also been shown by Tekgul et al., who studied 89 term infants with clinical neonatal seizures (Tekgul et al. 2006). These authors reported that neonates with abnormal neuroimaging studies were more likely to have a poor outcome than those with normal neuroimaging (36% vs. 1%, $p = 0.001$). Only one neonate with normal brain imaging had a poor outcome. Similar results have recently been published by Osmond and colleagues who evaluated 77 term neonates with seizures (Osmond et al. 2014) and found that the probability of developing neurodevelopmental impairment or recurrence of seizures was extremely low in the absence of major cerebral lesions on MRI.

Neonatal seizures, however, are caused by a highly heterogeneous group of aetiologies including HIE, PAIS, intracranial haemorrhages, central nervous system (CNS) infections, IEM, cerebral malformations, and early-onset epileptic syndromes due to genetic causes such as *KCNQ2* mutations. The aetiology of the neuropathological process underlying neonatal seizures is an important determinant of long-term prognosis. Neuroimaging narrows the differential diagnosis and may consequently serve as predictor of outcome.

In term neonates with HIE, 30–50% of newborn infants with basal ganglia and/or thalamic lesions (as seen on imaging, e.g. Fig. 10.6a–c) develop postnatal seizures including infantile spasms (Gano et al. 2013, Jung et al. 2015). In survivors of neonatal HIE, the occurrence of infantile spasms was also shown to be highly correlated with the presence of global brain injury, including brainstem injury and hypothalamic abnormalities on neonatal MRI studies (Gano et al. 2013, Jung et al. 2015). On the other hand, absence of subcortical involvement is associated with relative 'protection' for the development of postnatal seizures (Jung et al. 2015).

After HIE, PAIS is a common cause of neonatal seizures. Recently, Suppiej and colleagues reported postnatal epileptic seizures in 9 out of 55 (16.4%) children diagnosed with a PAIS (Fig. 10.6d–f; Suppiej et al. 2015). All patients but one had focal epilepsy with good seizure control after treatment with AEDs. The risk of developing epilepsy was shown to be higher in right middle cerebral artery stroke or when multiple arterial territories were involved.

Intracranial haemorrhages and intraventricular haemorrhages are more common in preterm than in term neonates. In very low birthweight neonates born between 24 and 36

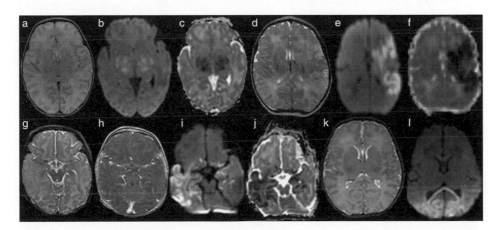

Figure 10.6. MRI features in infants with neonatal seizures of different aetiologies. Figure 10.6 a–c show abnormalities in hypoxic-ischaemic encephalopathy, d–f illustrate changes in perinatal arterial ischaemic stroke, g–j show changes seen in MRI in a neonate with herpes simplex virus encephalitis and k–l show MRI abnormalities associated with hypoglycaemia.

weeks of gestation, postnatal seizures occur in up to 20% of the children (Kohelet et al. 2006). The presence of grade II or grade III germinal matrix haemorrhages as well as periventricular haemorrhagic infarction and complicating post-haemorrhagic hydrocephalus is significantly correlated with the occurrence of postnatal seizures. In addition, neonates with thalamic infarction or haemorrhage due to thrombosis of the straight sinus have been shown to be at high risk of developing epilepsy and electrical status epilepticus in slow wave sleep (Kersbergen et al. 2013).

Any infection of the CNS can present with neonatal seizures. Both bacterial and viral CNS infections can occur in the neonatal period. In addition, neonates with congenital infections, which interfere with normal brain development, may present with seizures. In particular children with congenital cytomegalovirus (CMV) are at high risk of postnatal seizures (Suzuki et al. 2008). Suzuki and colleagues reviewed the clinical, laboratory and neuroimaging findings of 19 children with CMV infection. Seven patients developed seizures at a mean age of 20 months. The most common seizure type was partial seizures. The presence of ventriculomegaly and migrational abnormalities on neuroimaging studies was shown to be significantly correlated with the development of postnatal seizures. In neonatal herpes simplex encephalitis, bilateral, multifocal grey and white matter lesions identified on conventional magnetic resonance sequences and diffusion weighted imaging/diffusion tensor imaging have been associated with poor neurological outcome (Fig. 10.6g–j; Bajaj et al. 2014, Okanishi et al. 2015). Most likely, this pattern of neuroimaging findings is also a predictor of postnatal seizures in neonates with herpes simplex encephalitis. Other neonatal bacterial (e.g. group B Streptococci and *Escherichia coli*) and viral (e.g. parechovirus, enterovirus and rotavirus) CNS infections are linked to seizures. It is likely that cortical lesions identified on neuroimaging findings may be a predictor of the development of postnatal seizures in analogy with other infectious diseases.

Few data are available about the role of neuroimaging in predicting postnatal seizures in metabolic diseases and IEM. In non-ketotic hyperglycinemia, Hennermann et al. (2012) reported that the presence of morphological abnormalities on neonatal neuroimaging (e.g. hypoplasia of the corpus callosum, cerebral atrophy and hydrocephalus) is associated with a poor outcome including postnatal seizures. In neonatal hypoglycaemia, the duration and degree of hypoglycaemia are important predictors of poor neurological outcome including postnatal seizures and development of cerebral abnormalities on neuroimaging (Fig. 10.6k–l). Frequently, in significant neonatal hypoglycaemia the occipital and parietal cortex is predominantly affected on neuroimaging. However, some of the acute neuroimaging findings are transient and resolve on follow-up. Therefore, caution is needed in using only acute neuroimaging studies to predict outcome in neonatal hypoglycaemia (Kinnala et al. 1999).

Newborn infants with malformations of cortical development (e.g. lissencephaly, cobblestone lissencephaly, hemimegalencephaly and polymicrogyria) can present with neonatal seizures, but this is rather uncommon and most of the infants will develop seizures later in the first year of life. The presence of a malformation of cortical development may be just the tip of the malformative or syndromic iceberg and is per se an important risk factor for the occurrence of postnatal seizures and developmental disability. Refractory neonatal seizures may also be caused by an increasing number of identifiable underlying genetic aetiologies such as mutations in *KCNQ2*, *CDKL5* and *STXBP1*. Despite a poor long-term prognosis in terms of neurological development and occurrence of postnatal seizures, neuroimaging studies in neonates with epileptic encephalopathy caused by mutations in these genes may appear normal (Pavone et al. 2012). This observation emphasizes the role of identifying the underlying aetiology and the electroclinical syndrome in predicting the long-term prognosis in infants with neonatal seizures.

Evoked potentials

Somatosensory evoked potentials have been shown to be good prognostic indicators of outcome in children and adults with trauma and hypoxic ischaemic brain injury (Wijdicks et al. 2006, Carrai et al. 2010). Clinical and methodological factors have to be taken into consideration when undertaking somatosensory, auditory and visual evoked potentials (Vanhatalo and Lauronen 2006, Trollmann et al. 2010). Nevertheless evoked potentials appear to have potential value as early predictors of outcome in infants with neonatal HIE, the most common cause of neonatal seizures (Lori et al. 2011).

Chemical biomarkers as predictors of outcome

A number of biomarkers have been explored for predictive value. The usefulness of S100beta, creatine kinase-brain band, interleukin and other inflammatory cytokines, neuron specific enolase, and lactate in urine, blood or CSF in predicting long-term outcome appears to be questionable. Novel biomarkers such as glial fibrillary acidic protein, ubiquitin carboxyl terminal hydrolase L1 and phosphorylated axonal neurofilament heavy chain may play a role in prediction of neurodevelopmental outcomes (Merchant and Azzopardi 2015).

Combinations of clinical features and investigations as predictors

Combination of EEG, aetiology, MRI, clinical profile and other markers is thought to be a better or more powerful predictor of outcome in neonates with acute symptomatic seizures. In clinical practice, one automatically assesses all information available to prognosticate. Some studies provide combination scores to assist this.

Severity of HIE in infants with neonatal seizures influences the percentage of infants with adverse outcomes and the severity of the impairments. A combination of clinical variables such as low apgar scores, peripartum complications, foetal acidaemia, need for resuscitation and signs of neonatal encephalopathy helps prognosticate neurodevelopmental outcomes; absence of these indicates reduced probability of morbidity or mortality (Sarnat and Sarnat 1976, Merchant and Azzopardi 2015).

In infants with arterial ischemic stroke and neonatal seizures there is some suggestion that persistent amplitude asymmetry greater than 50% is associated with increased incidence of hemiparesis. A greater extent of MRI abnormality and a more abnormal EEG background increase the likelihood of a hemiparesis in the long term (Mercuri et al. 1999).

Combining the grade of clinically assessed encephalopathy with the grade of a-EEG abnormality is reported to improve predictive accuracy (Shalak et al. 2003). Head ultrasonography and clinical examination together have been reported to improve accuracy of predicted outcome (Jongeling et al. 2002). MRI, EEG and Sarnat scores (Sarnat and Sarnat 1976) were explored as prognostic indicators in one study. In the authors' opinion (El-Ayouty et al. 2007) the EEG background was the best predictor of outcome. In addition, severe injury of the basal ganglia was associated with poor outcome. Sarnat score had high specificity, but rather low sensitivity compared to EEG. Composite scoring systems for prognostication have been proposed by several groups (Ellison et al. 1981, Pisani et al. 2009, Garfinkle and Shevell 2011). Their usefulness needs to be validated and assessed.

Conclusion

In clinical practice, we intuitively evaluate all the information available before arriving at an estimate of the prognosis regarding neurodevelopmental outcome, including mortality. This is discussed with the team and the parents and important decisions regarding management options, including withdrawal of invasive care or move to palliative care, are made. The cause of the brain dysfunction that resulted in neonatal seizures and the EEG background continue to be the best prognostic indicators, with increasing contributions from neuroimaging. It is imperative that we are cognisant of the value of the clinical profile (antenatal, natal, postnatal history, family history, clinical examination, progress, response to medications), the EEG (ictal, interictal both at a point of time and sequential), the aetio-pathogenesis, the neuroimaging and other relevant investigations and information in prognostication.

REFERENCES

Bajaj M, Mody S, Natarajan G (2014) Clinical and neuroimaging findings in neonatal herpes simplex virus infection. *J Pediatr* 165: 404e1–407e1.

Beal JC, Cherian K, Moshe SL (2012) Early-onset epileptic encephalopathies: Ohtahara syndrome and early myoclonic encephalopathy. *Pediatr Neurol* 47: 317–323. doi: http://dx.doi.org/10.1016/j.pediatrneurol.2012.06.002.

Berfelo FJ, Kersbergen KJ, Van Ommen CH et al. (2010) Neonatal cerebral sinovenous thrombosis from symptom to outcome. *Stroke* 41: 1382–1388. doi: http://dx.doi.org/10.1161/STROKEAHA.110.583542.

Boylan G, Burgoyne L, Moore C, O'Flaherty B, Rennie J (2010) An international survey of EEG use in the neonatal intensive care unit. *Acta Paediatr* 99: 1150–1155. doi: http://dx.doi.org/10.1111/j.1651-2227.2010.01809.x.

Boylan GB (2011) EEG monitoring in the neonatal intensive care unit: A critical juncture. *Clin Neurophysiol: Official Journal of the International Federation of Clinical Neurophysiology* 122: 1905–1907. doi: http://dx.doi.org/10.1016/j.clinph.2011.03.015.

Boylan GB, Kharoshankaya L, Wusthoff CJ (2015) Seizures and hypothermia: Importance of electroencephalographic monitoring and considerations for treatment. *Semin Fetal Neonatal Med* 20: 103–108. doi: http://dx.doi.org/10.1016/j.siny.2015.01.001.

Boylan GB, Pressler RM, Rennie JM et al. (1999) Outcome of electroclinical, electrographic, and clinical seizures in the newborn infant. *Dev Med Child Neurol* 41: 819–825. doi: http://dx.doi.org/10.1111/j.1469-8749.1999.tb00548.x.

Brunquell PJ, Glennon CM, Dimario FJ Jr., Lerer T, Eisenfeld L (2002) Prediction of outcome based on clinical seizure type in newborn infants. *J Pediatr* 140: 707–712. doi: http://dx.doi.org/10.1067/mpd.2002.124773.

Bye AM, Cunningham CA, Chee KY, Flanagan D (1997) Outcome of neonates with electrographically identified seizures, or at risk of seizures. *Pediatr Neurol* 16: 225–231. doi: http://dx.doi.org/10.1016/S0887-8994(97)00019-2.

Carrai R, Grippo A, Lori S, Pinto F, Amantini A (2010) Prognostic value of somatosensory evoked potentials in comatose children: A systematic literature review. *Intensive Care Med* 36: 1112–1126. doi: http://dx.doi.org/10.1007/s00134-010-1884-7.

Cseko AJ, Bango M, Lakatos P, Kardasi J, Pusztai L, Szabo M (2013) Accuracy of amplitude-integrated electroencephalography in the prediction of neurodevelopmental outcome in asphyxiated infants receiving hypothermia treatment. *Acta Paediatr* 102: 707–711. doi: http://dx.doi.org/10.1111/apa.12226.

El-Ayouty M, Abdel-Hady H, El-Mogy S, Zaghlol H, El-Beltagy M, Aly H (2007) Relationship between electroencephalography and magnetic resonance imaging findings after hypoxic-ischemic encephalopathy at term. *Am J Perinatol* 24: 467–473. doi: http://dx.doi.org/10.1055/s-2007-986686.

Ellison PH, Largent JA, Bahr JP (1981) A scoring system to predict outcome following neonatal seizures. *J Pediatr* 99: 455–459. doi: http://dx.doi.org/10.1016/S0022-3476(81)80348-4.

Gano D, Sargent MA, Miller SP et al. (2013) MRI findings in infants with infantile spasms after neonatal hypoxic-ischemic encephalopathy. *Pediatr Neurol* 49: 401–405. doi: http://dx.doi.org/10.1016/j.pediatrneurol.2013.08.007.

Garcias Da Silva LF, Nunes ML, Da Costa JC (2004) Risk factors for developing epilepsy after neonatal seizures. *Pediatr Neurol* 30: 271–277. doi: http://dx.doi.org/10.1016/j.pediatrneurol.2003.09.015.

Garfinkle J, Shevell MI (2011) Prognostic factors and development of a scoring system for outcome of neonatal seizures in term infants. *European Journal of Paediatric Neurology : EJPN : Official Journal of the European Paediatric Neurology Society* 15: 222–229. doi: http://dx.doi.org/ 10.1016/j.ejpn.2010.11.002.

Glass HC, Glidden D, Jeremy RJ, Barkovich AJ, Ferriero DM, Miller SP (2009) Clinical neonatal seizures are independently associated with outcome in infants at risk for hypoxic-ischemic brain injury. *J Pediatr* 155: 318–323. doi: http://dx.doi.org/10.1016/j.jpeds.2009.03.040.

Guerin A, Aziz AS, Mutch C, Lewis J, Go CY, Mercimek-Mahmutoglu S (2015) Pyridox(am)ine-5-phosphate oxidase deficiency treatable cause of neonatal epileptic encephalopathy with burst suppression: Case report and review of the literature. *J Child Neurol* 30: 1218–1225. doi: 10.1177/0883073814550829.

Hellstrom-Westas L, Rosen I, Svenningsen NW (1995) Predictive value of early continuous amplitude integrated EEG recordings on outcome after severe birth asphyxia in full term infants. *Arch Dis Child Fetal Neonatal Ed* 72: F34–F38. doi: http://dx.doi.org/10.1136/fn.72.1.F34.

Hennermann JB, Berger JM, Grieben U, Scharer G, Van Hove JL, (2012) Prediction of long-term outcome in glycine encephalopathy: A clinical survey. *J Inherit Metab Dis* 35: 253–261. doi: http://dx.doi.org/10.1007/s10545-011-9398-1.

Holmes GL, Lombroso CT (1993) Prognostic value of background patterns in the neonatal EEG. *J Clin Neurophysiol: Official Publication of the American Electroencephalographic Society* 10: 323–352.

Jongeling BR, Badawi N, Kurinczuk JJ et al. (2002) Cranial ultrasound as a predictor of outcome in term newborn encephalopathy. *Pediatr Neurol* 26: 37–42. doi: http://dx.doi.org/10.1016/S0887-8994(01)00354-X.

Jung DE, Ritacco DG, Nordli DR, Koh S, Venkatesan C (2015) Early anatomical injury patterns predict epilepsy in head cooled neonates with hypoxic ischemic encephalopathy. *Pediatr Neurol* 53: 135–140. doi: http://dx.doi.org/10.1016/j.pediatrneurol.2015.04.009.

Kersbergen KJ, De Vries LS, Leijten FS et al. (2013) Neonatal thalamic hemorrhage is strongly associated with electrical status epilepticus in slow wave sleep. *Epilepsia* 54: 733–740. doi: http://dx.doi.org/10.1111/epi.12131.

Kersbergen KJ, Groenendaal F, Benders MJ, De Vries LS (2011) Neonatal cerebral sinovenous thrombosis: Neuroimaging and long-term follow-up. *J Child Neurol* 26: 1111–1120. doi: http://dx.doi.org/10.1177/0883073811408090.

Kinnala A, Rikalainen H, Lapinleimu H, Parkkola R, Kormano M, Kero P (1999) Cerebral magnetic resonance imaging and ultrasonography findings after neonatal hypoglycemia. *Pediatrics* 103: 724–729.

Kohelet D, Shochat R, Lusky A, Reichman B, Israel Neonatal N (2006) Risk factors for seizures in very low birthweight infants with periventricular leukomalacia. *J Child Neurol* 21: 965–970. doi: http://dx.doi.org/10.1177/08830738060210111301.

Koivisto M, Blanco-Sequeiros M, Krause U (1972) Neonatal symptomatic and asymptomatic hypoglycaemia: A follow-up study of 151 children. *Dev Med Child Neurol* 14: 603–614. doi: http://dx.doi.org/10.1111/j.1469-8749.1972.tb02642.x.

Laroia N, Guillet R, Burchfiel J, Mcbride MC (1998) EEG background as predictor of electrographic seizures in high-risk neonates. *Epilepsia* 39: 545–551. doi: http://dx.doi.org/10.1111/j.1528-1157.1998.tb01418.x.

Legido A, Clancy RR, Berman PH (1991) Neurologic outcome after electroencephalographically proven neonatal seizures. *Pediatrics* 88: 583–596.

Lin MC, Chi H, Chiu NC, Huang FY, Ho CS. (2012) Factors for poor prognosis of neonatal bacterial meningitis in a medical center in Northern Taiwan. *J Microbiol Immunol Infect.* 45(6):442–7. doi: 10.1016/j.jmii.2011.12.034. Epub 2012 May 7.

Lombroso CT (1983) Prognosis in neonatal seizures. *Adv Neurol* 34: 101–113.

Lombroso CT, Holmes GL (1993) Value of the EEG in neonatal seizures. *Epilepsy* 6: 39–70. doi: http://dx.doi.org/10.1016/S0896-6974(05)80010-6.

Lombroso CT, Matsumiya Y (1985) Stability in waking-sleep states in neonates as a predictor of long-term neurologic outcome. *Pediatrics* 76: 52–63.

Lori S, Bertini G, Molesti E et al. (2011) The prognostic role of evoked potentials in neonatal hypoxic-ischemic insult. *J Matern Fetal Neonatal Med* 24 (Suppl. 1): 69–71.

Mastrangelo M, Leuzzi V (2012) Genes of early-onset epileptic encephalopathies: From genotype to phenotype. *Pediatr Neurol* 46: 24–31. doi: http://dx.doi.org/10.1016/j.pediatrneurol.2011.11.003.

Mcbride MC, Laroia N, Guillet R (2000) Electrographic seizures in neonates correlate with poor neurodevelopmental outcome. *Neurology* 55: 506–513. doi: http://dx.doi.org/10.1212/WNL.55.4.506.

Menache CC, Bourgeois BF, Volpe JJ (2002) Prognostic value of neonatal discontinuous EEG. *Pediatr Neurol* 27: 93–101. doi: http://dx.doi.org/10.1016/S0887-8994(02)00396-X.

Menni F, De Lonlay P, Sevin C et al. (2001) Neurologic outcomes of 90 neonates and infants with persistent hyperinsulinemic hypoglycemia. *Pediatrics* 107: 476–479. doi: http://dx.doi.org/10.1542/peds.107.3.476.

Merchant N, Azzopardi D (2015) Early predictors of outcome in infants treated with hypothermia for hypoxic-ischaemic encephalopathy. *Dev Med Child Neurol* 57 (Suppl. 3): 8–16. doi: http://dx.doi.org/10.1111/dmcn.12726.

Mercuri E, Rutherford M, Cowan F et al. (1999) Early prognostic indicators of outcome in infants with neonatal cerebral infarction: A clinical, electroencephalogram, and magnetic resonance imaging study. *Pediatrics* 103: 39–46.

Mills PB, Camuzeaux SS, Footitt EJ et al. (2014) Epilepsy due to PNPO mutations: Genotype, environment and treatment affect presentation and outcome. *Brain* 137: 1350–1360. doi: http://dx.doi.org/10.1093/brain/awu051.

Mizrahi EM, Kellaway P (1987) Characterization and classification of neonatal seizures. *Neurology* 37: 1837–1844. doi: http://dx.doi.org/10.1212/WNL.37.12.1837.

Murray DM, Boylan GB, Ali I, Ryan CA, Murphy BP, Connolly S (2008) Defining the gap between electrographic seizure burden, clinical expression and staff recognition of neonatal seizures. *Arch Dis Child Fetal Neonatal Ed* 93: F187–F191. doi: http://dx.doi.org/10.1136/adc.2005.086314.

Nagarajan L, Ghosh S, Palumbo L (2011a) Ictal electroencephalograms in neonatal seizures: Characteristics and associations. *Pediatr Neurol* 45: 11–16. doi: http://dx.doi.org/10.1016/j.pediatrneurol.2011.01.009.

Nagarajan L, Ghosh S, Palumbo L, Akiyama T, Otsubo H (2011b) Fast activity during EEG seizures in neonates. *Epilepsy Res* 97: 162–169. doi: http://dx.doi.org/10.1016/j.eplepsyres.2011.08.003.

Nagarajan L, Palumbo L, Ghosh S (2010) Neurodevelopmental outcomes in neonates with seizures: A numerical score of background encephalography to help prognosticate. *J Child Neurol* 25: 961–968. doi: http://dx.doi.org/10.1177/0883073809355825.

Nagarajan L, Palumbo L, Ghosh S (2011c) Brief electroencephalography rhythmic discharges (BERDs) in the neonate with seizures: Their significance and prognostic implications. *J Child Neurol* 26: 1529–1533. doi: http://dx.doi.org/10.1177/0883073811409750.

Nagarajan L, Palumbo L, Ghosh S (2012) Classification of clinical semiology in epileptic seizures in neonates. *Eur J Paediatr Neurol* 16: 118–125. doi: http://dx.doi.org/10.1016/j.ejpn.2011.11.005.

Okanishi T, Yamamoto H, Hosokawa T et al. (2015) Diffusion-weighted MRI for early diagnosis of neonatal herpes simplex encephalitis. *Brain Dev* 37: 423–431. doi: http://dx.doi.org/10.1016/j.braindev.2014.07.006.

Oliveira AJ, Nunes ML, Da Costa JC (2000) Polysomnography in neonatal seizures. *Clin Neurophysiol* 111 (Suppl. 2): S74–S80. doi: http://dx.doi.org/10.1016/S1388-2457(00)00405-3.

Ortibus EL, Sum JM, Hahn JS (1996) Predictive value of EEG for outcome and epilepsy following neonatal seizures. *Electroencephalogr Clin Neurophysiol* 98: 175–185. doi: http://dx.doi.org/10.1016/0013-4694(95)00245-6.

Osmond E, Billetop A, Jary S, Likeman M, Thoresen M, Luyt K (2014) Neonatal seizures: Magnetic resonance imaging adds value in the diagnosis and prediction of neurodisability. *Acta Paediatr* 103: 820–826. doi: http://dx.doi.org/10.1111/apa.12583.

Painter MJ, Sun Q, Scher MS, Janosky J, Alvin J (2012) Neonates with seizures: What predicts development? *J Child Neurol* 27: 1022–1026. doi: http://dx.doi.org/10.1177/0883073811433845.

Pappas A, Shankaran S, Mcdonald SA et al. (2015) Cognitive outcomes after neonatal encephalopathy. *Pediatrics* 135: e624–e634. doi: http://dx.doi.org/10.1542/peds.2014-1566.

Pavone P, Spalice A, Polizzi A, Parisi P, Ruggieri M (2012) Ohtahara syndrome with emphasis on recent genetic discovery. *Brain Dev* 34: 459–468. doi: http://dx.doi.org/10.1016/j.braindev.2011.09.004.

Pisani F, Cerminara C, Fusco C, Sisti L (2007) Neonatal status epilepticus vs recurrent neonatal seizures: Clinical findings and outcome. *Neurology* 69: 2177–2185. doi: http://dx.doi.org/10.1212/01.wnl.0000295674.34193.9e.

Pisani F, Copioli C, Di Gioia C, Turco E, Sisti L (2008) Neonatal seizures: Relation of ictal video-electroencephalography (EEG) findings with neurodevelopmental outcome. *J Child Neurol* 23: 394–398. doi: http://dx.doi.org/10.1177/0883073807309253.

Pisani F, Sisti L, Seri S (2009) A scoring system for early prognostic assessment after neonatal seizures. *Pediatrics* 124: e580–e587. doi: http://dx.doi.org/10.1542/peds.2008-2087.

Ronen GM, Buckley D, Penney S, Streiner DL (2007) Long-term prognosis in children with neonatal seizures: A population-based study. *Neurology* 69: 1816–1822. doi: http://dx.doi.org/10.1212/01.wnl.0000279335.85797.2c.

Rutherford MA, Ramenghi LA, Cowan FM (2012) Neonatal stroke. *Arch Dis Child Fetal Neonatal Ed* 97: F377–F384. doi: http://dx.doi.org/10.1136/fetalneonatal-2010-196451.

Sankar R, Painter MJ (2005) Neonatal seizures: after all these years we still love what doesn't work. *Neurology*. 64(5): 776–7.

Sankar R, Rho JM (2007) Do seizures affect the developing brain? Lessons from the laboratory. *J Child Neurol* 22(5 Suppl): 21S–9S.

Sarnat HB, Sarnat MS (1976). Neonatal encephalopathy following fetal distress: A clinical and electroencephalographic study. *Arch Neurol* 33: 696–705. doi: http://dx.doi.org/10.1001/archneur.1976.00500100030012.

Shah DK, Boylan GB, Rennie JM (2012) Monitoring of seizures in the newborn. *Arch Dis Child Fetal Neonatal Ed* 97: F65–F69. doi: http://dx.doi.org/10.1136/adc.2009.169508.

Shah DK, Wusthoff CJ, Clarke P et al. (2014) Electrographic seizures are associated with brain injury in newborns undergoing therapeutic hypothermia. *Arch Dis Child Fetal Neonatal Ed* 99: F219–F224. doi: http://dx.doi.org/10.1136/archdischild-2013-305206.

Shah NA, Wusthoff CJ (2015) How to use: Amplitude-integrated EEG (aEEG). *Arch Dis Child Educ Pract Ed* 100: 75–81. doi: http://dx.doi.org/10.1136/archdischild-2013-305676.

Shalak LF, Laptook AR, Velaphi SC, Perlman JM (2003) Amplitude-integrated electroencephalography coupled with an early neurologic examination enhances prediction of term infants at risk for persistent encephalopathy. *Pediatrics* 111: 351–357. doi: http://dx.doi.org/10.1542/peds.111.2.351.

Shankaran S (2014) Outcomes of hypoxic-ischemic encephalopathy in neonates treated with hypothermia. *Clin Perinatol* 41: 149–159. doi: http://dx.doi.org/10.1016/j.clp.2013.10.008.

Shellhaas RA, Chang T, Tsuchida T et al. (2011) The American clinical neurophysiology society's guideline on continuous electroencephalography monitoring in neonates. *J Clin Neurophysiol* 28: 611–617. doi: http://dx.doi.org/10.1097/WNP.0b013e31823e96d7.

Shewmon DA (1990) What is a neonatal seizure? Problems in definition and quantification for investigative and clinical purposes. *J Clin Neurophysiol: Official Publication of the American Electroencephalographic Society* 7: 315–368.

Silverstein FS, Jensen FE, Inder T, Hellstrom-Westas L, Hirtz D, Ferriero DM (2008) Improving the treatment of neonatal seizures: National institute of neurological disorders and stroke workshop report. *J Pediatr* 153: 12–15. doi: http://dx.doi.org/10.1016/j.jpeds.2008.01.041.

Stockler S, Plecko B, Gospe SM Jr. et al. (2011) Pyridoxine dependent epilepsy and antiquitin deficiency: Clinical and molecular characteristics and recommendations for diagnosis, treatment and follow-up. *Mol Genet Metab* 104: 48–60. doi: http://dx.doi.org/10.1016/j.ymgme.2011.05.014.

Suppiej A, Mastrangelo M, Mastella L et al. (2016) Pediatric epilepsy following neonatal seizures symptomatic of stroke. *Brain Dev* 38: 27–31. doi: http://dx.doi.org/10.1016/j.braindev.2015.05.010.

Suzuki Y, Toribe Y, Mogami Y, Yanagihara K, Nishikawa M (2008) Epilepsy in patients with congenital cytomegalovirus infection. *Brain Dev* 30: 420–424. doi: http://dx.doi.org/10.1016/j.braindev.2007.12.004.

Tekgul H, Gauvreau K, Soul J et al. (2006) The current etiologic profile and neurodevelopmental outcome of seizures in term newborn infants. *Pediatrics* 117: 1270–1280. doi: http://dx.doi.org/10.1542/peds.2005-1178.

Tharp BR, Cukier F, Monod N (1981) The prognostic value of the electroencephalogram in premature infants. *Electroencephalogr Clin Neurophysiol* 51: 219–236. doi: http://dx.doi.org/10.1016/0013-4694(81)90136-X.

Thoresen M, Hellstrom-Westas L, Liu X, De Vries LS (2010) Effect of hypothermia on amplitude-integrated electroencephalogram in infants with asphyxia. *Pediatrics* 126: e131–e139. doi: http://dx.doi.org/10.1542/peds.2009-2938.

Toet MC, Groenendaal F, Osredkar D, Van Huffelen AC, De Vries LS (2005) Postneonatal epilepsy following amplitude-integrated EEG-detected neonatal seizures. *Pediatr Neurol* 32: 241–247. doi: http://dx.doi.org/10.1016/j.pediatrneurol.2004.11.005.

Trollmann R, Nusken E, Wenzel D (2010) Neonatal somatosensory evoked potentials: Maturational aspects and prognostic value. *Pediatr Neurol* 42: 427–433. doi: http://dx.doi.org/10.1016/j.pediatrneurol.2009.12.007.

Uria-Avellanal C, Marlow N, Rennie JM (2013) Outcome following neonatal seizures. *Semin Fetal Neonatal Med* 18: 224–232. doi: http://dx.doi.org/10.1016/j.siny.2013.01.002.

Van Der Heide MJ, Roze E, Van Der Veere CN, Ter Horst HJ, Brouwer OF, Bos AF (2012) Long-term neurological outcome of term-born children treated with two or more anti-epileptic drugs during the neonatal period. *Early Hum Dev* 88: 33–38. doi: http://dx.doi.org/10.1016/j.earlhumdev.2011.06.012.

Van Rooij LG, Toet MC, Van Huffelen AC et al. (2010) Effect of treatment of subclinical neonatal seizures detected with aEEG: Randomized, controlled trial. *Pediatrics* 125: e358–e366. doi: http://dx.doi.org/10.1542/peds.2009-0136.

Vanhatalo S, Lauronen L (2006) Neonatal SEP – back to bedside with basic science. *Semin Fetal Neonatal Med* 11: 464–470. doi: http://dx.doi.org/10.1016/j.siny.2006.07.009.

Volpe JJ (2008) Neurology of the newborn. In: Volpe JJ, editor. *Neonatal Seizures,* 5th ed. Philadelphia, PA: WB Saunders Elsevier.

Watanabe K, Miyazaki S, Hara K, Hakamada S (1980) Behavioral state cycles, background EEGs and prognosis of newborns with perinatal hypoxia. *Electroencephalogr Clin Neurophysiol* 49: 618–625. doi: http://dx.doi.org/10.1016/0013-4694(80)90402-2.

West CR, Harding JE, Williams CE, Nolan M, Battin MR (2011) Cot-side electroencephalography for outcome prediction in preterm infants: Ostudy. *Arch Dis Child Fetal Neonatal Ed* 96: F108–F113. doi: http://dx.doi.org/10.1136/adc.2009.180539.

Wijdicks EF, Hijdra A, Young GB, Bassetti CL, Wiebe S, Quality Standards Subcommittee of the American Academy of Neurology (2006) Practice parameter: Prediction of outcome in comatose survivors after cardiopulmonary resuscitation (an evidence-based review): Report of the Quality Standards Subcommittee of the American Academy of Neurology. *Neurology* 67: 203–210. doi: http://dx.doi.org/10.1212/01.wnl.0000227183.21314.cd.

Zara F, Specchio N, Striano P et al. (2013) Genetic testing in benign familial epilepsies of the first year of life: Clinical and diagnostic significance. *Epilepsia* 54: 425–436. doi: http://dx.doi.org/10.1111/epi.12089.

Zhang D, Ding H, Liu L et al. (2013) The prognostic value of amplitude-integrated EEG in full-term neonates with seizures. *PLoS One* 8: e78960. doi: http://dx.doi.org/10.1371/journal.pone.0078960.

11
NEURODEVELOPMENTAL OUTCOMES OF NEONATES WITH SEIZURES

Jarred Garfinkle and Michael I Shevell

Seizures are the most common acute manifestation of injury to the neonatal brain. Cerebral palsy, global developmental delay, intellectual disability, and epilepsy are some of the more common later manifestations of this injury (Fig. 11.1). Alongside significant improvements in the diagnosis, investigation, and treatment of neonatal seizures, there have been advances in our understanding of their long-term neurodevelopmental consequences. Neonates with seizures that are the result of the most severe underlying acquired brain injuries can die in the neonatal intensive care unit (NICU) or in the months following their discharge. Recent studies report a mortality of 7–25% in term neonates with seizures (McBride et al. 2000, Tekgul et al. 2006, Pisani et al. 2007, Ronen et al. 2007, Garfinkle and Shevell 2011b). The mortality of preterm neonates with seizures is higher at 22–58% and is related to lower gestational age (Scher et al. 1993, Ronen et al. 2007, Pisani et al. 2007, Davis et al. 2010, Shah et al. 2010). Of those who survive their acute injury, 25–70% will go on to have subsequent neurodevelopmental impairments (Tekgul et al. 2006, Nagarajan et al. 2010, Uria-Avellanal et al. 2013).

While neonatal seizures are the most common and perhaps most spectacular acute manifestation of injury to the neonatal brain (Volpe 2008), other acute manifestations of injury to the neonatal brain – such as lethargy or coma, abnormal posture and/or tone, and autonomic instability, to name a few – can occur in the absence of seizures. Together, these acute manifestations encompass 'neonatal encephalopathy', a term that was coined in 1976 and is still very much in use (Sarnat and Sarnat 1976, Shankaran et al. 2005). Moreover, injuries to the neonatal brain – such as hypoxic-ischemic encephalopathy (HIE; an encephalopathy attributable with a high degree of certainty to hypoxia-ischemia or asphyxia) and arterial and venous strokes – can lead to late neurodevelopmental consequences in the absence of overt clinically diagnosable neonatal seizures (Sarnat and Sarnat 1976, Wusthoff et al. 2011, Volpe 2012). The contribution of neonatal seizures in and of themselves to these later outcomes is still uncertain, although some evidence suggests that neonatal seizures themselves, especially if frequent, intractable or prolonged, are independently associated with further hypoxic-ischemic brain injury as measured by magnetic resonance spectroscopy and with later neurodevelopmental impairment (Miller et al. 2002, Glass et al. 2009). On the other hand, a secondary analysis of data collected for one of the trials of therapeutic hypothermia found that after adjusting for the objective

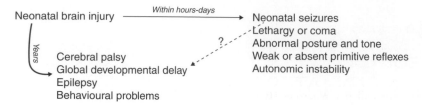

Figure 11.1. Acute and later manifestations of injury to the neonatal brain.

severity of encephalopathy and treatment, neonatal seizures were not independently associated with later outcomes. The debate as to whether neonatal seizures are mere epiphenomena of brain injury or additional contributors to brain injury remains presently unsettled and an obvious focus of current and future research efforts (Glass et al. 2011a, Shetty 2015).

An understanding of the various neurodevelopmental outcomes of neonates with seizures and the identification of reliable prognostic indicators for these outcomes could facilitate clinician decision-making, assist initial family counselling, and more efficiently target ongoing intervention efforts. In addition, a better understanding of epilepsy subsequent to neonatal seizures could encourage the development of rational treatment guidelines for neonatal seizures, which are currently lacking (Glass et al. 2012, Shetty 2015). In this chapter we will discuss the most important subsequent neurological outcomes of neonatal seizures, including epilepsy, cerebral palsy, global developmental delay/intellectual disability, and behavioral disorders. In addition, we will review the neonatal prognostic markers of these disorders to the extent currently possible.

Epilepsy

Based on the available evidence, the frequency of epilepsy following neonatal seizures is between 10% and 30% (Hellström-Westas et al. 1995, Toet et al. 2005, Tekgul et al. 2006, Guillet and Kwon 2007, Ronen et al. 2007, Pisani et al. 2007, Garfinkle and Shevell 2011b, Glass et al. 2011b, Uria-Avellanal et al. 2013). A recent review by Pisani et al. (2015) detailed a relatively exhaustive list of studies that investigated later epilepsy after neonatal seizures. From a total of 44 studies published between 1954 and 2013 corresponding to 4538 infants with neonatal seizures, the frequency of later epilepsy was 16.8%. Among these studies, the frequency of later epilepsy mostly ranged from 10% to 30%. When patients who were lost to follow-up (minimum follow-up was 2 months–12 years) were excluded, the frequency was 17.9% (Pisani et al. 2015). In addition, most children who develop epilepsy following neonatal seizures do so in conjunction with other concurrent neurodevelopmental impairments (Pisani et al. 2015). In one study of 120 children who were followed by a single neurologist after neonatal seizures, 29 children (27%) had epilepsy. Of those 29 children, only 5 (17%) had epilepsy in the absence of other concurrent neurodevelopmental impairments (Garfinkle and Shevell 2011b).

The definition of epilepsy varies amongst the studies thus far undertaken on this topic and unfortunately, in some studies is left undefined. In 2014, the International League against Epilepsy defined epilepsy as a disease of the brain characterized by any of the following: (1) at least two unprovoked seizures occurring at least 24 hours apart; or (2) one unprovoked seizure and a probability of further seizures of at least 60%; or (3) the diagnosis of a specific epilepsy syndrome (Berg et al. 2010, Fisher et al. 2014). Based on this definition, very few neonates with seizures would qualify for a diagnosis of epilepsy upon discharge from the NICU.

The onset of later epilepsy is difficult to discern because most studies do not specifically report it. In addition, the onset of epilepsy is highly dependent on whether, and at what point, the treating physician decides to taper the initial antiepileptic medications that were started during the newborn period (Clancy and Legido 1991, Pisani et al. 2012). In a more recent prospective study, the parents of term children enrolled in a longitudinal cohort study of neonates admitted to a single academic NICU were administered a structured seizure questionnaire. The median age of follow-up was 6 years. Thirteen of the 129 (10%) evaluated children had epilepsy. The age at epilepsy onset ranged from 0 to 5 years; half had an onset within the first year of life (Glass et al. 2011b). Interestingly, epilepsy subsequent to neonatal seizures in the context of perinatal arterial stroke may have a later onset (Suppiej et al. 2015).

Several risk factors for the development of epilepsy following neonatal seizures have been delineated. Neonatal status epilepticus is highly predictive of later epilepsy. In the two studies that evaluated status epilepticus, 42–83% of neonates who were diagnosed with status epilepticus later developed epilepsy (Glass et al. 2011b, Pisani et al. 2012). The success of controlling status epilepticus with antiepileptic drugs (AEDs) may however not be associated with later epilepsy (van Rooij et al. 2007). Evidence from animal studies supports the principle that long-lasting seizures can permanently disrupt neuronal development, induce synaptic reorganization, and produce a reduction in the threshold necessary for later overt seizures, but they do not necessarily result in epilepsy (Liu et al. 1999, Ben-Ari and Holmes 2006).

The use of more than a single antiepileptic medication to adequately control the acute neonatal seizures is also a predictor of later epilepsy (Toet et al. 2005, Garfinkle and Shevell 2011a, Pisani et al. 2012). In the setting of HIE, severe or near-total brain injury on magnetic resonance imaging (MRI) has been shown to be predictive of later epilepsy (Glass et al. 2011b). Other risk factors include the persistence of seizures beyond 48 hours of life (Toet et al. 2005) and a severely abnormal electroencephalography (EEG) background (Garcias Da Silva et al. 2004, Khan et al. 2008, Nagarajan et al. 2010, Garfinkle and Shevell 2011a, Pisani et al. 2012). Seizure semiology has also been studied in order to correlate specific seizure types with later outcomes. One study found that seizure types other than the focal clonic variant, which is typically associated with either a focal stroke or hemorrhage as the underlying pathology, were associated with later epilepsy (Mizrahi and Kellaway 1987, Garfinkle and Shevell 2011a). No single etiology has been consistently associated with the development of epilepsy subsequent to neonatal seizures (Toet et al. 2005, Suppiej et al. 2015). The utility of the standardized neonatal neurological examination as a later predictor has not been demonstrated thus far (Pisani et al. 2012). The tremendous variability in risk factors thus far identified may reflect variation in study population and definitions of what constitutes both a neonatal seizure and later epilepsy. For instance, Soltirovska-Salamon et al. (2014) attempted to apply predictors from the 'Garfinkle-Shevell scoring system' to their own population; of the five potential risk factors, only two were predictive of later epilepsy (Garfinkle and Shevell 2011b). The limitation observed may be a product of applying a scoring system derived for term newborn infants to both preterm and term newborn infants.

Interestingly, one group has invoked the 'two-hit' hypothesis for the development of epilepsy subsequent to neonatal seizures. They described two children who had had neonatal seizures who only developed epilepsy after the occurrence of a febrile status epilepticus. They speculated that seizures in the neonatal period result in epileptogenic disturbances that cause the more mature brain to be especially prone to later seizure-induced injury (Spagnoli et al. 2015).

Implications for the continuation of antiepileptic drugs

The continuation of antiepileptic treatment in newborn infants after their seizures have stopped is highly variable and the best time to stop daily medication administration is still not clear. A recent survey of American pediatric neurologists and neonatologists reported that most physicians continue to prescribe maintenance phenobarbital to newborn infants with seizures after they leave the NICU (Guillet and Kwon 2008). It is, however, unknown if continuing phenobarbital treatment for up to several months is helpful or harmful in the long term (van Rooij et al. 2013).

The presence, frequency, and duration of seizure activity may contribute to further brain damage, which may lead to later neurodevelopmental impairment and epilepsy (Miller et al. 2002, Glass et al. 2009). Therefore, neonatal seizures warrant prompt treatment. Once the acute injury abates, however, the risk for ongoing seizures, and thus further acquired impairment, is low. The rationale for using AEDs at discharge is to decrease the likelihood of seizure recurrence. Thus a low risk for further seizures beyond discharge must be balanced against the potential deleterious effects of medication use.

Importantly, there are theoretical concerns that some treatment strategies for neonatal seizures could be detrimental to the developing brain. AEDs can cause apoptotic neurodegeneration in the developing rat brain at plasma concentrations used for seizure control in humans (Bittigau et al. 2002, Ikonomidou and Turski 2010). In a randomized controlled trial published in 1990, children with febrile seizures randomized to phenobarbital demonstrated depressed cognitive function that outlasted the administration of the drug (Farwell et al. 1990).

Therefore, the decision regarding maintenance antiepileptic medications after NICU discharge relates mostly to balancing the likelihood of post-neonatal epilepsy versus the potential long-term neurodevelopmental toxicity of the therapy. To date, there exists one published recommendation regarding the discontinuation of AEDs after neonatal seizures. The World Health Organization recommends that in neonates with a normal neurological examination or EEG, AEDs could be stopped if the neonate if seizure-free for at least 72 hours (weak recommendation; World Health Organization 2011). This is an important gap in treatment evidence and future research efforts should investigate the effects of the continuation or discontinuation of antiepileptic drug use once the acute neonatal seizures have abated.

INFANTILE SPASMS

Compared to the general population, infantile spasms make up a high proportion of the epilepsy that follows neonatal seizures (Clancy and Legido 1991, Gano et al. 2013, Inoue et al. 2014, Jung da et al. 2015). In a population of neonates with HIE submitted to therapeutic hypothermia, 8 of the 13 children with later epilepsy experienced infantile spasms. In addition, all of the survivors who had brainstem injury on MRI developed later infantile spasms (Jung da et al. 2015). This supports the notion that the pathogenesis of infantile spasms may involve subcortical structures and 'brainstem release' phenomena (Lado and Moshe 2002).

Cerebral palsy

Cerebral palsy is a clinical diagnosis of a nonprogressive motor impairment resulting from a presumably early insult to the developing brain (Rosenbaum et al. 2007). It remains a major cause of childhood disability, affecting 2 per 1000 live-born children (Himmelmann and Uvebrant 2014). Despite changes in neonatal mortality and advances in perinatal care, the overall frequency of cerebral palsy has been largely unaffected over the past decades, perhaps reflecting the increasing probability of survival at low gestational ages (Himmelmann and Uvebrant 2014). The frequency of cerebral palsy following neonatal seizures ranges from 25% to 43%, but has been reported as low as 3% (Brunquell et al. 2002, Pisani et al. 2007, Ronen et al. 2007, Nagarajan et al. 2011, Garfinkle and Shevell 2011b, Lai et al. 2013).

A recent systematic review of risk factors for cerebral palsy in developed countries found that amongst the neonatal variables, the presence of neonatal seizures was the strongest risk factor across all gestational ages (McIntyre et al. 2013). In term-born children, the range of point estimates of measures of relative risk was 3.7–63 across three studies (McIntyre et al. 2013). In one population-based case control study of 271 singletons with spastic cerebral palsy, those with neonatal seizures were significantly more likely to develop cerebral palsy (OR 5.6; 95% CI 2.5, 12.8; Nielsen et al. 2008).

Several risk factors for the development of cerebral palsy following neonatal seizures have been identified. In one study, seizure semiology, seizure onset, EEG background findings, and the 5-minute apgar score (but not actual seizure etiology) were associated with later cerebral palsy (Garfinkle and Shevell 2011a). In another, the cumulative dose of phenobarbital, but not that of levetiracetam, predicted the later development of cerebral palsy (Maitre et al. 2013).

Intellectual disability

Few studies have examined the long-term cognitive outcomes of cohorts of neonates with seizures. One such recent study with a median follow-up of 10 years found that 32% of survivors of neonatal seizures had an intellectual disability, although the exact definition of intellectual disability was not provided (Ronen et al. 2007).

Many more studies have evaluated neurodevelopment at an earlier age, but the terminology and definitions utilized varies. One study that followed children with neonatal seizures to a median age of 3.5 years found that 40% of them were intellectually disabled (Brunquell et al. 2002). In another cohort of children with neonatal seizures, 27% of such children had marked cognitive impairment defined as a score of 70 or below on the Mental Development Index of the Bayley Scales of Infant Development II (Tekgul et al. 2006). Another cohort study found that 38% of children with neonatal seizures had global developmental delay (Garfinkle and Shevell 2011b). Global developmental delay is a subset of developmental disabilities defined as significant delay in two or more of the following developmental domains: gross/fine motor, speech/language, cognition, social/personal, and activities of daily living (Shevell et al. 2003). The term 'global developmental delay' is usually reserved for younger children, whereas the term 'intellectual disability' is applied to older children when IQ testing is more valid.

Behavior

The association of neonatal seizures with later neurobehavioral disorders has not yet been properly addressed. Although the long-term behavioral outcomes of cohorts of neonates with HIE and those born preterm have been explored, restricted well-defined cohorts of children who had neonatal seizures have not been similarly followed (Lindstrom et al. 2006, Hack et al. 2009).

Preclinical animal studies have shed some light on the long-term behavioral effects of neonatal seizures (Stafstrom 2002). In one study, rats submitted to experimentally induced neonatal status epilepticus showed impaired later social behavior (Castelhano et al. 2015). In addition, other preclinical animal studies have suggested that AEDs also impact on the developing brain. For instance, neonatal exposure to phenobarbital was shown to potentiate schizophrenia-like behavioral outcomes in rats (Bhardwaj et al. 2012).

Conclusion

Children who survive neonatal seizures are at high risk for later neurodevelopmental sequelae such as epilepsy, cerebral palsy and intellectual disability. Less is known about their later neurobehavioral outcomes. Although some risk factors have been identified for these outcomes, the heterogeneity of the populations and specific outcome measures precludes the development of accurate scoring systems that may enable better prediction of later outcomes. The prediction of later epilepsy, in particular, would help with informing therapeutic decisions regarding the continuation or withdrawal of AEDs before discharge from the NICU. Better prediction of later developmental and intellectual impairments would facilitate early intervention efforts that make the best use of limited rehabilitation resources. Further work is needed to better characterize these outcomes and understand how they relate to neonatal seizures.

REFERENCES

Ben-Ari Y, Holmes GL (2006) Effects of seizures on developmental processes in the immature brain. *Lancet Neurol* 5: 1055–1063. doi: http://dx.doi.org/10.1016/S1474-4422(06)70626-3.

Berg AT, Berkovic SF, Brodie MJ et al. (2010) Revised terminology and concepts for organization of seizures and epilepsies: Report of the ILAE commission on classification and terminology, 2005–2009. *Epilepsia* 51: 676–685. doi: http://dx.doi.org/10.1111/j.1528-1167.2010.02522.x.

Bhardwaj SK, Forcelli PA, Palchik G, Gale K, Srivastava LK, Kondratyev A (2012) Neonatal exposure to phenobarbital potentiates schizophrenia-like behavioral outcomes in the rat. *Neuropharmacology* 62: 2337–2345. doi: http://dx.doi.org/10.1016/j.neuropharm.2012.02.001.

Bittigau P, Sifringer M, Genz K et al. (2002) Antiepileptic drugs and apoptotic neurodegeneration in the developing brain. *Proc Natl Acad Sci USA* 99: 15089–15094. doi: http://dx.doi.org/10.1073/pnas.222550499.

Brunquell PJ, Glennon CM, Dimario FJ Jr., Lerer T, Eisenfeld L (2002) Prediction of outcome based on clinical seizure type in newborn infants. *J Pediatr* 140: 707–712. doi: http://dx.doi.org/10.1067/mpd. 2002.124773.

Castelhano AS, Ramos FO, Scorza FA, Cysneiros RM (2015) Early life seizures in female rats lead to anxiety-related behavior and abnormal social behavior characterized by reduced motivation to novelty and deficit in social discrimination. *J Neural Transm* 122: 349–355. doi: http://dx.doi.org/10.1007/s00702-014-1291-2.

Clancy RR, Legido A (1991) Postnatal epilepsy after EEG-confirmed neonatal seizures. *Epilepsia* 32: 69–76. doi: http://dx.doi.org/10.1111/j.1528-1157.1991.tb05614.x.

Davis AS, Hintz SR, Van Meurs KP et al. (2010) Seizures in extremely low birth weight infants are associated with adverse outcome. *J Pediatr* 157: 720–725. e1–e2.

Farwell JR, Lee YJ, Hirtz DG, Sulzbacher SI, Ellenberg JH, Nelson KB (1990) Phenobarbital for febrile seizures–effects on intelligence and on seizure recurrence. *N Engl J Med* 322: 364–369. doi: http://dx.doi.org/10.1056/NEJM199002083220604.

Fisher RS, Acevedo C, Arzimanoglou A et al. (2014) ILAE official report: A practical clinical definition of epilepsy. *Epilepsia* 55: 475–482. doi: http://dx.doi.org/10.1111/epi.12550.

Gano D, Sargent MA, Miller SP et al. (2013) MRI findings in infants with infantile spasms after neonatal hypoxic-ischemic encephalopathy. *Pediatr Neurol* 49: 401–405. doi: http://dx.doi.org/10.1016/j.pediatrneurol.2013.08.007.

Garcias Da Silva LF, Nunes ML, Da Costa JC (2004) Risk factors for developing epilepsy after neonatal seizures. *Pediatr Neurol* 30: 271–277. doi: http://dx.doi.org/10.1016/j.pediatrneurol.2003.09.015.

Garfinkle J, Shevell M (2011a) Cerebral palsy, developmental delay, and epilepsy after neonatal seizures. *Pediatric neurology* 44: 88–96. doi: http://dx.doi.org/10.1016/j.pediatrneurol.2010.09.001.

Garfinkle J, Shevell M (2011b) Prognostic factors and development of a scoring system for outcome of neonatal seizures in term infants. *Eur J Paediatr Neurol: EJPN: Official Journal of the European Paediatric Neurology Society* 15: 222–229.

Glass H, Glidden D, Jeremy R, Barkovich A, Ferriero D, Miller S (2009) Clinical neonatal seizures are independently associated with outcome in infants at risk for hypoxic-ischemic brain injury. *J Pediatr* 155: 318–323. doi: http://dx.doi.org/10.1016/j.jpeds.2009.03.040.

Glass HC, Ferriero DM, Miller SP (2011a) Correspondence on 'clinical seizures in neonatal hypoxic-ischemic encephalopathy have no independent impact on neurodevelopmental outcome: Secondary analyses of data from the neonatal research network hypothermia trial'. *J Child Neurol* 26: 532; author reply 533–534. doi: http://dx.doi.org/10.1177/0883073811399801.

Glass HC, Hong KJ, Rogers EE et al. (2011b) Risk factors for epilepsy in children with neonatal encephalopathy. *Pediatr Res* 70: 535–540. doi: http://dx.doi.org/10.1203/PDR.0b013e31822f24c7.

Glass HC, Kan J, Bonifacio SL, Ferriero DM (2012) Neonatal seizures: Treatment practices among term and preterm infants. *Pediatr Neurol* 46: 111–115. doi: http://dx.doi.org/10.1016/j.pediatrneurol. 2011.11.006.

Guillet R, Kwon J (2007) Seizure recurrence and developmental disabilities after neonatal seizures: Outcomes are unrelated to use of phenobarbital prophylaxis. *J Child Neurol* 22: 389–395. doi: http://dx.doi.org/10.1177/0883073807301917.

Guillet R, Kwon J (2008) Prophylactic phenobarbital administration after resolution of neonatal seizures: Survey of current practice. *Pediatrics* 122: 731–735. doi: http://dx.doi.org/10.1542/peds.2007-3278.

Hack M, Taylor HG, Schluchter M, Andreias L, Drotar D, Klein N (2009) Behavioral outcomes of extremely low birth weight children at age 8 years. *J Dev Behav Pediatr* 30: 122–130. doi: http://dx.doi.org/10.1097/DBP.0b013e31819e6a16.

Hellström-Westas L, Blennow G, Lindroth M, Rosén I, Svenningsen N (1995) Low risk of seizure recurrence after early withdrawal of antiepileptic treatment in the neonatal period. *Arch Dis Child Fetal Neonatal Ed* 72: 101. doi: http://dx.doi.org/10.1136/fn.72.2.F97.

Himmelmann K, Uvebrant P (2014) The panorama of cerebral palsy in Sweden. XI. Changing patterns in the birth-year period 2003–2006. *Acta Paediatr* 103: 618–624. doi: http://dx.doi.org/10.1111/apa.12614.

Ikonomidou C, Turski L (2010) Antiepileptic drugs and brain development. *Epilepsy Res* 88: 11–22. doi: http://dx.doi.org/10.1016/j.eplepsyres.2009.09.019.

Inoue T, Shimizu M, Hamano SI, Murakami N, Nagai T, Sakuta R (2014) Epilepsy and West syndrome in neonates with hypoxic–ischemic encephalopathy. *Pediatr Int* 56: 369–372. doi: http://dx.doi.org/10.1111/ped.12257.

Jung Da E, Ritacco DG, Nordli DR, Koh S, Venkatesan C (2015) Early anatomical injury patterns predict epilepsy in head cooled neonates with hypoxic-ischemic encephalopathy. *Pediatr Neurol* 53: 135–140. doi: http://dx.doi.org/10.1016/j.pediatrneurol.2015.04.009.

Khan RL, Nunes ML, Garcias Da Silva LF, Da Costa JC (2008) Predictive value of sequential electroencephalogram (EEG) in neonates with seizures and its relation to neurological outcome. *J Child Neurol* 23: 144–150. doi: http://dx.doi.org/10.1177/0883073807308711.

Lado F, Moshe S (2002) Role of subcortical structures in the pathogenesis of infantile spasms: What are possible subcortical mediators? *Int Rev Neurobiol* 49: 115–140. doi: http://dx.doi.org/10.1016/S0074-7742(02)49010-1.

Lai YH, Ho CS, Chiu NC, Tseng CF, Huang YL (2013) Prognostic factors of developmental outcome in neonatal seizures in term infants. *Pediatr Neonatol* 54: 166–172. doi: http://dx.doi.org/10.1016/j.pedneo.2013.01.001.

Lindstrom K, Lagerroos P, Gillberg C, Fernell E (2006) Teenage outcome after being born at term with moderate neonatal encephalopathy. *Pediatr Neurol* 35: 268–274. doi: http://dx.doi.org/10.1016/j.pediatrneurol.2006.05.003.

Liu Z, Yang Y, Silveira DC et al. (1999) Consequences of recurrent seizures during early brain development. *Neuroscience* 92: 1443–1454. doi: http://dx.doi.org/10.1016/S0306-4522(99)00064-0.

Maitre NL, Smolinsky C, Slaughter JC, Stark AR (2013) Adverse neurodevelopmental outcomes after exposure to phenobarbital and levetiracetam for the treatment of neonatal seizures. *J Perinatol* 33: 841–846. doi: http://dx.doi.org/10.1038/jp.2013.116.

Mcbride MC, Laroia N, Guillet R (2000) Electrographic seizures in neonates correlate with poor neurodevelopmental outcome. *Neurology* 55: 506–513. doi: http://dx.doi.org/10.1212/WNL.55.4.506.

Mcintyre S, Taitz D, Keogh J, Goldsmith S, Badawi N, Blair E (2013) A systematic review of risk factors for cerebral palsy in children born at term in developed countries. *Dev Med Child Neurol* 55: 499–508. doi: http://dx.doi.org/10.1111/dmcn.12017.

Miller S, Weiss J, Barnwell A et al. (2002) Seizure-associated brain injury in term newborns with perinatal asphyxia. *Neurology* 58: 542–548. doi: http://dx.doi.org/10.1212/WNL.58.4.542.

Mizrahi EM, Kellaway P (1987) Characterization and classification of neonatal seizures. *Neurology* 37: 1837–1844. doi: http://dx.doi.org/10.1212/WNL.37.12.1837.

Nagarajan L, Ghosh S, Palumbo L (2011) Ictal electroencephalograms in neonatal seizures: Characteristics and associations. *Pediatr Neurol* 45: 11–16. doi: http://dx.doi.org/10.1016/j.pediatrneurol.2011.01.009.

Nagarajan L, Palumbo L, Ghosh S (2010) Neurodevelopmental outcomes in neonates with seizures: A numerical score of background encephalography to help prognosticate. *J Child Neurol* 25: 961–968. doi: http://dx.doi.org/10.1177/0883073809355825.

Nielsen LF, Schendel D, Grove J et al. (2008) Asphyxia-related risk factors and their timing in spastic cerebral palsy. *BJOG* 115: 1518–1528. doi: http://dx.doi.org/10.1111/j.1471-0528.2008.01896.x.

Pisani F, Cerminara C, Fusco C, Sisti L (2007) Neonatal status epilepticus vs recurrent neonatal seizures: Clinical findings and outcome. *Neurology* 69: 2177–2185. doi: http://dx.doi.org/10.1212/01.wnl.0000295674.34193.9e.

Pisani F, Facini C, Pavlidis E, Spagnoli C, Boylan G (2015) Epilepsy after neonatal seizures: Literature review. *Eur J Paediatr Neurol* 19: 6–14. doi: http://dx.doi.org/10.1016/j.ejpn.2014.10.001.

Pisani F, Piccolo B, Cantalupo G et al. (2012) Neonatal seizures and postneonatal epilepsy: A 7-y follow-up study. *Pediatr Res* 72: 186–193. doi: http://dx.doi.org/10.1038/pr.2012.66.

Ronen G, Buckley D, Penney S, Streiner D (2007) Long-term prognosis in children with neonatal seizures: A population-based study. *Neurology* 69: 1816–1822. doi: http://dx.doi.org/10.1212/01.wnl. 0000279335.85797.2c.

Rosenbaum P, Paneth N, Leviton A et al. (2007) A report: The definition and classification of cerebral palsy April 2006. *Dev Med Child Neurol Suppl* 109: 8–14.

Sarnat HB, Sarnat MS (1976) Neonatal encephalopathy following fetal distress. A clinical and electroencephalographic study. *Arch Neurol* 33: 696–705. doi: http://dx.doi.org/10.1001/archneur.1976. 00500100030012.

Scher MS, Aso K, Beggarly ME, Hamid MY, Steppe DA, Painter MJ (1993) Electrographic seizures in preterm and full-term neonates: Clinical correlates, associated brain lesions, and risk for neurologic sequelae. *Pediatrics* 91: 128–134.

Shah DK, Zempel J, Barton T, Lukas K, Inder TE (2010) Electrographic seizures in preterm infants during the first week of life are associated with cerebral injury. *Pediatr Res* 67: 102–106. doi: http://dx.doi. org/10.1203/PDR.0b013e3181bf5914.

Shankaran S, Laptook AR, Ehrenkranz RA et al. (2005) Whole-body hypothermia for neonates with hypoxic-ischemic encephalopathy. *N Engl J Med* 353: 1574–1584. doi: http://dx.doi.org/10.1056/NEJMcps050929.

Shetty J (2015) Neonatal seizures in hypoxic-ischaemic encephalopathy–risks and benefits of anticonvulsant therapy. *Dev Med Child Neurol* 57 (Suppl. 3): 40–43. doi: http://dx.doi.org/10.1111/dmcn.12724.

Shevell M, Ashwal S, Donley D et al. (2003) Practice parameter: Evaluation of the child with global developmental delay: Report of the Quality Standards Subcommittee of the American Academy of Neurology and the Practice Committee of the Child Neurology Society. *Neurology* 60: 367–380. doi: http://dx.doi. org/10.1212/01.WNL.0000031431.81555.16.

Soltirovska-Salamon A, Neubauer D, Petrovcic A, Paro-Panjan D (2014) Risk factors and scoring system as a prognostic tool for epilepsy after neonatal seizures. *Pediatr Neurol* 50: 77–84. doi: http://dx.doi. org/10.1016/j.pediatrneurol.2013.08.010.

Spagnoli C, Cilio MR, Pavlidis E, Pisani F (2015) Symptomatic neonatal seizures followed by febrile status epilepticus: The two-hit hypothesis for the subsequent development of epilepsy. *J Child Neurol* 30: 615–618. doi: http://dx.doi.org/10.1177/0883073814533004.

Stafstrom CE (2002) Assessing the behavioral and cognitive effects of seizures on the developing brain. *Prog Brain Res* 135: 377–390. doi: http://dx.doi.org/10.1016/S0079-6123(02)35034-9.

Suppiej A, Mastrangelo M, Mastella L et al. (2015). Pediatric epilepsy following neonatal seizures symptomatic of stroke. *Brain Dev* 38: 27–31. doi: http://dx.doi.org/10.1016/j.braindev.2015.05.010.

Tekgul H, Gauvreau K, Soul J et al. (2006) The current etiologic profile and neurodevelopmental outcome of seizures in term newborn infants. *Pediatrics* 117: 1270–1280. doi: http://dx.doi.org/10.1542/ peds.2005-1178.

Toet M, Groenendaal F, Osredkar D, Van Huffelen A, De Vries L, (2005) Postneonatal epilepsy following amplitude-integrated EEG-detected neonatal seizures. *Pediatr Neurol* 32: 241–247. doi: http://dx.doi. org/10.1016/j.pediatrneurol.2004.11.005.

Uria-Avellanal C, Marlow N, Rennie J (2013) Outcome following neonatal seizures. *Semin Fetal Neonatal Med* 18: 224–232. doi: http://dx.doi.org/10.1016/j.siny.2013.01.002.

Van Rooij L, De Vries L, Handryastuti S et al. (2007) Neurodevelopmental outcome in term infants with status epilepticus detected with amplitude-integrated electroencephalography. *Pediatrics* 120: 63. doi: http://dx.doi.org/10.1542/peds.2006-3007.

Van Rooij L, Hellström-Westas L, De Vries L (2013) Treatment of neonatal seizures. *Semin Fetal Neonatal Med* 18: 209–215. doi: http://dx.doi.org/10.1016/j.siny.2013.01.001.

Volpe JJ (2008) *Neurology of the Newborn.* Philadelphia: WB Saunders.

Volpe JJ (2012) Neonatal encephalopathy: An inadequate term for hypoxic-ischemic encephalopathy. *Ann Neurol* 72: 156–166. doi: http://dx.doi.org/10.1002/ana.23647.

World Health Organization (2011) *Guidelines on Neonatal Seizures.* Geneva, Switzerland: World Health Organization.

Wusthoff CJ, Kessler SK, Vossough A et al. (2011) Risk of later seizure after perinatal arterial ischemic stroke: A prospective cohort study. *Pediatrics* 127: e1550–e1557.

12
NEUROPROTECTIVE STRATEGIES FOR NEONATES WITH SEIZURES

Shilpa D. Kadam, Xiaohe Yu and Michael V. Johnston

Neonatal seizures, especially refractory neonatal seizures, frequent recurrent seizures, and status epilepticus can be associated with later neurological dysfunction with survivors experiencing higher rates of post-neonatal epilepsy and motor and cognitive deficits (Scher 2003, Scher et al. 2003). The debate whether prolonged neonatal seizures can cause brain injury themselves or whether they simply reflect the effects of underlying brain pathology such as hypoxia-ischemia, stroke, or hypoglycemia continues (Thibeault-Eybalin et al. 2009). Experiments in rodents have shown that repeated seizures produced by drugs such as flurothyl or pentylenetetrazol in the neonatal period can produce impaired learning as well as a lower seizure threshold in later life (Holmes et al. 1998). Clinical studies of neonates with hypoxia-ischemia and seizures suggest that full-scale intelligence and neuromotor scores are lower in those with severe seizures (Thibeault-Eybalin et al. 2009), confounded by the fact that seizure severity can simply be a marker for greater severity of the initial insult. Feng et al. (2008) reported that experimental pilocarpine-induced status epilepticus is associated with allosteric changes in γ-Aminobutyric acid (GABA) receptors that lead to impaired postsynaptic inhibition. Hence, the search for novel antiepileptic drugs (AEDs) and neuroprotective therapeutic strategies is particularly important in the case of neonatal seizures (Helmy et al. 2011). Taken together, it is important to develop therapies that not only stop the seizures but also protect the brain, if possible.

Neuroprotection in the context of neonatology refers to interventions that can be applied either prenatally or postnatally to prevent or interrupt injury from insults including hypoxia-ischemia, stroke, hypoglycemia, or status epilepticus (Johnston et al. 2011). Probably the first use of neuroprotection for neonates was total body cooling prior to surgery for complex congenital heart disorders such as transposition of the great vessels in the 1950s (Zavanella and Subramanian 1978). Cooling was also used in preterm infants in the 1950s but an increased death rate led to discontinuation of this approach (Silverman et al. 1958), and it was not until the 1990s that clinical research on cooling for perinatal asphyxia in term infants re-emerged (Amess et al. 1997, Thoresen et al. 1997).

The modern era for the use of cooling as a neuroprotective strategy had its roots in the basic studies of Vannucci and others in the 1980s with the development of a simple but useful model of hypoxia-ischemia in the 7–day-old rat pup (Rice et al. 1981). Prior to that time, neonatal studies of primates with asphyxia by Myers (1972) yielded information about the causation and pathogenesis of asphyxia but it was difficult to examine therapies because of problems with prolonged survival and expense of the model. The Rice and Vannucci model is still widely used to explore the effects of potential neuroprotective compounds and the pathogenesis of seizures due to hypoxia-ischemia (Yager et al. 2002). The first *in vivo* evidence of protection by the N-methyl-D-aspartate (NMDA) glutamate channel blocker dizocilpine (MK-801) against perinatal hypoxia-ischemia when given prior to or shortly after onset of the hypoxic-ischemic insult (McDonald et al. 1987, McDonald and Johnston 1990) was performed in this model. The compound was never approved for use in humans by the Federal Drugs Administration because of the side effects seen in studies of stroke in adult patients. Opening of NMDA glutamate receptors activated by membrane depolarization and glutamate flooding due to impaired function of glutamate re-uptake pumps (Johnston et al. 2011) leads to activation of extra-synaptic NMDA receptor channels (Brassai et al. 2015) that have been shown to initiate toxic effects different from the synaptic receptors.

Cascade of injury from seizures and hypoxia-ischemia
Neuroprotection is based on an understanding of the delayed cascade of injury that characterizes the response to seizures and hypoxia-ischemia in the brain (Fig. 12.1). The initial response to injury is a reaction to loss of energy substrates, such as that occurs in hypoxia-ischemia and/or the mismatch that occurs between increased demands for energy during seizures and limited energy delivery. When this occurs, restricted delivery of oxygen and glucose can lead to reduced uptake of glutamate via specific glial glutamate transporters, which in turn leads to overstimulation of excitatory glutamate synaptic and extrasynaptic receptors. Entry of calcium through NMDA receptor channels also leads to activation of nitric oxide synthase (nNOS), which causes oxidative stress within neurons. These changes put pressure on mitochondria to keep up with energy supplies and oxidative stress within mitochondria leads to damage of the oxidative phosphorylation machinery. Stressed mitochondria can send two major types of signals to the nucleus that begin to degrade DNA: one that is known as apoptosis inducing factor (AIF) that is released from mitochondria and travels to the nucleus, and another protein known as cytochrome C that is released from mitochondria and activates caspase 3, a cysteine protease that can also lead to DNA degradation. These pathways are generally known as caspase-dependent and caspase independent pathways for cell death. Interestingly it has been shown that there are some sex differences in these pathways and the caspase-dependent system is more active in females than males and the caspase independent pathway is more active in males. There also do seem to be some sex differences between males and females clinically, as males appear to be overrepresented in children with cerebral palsy (Johnston and Hagberg 2007). Another interesting developmental feature is that in rodents, caspase is more abundant in the perinatal brain than in older adults, and so cell death pathways may be more activated in infants. Additionally, it is known that refractoriness to first line antiseizure drugs emerges with increasing number of seizure events that go untreated, indicating that seizure events by themselves may contribute to the phenomenon. Therefore, early and efficacious seizure suppression may be desirable as a neuroprotective strategy (Boylan and Pressler 2013).

Increased seizure susceptibility in the immature brain

The neonatal period is one of heightened synaptic plasticity and synaptogenesis during brain development. Glutamate is the predominant excitatory amino acid neurotransmitter in neurons, and glutamate receptors (GluRs) are developmentally regulated in neurons and glia (Johnston 2005). GluR subunits are differentially expressed during development. Excitatory ionotropic glutamate receptors (iGluRs) are expressed at higher levels in newborn infants than in old children and adults. GluR-mediated excitation is enhanced in the immature brain. GABA is the major inhibitory neurotransmitter in the adult brain, but in early development GABA action can be excitatory where it may function as a trophic signal. In addition, the expression of GABA receptors is significantly lower than in adults. Brooks-Kayal et al. (2001) reported that GABA receptors do not achieve maximal expression levels until the fourth postnatal week (Brooks-Kayal et al. 2001). In the immature brain excitation predominates over inhibition. This tendency toward hyperexcitability renders neonates more susceptible to seizures (Sanchez and Jensen 2001, Rakhade and Jensen 2009).

Excitatory ionotropic glutamate receptors and therapeutic targets of neonatal seizure

Glutamate is the most abundant neurotransmitter in the brain. It is synthesized from glutamine in presynaptic terminals by glutaminase. Upon activation by glutamate, ionotropic receptors (iGluRs) directly allow the flow of ions across the neuronal membrane. iGluRs are further subdivided into three groups based on the agonist which preferentially activates the receptor subtypes (1)N-methyl-D-aspartate receptors (NMDARs), (2) alpha-amino-3-hydroxy-5-methyl-4-isoxazole propionate receptors (AMPARs), and (3) kainate receptors (Table 12.1):. NMDARs consist of eight different NMDAR1 (NR1) subunits in combination with NR2A, NR2B, NR2C, NR2D, and/or NR3A, NR3A subunits (Paoletti and Neyton 2007). In the immature brain, neuronal NMDARs contain high levels of the NR2B, NR2A, and NR3A subunits. Such elevated levels of NR2B subunits result in extended current decay times; the high levels of NR2D and NR3A subunits reduce the sensitivity of NMDARs to magnesium ions. The overexpression of NR2B, NR2D, and NR3A subunits in the immature brain all contribute to increased NMDAR-mediated calcium influx and promote hyperexcitability (Paoletti and Neyton 2007, Henson et al. 2010).

TABLE 12.1
Features of neurotransmitter receptors in immature neurons

Receptors	Molecular differences	Functional differences
NMDA	Elevated levels of NR2B subunit	Extended current decay times
	Increase in NR2D, NR3A subunit	Less sensitive to action of magnesium
Mg^{2+}		
AMPA	Absence of GluR2 subunit	High permeability for Ca^{2+}
GABA$_A$	Stable NKCC1 expression and	Opening produces depolarization
	KCC2 delayed expression	Less sensitive to augmentation by benzodiazepines

NMDA, N-methyl-D-aspartate; AMPA, alpha-amino-3-hydroxy-5-methyl-4-isoxazole propionate; GABA, gamma-aminobutyric acid; NR2, NR3, NMDA receptor subunits; NKCC, sodium-potassium chloride co-transporter.

Antagonists of NMDA receptors exhibit an excellent anticonvulsant action in adult and developing animals (Mares et al. 2004, Mares and Mikulecka 2009) but also have serious side effects such as hyper locomotion and derangement of cognitive processes (Rezvani 2006, Mares and Mikulecka 2009). Attention is now focused on low-affinity NMDA receptor antagonists like memantine and felbamate, and on subunit-specific antagonists (Ghasemi and Schachter 2011). Memantine and felbamate are neuroprotective in immature rodent models (Mares and Mikulecka 2009), but their clinical use as anticonvulsants is limited because of the side effects and the not yet explained pro-convulsant activity in some seizure models. Ifenprodil, the first drug found to be a specific NR2B-selective NMDA antagonist (Williams 1993), is more promising. Its anticonvulsant action was described in both mature and immature brain models of epileptic seizures (Hrncic et al. 2009, Paoletti et al. 2013). The anticonvulsant effect of ifenprodil was found in 12-, 15-, and 18-day-old rats without serious side effects on motor performance; however, no effect was observed in 25-day-old animals, indicating that its anticonvulsant action in rat pups was age-dependent (Mares 2014). The NR2B subunit is dominant at early development stages (Wyllie et al. 2013) so ifenprodil may be useful in the treatment of age-specific epileptic syndromes.

AMPARs are composed of combinations of GluR1, GluR2, GluR3, and/or GluR4 subunits. AMPARs are also maturationally regulated. There is a higher prevalence of GluR2 subunit-deficient receptors in the immature brain than in the adult brain, which leads to increased calcium influx (Talos et al. 2006a, 2006b, Shepherd and Huganir 2007, Rakhade and Jensen 2009). These changes correspond to an increased risk of excitotoxic cellular injury due to hypoxia-ischemia. Knockout models of the GluR2 subunit lead to a reduced seizure threshold which also supports the hypothesis that α-amino-3-hydroxy-5-methyl-4-isoxazolepropionic acid (AMPA) receptors without the GluR2 subunit promote hyperexcitability (Friedman and Koudinov 1999). The AMPAR antagonist, topiramate, has demonstrated efficacy in neonatal seizures. The specific AMPAR antagonist talampanel was also shown to protect against neonatal seizures in a rodent model (Aujla et al. 2009).

Kainate receptors are heteromeric combinations of GluR5, GluR6, GluR7, KA1, and/or KA2 subunits. NMDARs are always permeable to calcium, whereas the divalent cation permeability of AMPARs and kainite receptors depends on the subunit composition of the receptor. Kainate receptors become more permeable to calcium when the GluR5 or GluR6 subunits are absent (Fig. 12.1; Table 12.2).

GABA$_A$ receptors and the co-transporters of chloride

GABA$_A$ receptors (GABA$_A$Rs) are ligand-gated chloride channels. The electrochemical gradient of Cl$^-$ across the neuronal plasma membrane is controlled by cation-chloride cotransporters (CCCs) (Blaesse et al. 2009). CCCs are secondary active transporters that drive net Cl$^-$ extrusion (K-Cl co-transporters, KCCs) or uptake (Na-K-2Cl co-transporters, NKCCs) by using the K$^+$ and Na$^+$ gradients which, in turn, are generated by the Na-K ATPase In early development brain, GABA mediates much of the excitatory neurotransmission, while in adult brain GABA acts as the major inhibitory neurotransmitter. In the adult brain, activation of GABA$_A$ receptors results in membrane hyperpolarization due to Cl$^-$ influx through its ion channel, and hence is inhibitory. In immature neurons, however, GABA agonists can cause depolarization due to a

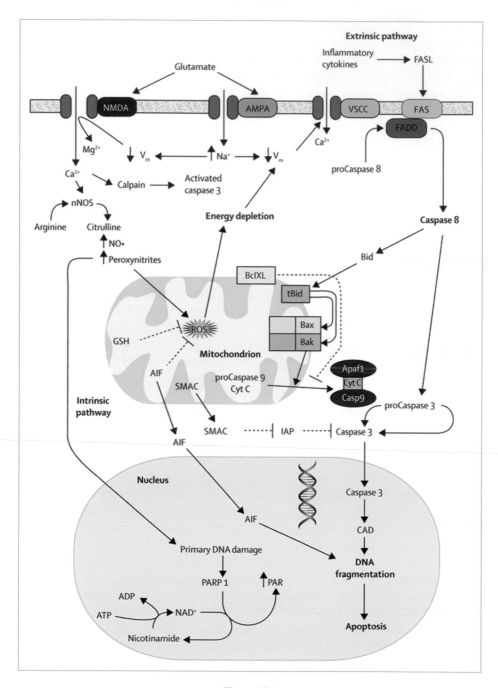

Figure 12.1

Figure 12.1. Downstream signaling pathways that mediate the apoptosis–necrosis continuum. Delayed cell death signaling pathways mediate the effects of hypoxia-ischemia in the brain. The extrinsic pathway mirrors the cells' external environment and begins when inflammatory cytokines (to the right of the figure at the cell surface) bind to and activate Fas-cell death receptors, whereas the intrinsic pathway is activated when signals released from within stressed mitochondria activate caspase and non-caspase-mediated-cell-death pathways within the nucleus. These two cell-death pathways activate common signaling networks within the mitochondria and the nucleus. Mitochondria exposed to caspase-induced stress can release cytochrome C through channels formed by the Bax and Bak proteins in the outer mitochondrial membrane (caspase-mediated cell death) or can release (AIF, which activates DNA fragmentation directly (non-caspase pathway). Cytochrome C can combine with Apaf1 and caspase 9 to form the apoptosome, which triggers activation of caspase 3. DNA breaks mediated by free radicals such as nitric oxide (NO) and peroxynitrite activate poly-ADP-ribose polymerase 1 (PARP1), which consumes NAD+ and worsens the energy shortage for mitochondria (shown within the nucleus). Convergence of signaling for the extrinsic (Fas) and intrinsic cell-death pathways is responsible for the interaction between infection (endotoxin) and hypoxia-ischaemia that increases cell death. Vm – membrane potential; VSSC – voltage sensitive calcium channel; Fas – death receptor in tumor necrosis factor family; FADD – Fas adaptor death domain protein; BclXL – antiapoptotic proteins in the Bcl2 family of proteins; Bax and Bak – proapoptotic proteins that form channels in outer mitochondrial membrane releasing cytochorome C to trigger apoptosis; tBid – truncated BH3-only proapoptotic protein; Apaf1 – apoptotic protein activating factor 1; SMAC – antagonist of inhibitor of apoptosis; IAP – inhibitor of apoptosis; CAD – caspase activating DNAse; Cyt C – cytochrome C; nNOS – neuronal nitric oxide synthase; NO – nitric oxide; ROS – reactive oxygen species; PARP1 – poly-ADP-ribose polymerase 1; PAR – poly-ADP ribose formed by ribosylation of DNA and proteins; GSH – glutathione, an antioxidant; AIF – apoptosis-inducing factor; Bid – BH3 interacting domain proapoptotic protein; NAD – nicotinamide adenine dinucleotide; FASL – Fas death receptor ligand. (Reproduced from *Lancet Neurology* . Johnston, et al, Treatment advances in neonatal neuroprotection and neurointensive care. **10**: 372–382, © 2011, with kind permission of the Lancet Publishing Group.)

TABLE 12.2
Potential targets of therapy for neonatal seizures

Mechanism targeted	*Potential therapeutic*
NMDAR	NMDAR inhibitors (memantine, felbamate); NR2B-specific inhibitors (ifenprodil)
AMPAR	AMPAR antagonists (topiramate, talampanel)
NKCC1	NKCC1 inhibitor (bumetanide and its pro-drug)
GABA$_A$	GABA$_A$R agonists (phenobarbital, benzodiazepines)
Inflammation	Anti-inflammatory compounds (ACTH, steroids, IVIg)
Neuronal injury	Erythropoietin, Melatonin, Xenon

Abbreviations: NMDAR, N-methyl-d-aspartate receptor; NR2B, NMDAR subunit 2B; AMPAR, alpha -amino-3-hydroxy-5-methyl-4-isoxazole propionate receptor; NKCC1, sodium–potassium–chloride co-transporter 1; GABA$_A$R, gamma -aminobutyric acid receptor A.

net efflux of Cl$^-$ through the GABA receptor ion channel, resulting in neuronal excitation. This switch was thought to be in part due to developmental changes in the expression of the Na$^+$-K$^+$-2 Cl$^-$ cotransporter isoform 1 (NKCC1) and the K$^+$-Cl$^-$ cotransporter isoform 2 (KCC2) (Fig. 12.2; Table 12.3). In the immature brain, neuronal intracellular Cl$^-$ concentrations are

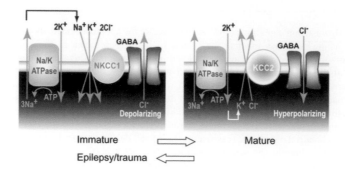

Figure 12.2. A shift from depolarizing to hyperpolarizing GABA$_A$ receptor-mediated Cl⁻currents takes place during neuronal development, and an opposite effect is often seen following epilepsy and trauma. In cortical and hippocampal neurons, the NKCC1 mediates Cl⁻uptake, while the KCC2 extrudes Cl⁻. The energy for both of these electrically neutral ion-transport processes is derived from the ion gradients generated by the Na⁻K ATPase: NKCC1 is driven by the Na⁺ concentration gradient and KCC2 by the K⁺ gradient. In immature neurons (left) GABA$_A$ receptor-mediated Cl⁻currents are depolarizing. During neuronal development, upregulation of KCC2 (rightward arrow) renders GABA$_A$ receptor-mediated Cl⁻currents hyperpolarizing (right). Recurrent seizures and other traumatic insults can lead to the downregulation of KCC2 and to a reestablishment of NKCC1-dependent depolarizing GABAergic signaling. GABAA, gamma-aminobutyric acid; NKCC1, sodium-potassium-chloride co-transporter 1; ATPase, adenylpyrophosphatase. (Reproduced from *Neuropharmacology,* Walker MC, Puskarjov M, Kaila K. Citation-chloride cotransportersNKCC1 and KCC2 as potential targets for novel antiepileptic and antiepileptogenic treatments. 69: 62–74. © 2013, with kind permission of Elsevier.)

higher than in the adult due to a reported high NKCC1 expression (Dzhala et al. 2005, Talos et al. 2006a, 2006b) coincident with a low KCC2 expression, relative to normal adult expression patterns. The expression of NKCC1 mRNA was also reported to be increased in human forebrain neurons during the perinatal period, relative to later life. In humans, this switch was thought to occur in utero after NKCC1 peaks between 31 and 41 weeks postconception. Recently, inhibitors of cation-chloride cotransporters NKCC1 and KCC2 such as furosemide and, especially, bumetanide (BTN) have attracted much interest as putative AEDs.

Recent human studies in developing brains have reported a sustained expression of NKCC1 in the maturing brain (Morita et al. 2014) associated with increasing KCC2 expression as the brain matures. The contradictory results between recent human brain findings and previous reports from both human and animal model reports that showed decrease in NKCC1 eVion with age may have occurred because of the inability of the previous NKCC1 probes to detect both the spice variants of NKCC1 (a and b) present in the brain. The availability of a reliable pan NKCC1 probe which can detect both the spice variants does not currently exist. Once available, however, it will allow for better evaluation of the developmental profile of NKCC1 expression and its role in determining intracellular chloride gradients in maturing brains. However, the developmental profile of KCC2 by itself can explain the developmental depolarizing to hyperpolarizing switch in GABA action as proposed by several investigators. (Deisz et al. 2011, 2014, Khanna et al. 2013, Kaila et al. 2014).

Basic research has helped us understand why neonatal seizures are so very different than seizures in older children and adults by also highlighting the role of Cl⁻ co-transporters

TABLE 12.3
Mechanism of therapeutic targets of neonatal seizures

Therapeutic targets	*Mechanism of action*
Antiepileptic drugs:	
Phenobarbital	Enhance GABA inhibition
Phenytoin	Inhibit voltage-dependent sodium channels
Benzodiazepines	Enhance GABA inhibition
Lidocaine	Inhibit voltage-dependent sodium channels
Pyridoxine	Co-factor for multiple enzymatic process for neurotransmitters
Levetiracetam	Regulation of excitatory synaptic transmission mediated by AMPA and NMDA receptors
Topiramate	Modulation of AMPA and kainite receptors, sodium, GABA channels
Others therapeutic strategies:	
Therapeutic hypothermia	Numerous potential mechanisms
Xenon	NMDA antagonist
Bumetanide	Inhibits NKCC1 transporter
Erythropoietin	Antioxidant
Melatonin	Antioxidant, anti-inflammation, free radical scavenging
Anti-inflammation drugs	Blockade of specific inflammatory molecules and pathways

AMPA, alpha -amino-3-hydroxy-5-methyl-4-isoxazolepropioninc acid; NMDA, N-methyl-d-aspartate; GABA, gamma-amino-butyric acid.; NKCC1, sodium–potassium–chloride co-transporter 1.

in neonatal seizure susceptibilities (Ben-Ari et al. 2012). Early in development, the depolar-izing GABAergic signaling that is instrumental in normal neuronal differentiation and migration was shown to be responsible for the inefficacy of GABA agonists like pheno-barbital (Dzhala and Staley 2003, Staley 2004, Dzhala et al. 2005, Kaila et al. 2014). NKCC1 is expressed in neurons and astrocytes throughout the brain and plays an important role in regulating neuronal volume and ion homeostasis (Kahle and Staley 2008). In contrast KCC2 is neuron-specific and a critical mediator of synaptic inhibition, and cellular protec-tion against excitotoxicity (Kahle et al. 2013). The expression level of KCC2 increases exponentially with conceptional age, especially perinatally, starting in the second half of gestation in humans, to reach the significantly higher and stable adult levels (Morita et al. 2014). The lower KCC2 expression in neonates compared to adult brains reverses the transmembrane chloride gradient due to the predominant action of NKCC1, leading to higher intracellular levels compared to extracellular levels. Therefore, opening of GABA channels leads to the chloride moving out of the cell along its concentration gradient and thus depolarizing the cell (Ben-Ari 2002). This has been suggested as the reason for the frequently reported inefficacy of GABA agonists like phenobarbital in curbing recurrent neonatal seizures. The ability to curb these refractory seizures using drugs that modulate Cl co-transporter function (Kaila et al. 2014, Puskarjov et al. 2014) has the potential to provide neuroprotection in syndromes like hypoxic-ischaemic encephalopathy (HIE) with their severe status-like seizure burdens (Boylan and Pressler 2013).

Inflammatory and immune responses in epilepsy

Clinical and neuropathological evidence suggest that inflammation probably plays an important role in seizure disorders (Table 12.4), and injury from status epilepticus as it does in hypoxic-ischemic injuries. Increased expression of cytokines (such as Interleukin [IL]-6, Tumor Necrosis Factor [TNF]-α and IL-1β) and immune cells have been observed in patients with epilepsy and in animal models. Cytokines are soluble mediators of cell communication that are critical in immune regulation, and studies have shown that epileptic seizures can induce the production of cytokines, which in turn influence the pathogenesis and course of epilepsies. Brain inflammation might be a consequence as well as a cause of seizure/epilepsy. IL-1β and high-mobility group box 1 (HMGB1) protein is released from astrocytes and microglia after seizures. This signaling occurs through activation of the IL-1receptor/Toll-like receptor (IL1R/TLR) system. IL1R/TLR signaling in turn can activate the Src kinase-mediated phosphorylation of NMDA receptor subunit 2B (NR2B).

TABLE 12.4
Inflammation in human epilepsies and convulsive disorders

Epileptic syndrome convulsive disorder	Inflammatory markers		Anti-inflammatory treatments
	Plasma or CSF	*Brain tissue*	
Rasmussen encephalitis	GluR3 Ab, Munc-18 Ab	GluR3 Ab	ACTH, steroids, IVIg
		CD-8⁺ lymphocytes GrB; MAC; cytokines	PEX, PAI, immunosuppressant
West syndrome	IFN- α, TNF- α, IL2	n.d	ACTH, steroids, IVIg
Lennox–Gastaut syndrome	n.d.	n.d.	ACTH, steroids, IVIg
Landau Kleffner syndrome	n.d.	n.d.	ACTH, steroids, IVIg
Febrile seizures	IL-1β, IL-1Ra, IL-6, IL-10, TNF- α	n.d	n.d
TLE	IL-6, IL-1 β, IL-1Ra	IL-1, NF-kB[a]	n.d.
Tonic-clonic seizures	IL-6, IL-1 α, IL-1 β	n.d.	n.d.
Tuberous Sclerosis	n.d.	CD-68 macrophages ICAM-1, TNF- α, NF-kB, MAPK	n.d.

[a]Only in patients with MTLE and HS. Cerebrospinal fluid; n.d., not determined; PEX; plasma exchange; PAI; protein A immunoabsortion; IVIg, intravenous immunoglobulin; MAPK, mitogen activated protein kinase.

Reproduced from *Epilepsia* Vezzani A, Granata T. Brain Inflammation in Epilepsy: Experimental and Clinical Evidence p20 © 2005, with kind permission of John Wiley and Sons.

Consequently, NMDA mediated $Ca2^+$ influx can enhance depolarization in neurons, leading to increased neuronal excitability and excitotoxicity. In mice, activation of IL1R/TLR signaling promotes seizure onset and recurrence, whereas its pharmacological blockade or genetic deletions of IL-1R1 gene drastically delay the onset of seizures (Vezzani 2005). TNF-α is mainly released by microglia in the brain, and it can stimulate astrocytes to reduce glutamate uptake at synapse as well as release glutamate. Extracellular flooding of glutamate leads to the activation toxic extra-synaptic NMDA glutamate receptors. In addition, brain inflammation may contribute to blood-brain barrier (BBB) breakdown. This breakdown leads to BBB leakage and the entry of albumin into the brain. Albumin has been shown to induce long-lasting hyper-excitability by impairing astrocyte capacity to buffer extracellular potassium and glutamate via activation of the transforming growth factor (TGF)-β pathway, which results in downregulation of the glutamate transporter. Consequently, epileptic seizures and inflammatory mediators can form a positive feedback loop, reinforcing each other.

Therapeutic targets of neonatal seizures

ANTIEPILEPTIC DRUGS

Phenobarbital and phenytoin are standard AEDs (Table 12.3) that work by somewhat different but complementary actions to reduce neuronal excitability. Phenobarbital acts on the GABA-benzodiazepine receptor to enhance the effects of GABA to open the channel and allow chloride to flux through it. On the other hand phenytoin blocks actively opening and closing sodium channels on neuronal membranes and it is able to block sustained repetitive firing that occurs during seizures. It is a useful drug for stopping seizures in some cases but its neuroprotective effect is limited. Activation of the GABA benzodiazepine receptor is a reasonable way to stop seizures but as described in this chapter, its activity is limited somewhat by the developmental program for chloride transporters (Dzhala et al. 2005) and therefore less effective in suppressing seizures in neonates than in older children and adults (Bartha et al. 2007).

Phenobarbital has been shown to augment the neuroprotective effect of hypothermia in similar rodent models (Barks et al. 2010). However, phenobarbital was also shown to be ineffective in controlling electrographic seizures in noncooled neonates (Sarkar et al. 2012). Early in development, the depolarizing GABAAergic signaling is partly responsible for the inefficacy of GABA agonists like phenobarbital as described above (Dzhala and Staley 2003, Staley 2004, Dzhala et al. 2005b, Kaila et al. 2014a, Kang et al. 2015). Electroclinical dissociation is now a fairly well-understood concept in the human neonate wherein GABA agonists are able to block the clinical manifestations of seizures; however, as detected with electrographic monitoring, the brain continues to seize (Scher and Painter 1989, Weiner et al. 1991, Evans and Levene 1998, Rakhade and Jensen 2009).

Phenobarbital has also been reported to induce neuronal apoptosis in the developing rodent brain (Bittigau et al. 2003, Gonzalez and Ferriero 2009). However, comparing the very short period of brain growth in mice to the much longer period of development in humans is always a barrier for direct extrapolation from rodent model findings. Additionally, apoptosis is normal during the period of brain growth in humans. In summary, phenobarbital may be a reasonable drug to give to infants with seizures undergoing therapeutic hypothermia to help improve neuroprotection.

In contrast to phenobarbital and phenytoin, levetiracetam and topiramate do not appear to cause neuronal apoptosis in the developing animal models and may have neuroprotective and antiepileptogenic effects (Koh et al. 2004, Schubert et al. 2005, Kim et al. 2007). Levetiracetam regulates excitatory activity primarily by binding to presynaptic vesicles in excitatory synapses that contain glutamate, and thus complements the postsynaptic actions of barbiturates and phenytoin. The anticonvulsant effects of topiramate seem to be mediated through multiple mechanisms, including inhibition of carbonic anhydrase isozymes, blockade of non-NMDA glutamate receptors including AMPA and kainate receptors, as well as $GABA_A$R-activated ion channels, and voltage-activated Na^+ and $Ca2^+$ channels (Herrero et al. 2002).

Valproic acid is another anticonvulsant that has been shown to have neuroprotective effects in animal models (Suda et al. 2013, 2014). It acts by several mechanisms including stimulating GABAergic receptors and inhibiting rapidly firing sodium channels. Valproic acid has also been shown to attenuate ischemic injury through anti-inflammatory and anti-apoptotic mechanisms as well as through inhibition of histone deacetylase (Hasan et al. 2013, Kimura et al. 2015). However there are no trials to support using valproate acid for this purpose in newborn infants.

OTHER THERAPEUTIC STRATEGIES

Hypothermia

HIE is one of the most important causes of neonatal seizures in term infants and the severity of seizures seems to correlate with the severity of encephalopathy although it remains unclear how much seizures contribute to cell death. Therapeutic hypothermia is the first neuroprotective strategy that has demonstrated efficacy for neonatal HIE in multiple randomized controlled trials. Prior to the introduction of therapeutic hypothermia, electrographic seizures were reported in more than 50% of neonates with HIE; status epilepticus was a frequent occurrence, and the overall seizure burden was high (Lynch et al. 2012). Therapeutic hypothermia is likely to modulate multiple neurotoxic processes, including decreased cerebral metabolism, ion pump dysfunction, formation of cytotoxic edema, free radical formation, and neuro-inflammation (Fig. 12.1). Studies by Thoresen and colleagues in piglets indicated that the protective effects of hypothermia are mediated by a reduction in the release in excitotoxic amino acids including glutamate in the brain as well as nitric oxide which is formed by calcium passing through the NMDA glutamate receptor (Thoresen et al. 1997). D'Ambrosio studies show cooling by 0.5°C to 2°C inhibited the onset of post-traumatic epileptic seizures (D'Ambrosio et al. 2013). Surface cooling of the brain has also been shown to reduce seizures in adult humans and animals (Rothman 2009, Smyth et al. 2015). Infants with moderate HIE, treated with whole-body cooling, have a significantly lower electrographic seizure burden than noncooled neonates (Low et al. 2012, Srinivasakumar et al. 2013). Khadrawy et al. reported in experimental status epilepticus in rats, the anticonvulsant effect of cooling appeared to be mediated by a reduction in nitric oxide levels Giles et al. reported a term male infant who was cooled for HIE, but developed new onset seizures during the rewarming phase of therapeutic hypothermia (Kendall et al. 2012). These seizures stopped within 30 minutes of a return to hypothermia without anticonvulsant medication. They continued cooling for an additional 24 hours, after which seizures remained in remission upon rewarming. However, there is limited evidence that cooling leads to the cessation of seizures. Caution must be used in the interpretation of a single case report, but it does appear warranted to pursue further research into the antiepileptic properties of hypothermia. In addition, therapeutic hypothermia also makes seizures more difficult to detect. As a result, continuous EEG monitoring is advocated for both seizure detection and monitoring of treatment.

Xenon and xenon in combination with hypothermia

Hypothermia improves HIE outcomes and it is the current standard of care. Yet, clinical trials suggest that 44~53% of infants who receive hypothermia will die or have moderate to severe neurological disability. Novel neuroprotective therapies are needed to further reduce the rate and severity of neurodevelopmental disabilities resulting from HIE. Xenon, used as a general anesthetic in Europe, is a monoatomic gas with very high tissue solubility, and a specific NMDA glutamate receptor antagonist. The noble gas has received increasing interest as a neuroprotectant over the last decade. Xenon combined with therapeutic hypothermia has been shown to offer additional neuroprotection in animal models of neonatal encephalopathy with minimal adverse effects (Banks et al. 2010, Chakkarapani et al. 2010, Liu et al. 2015). Randomized trials are currently investigating whether xenon combined with cooling offers additional neuro-protection compared to cooling alone. Xenon may be expected to have anticonvulsant effects through glutamate receptor blockade. Azzopardi et al. (2013) examined seizure activity on the real time and amplitude-integrated EEG records of 14 term infants with HIE treated within 12 hours of birth with 30% inhaled xenon for 24 hours combined with 72 hours of moderate systemic hypothermia. Seizures were identified on 5 of 14 infants. Seizures stopped during xenon therapy but recurred within a few minutes of withdrawing xenon and stopped again after xenon was restarted. These data show that inhaled xenon has anticonvulsant and EEG suppressant effects in infants with HIE. Inhaled xenon may be a valuable new therapy in this hard-to-treat population.

Bumetanide

Bumetanide has been used in newborn infants which is a loop diuretic because it is actively concentrated by organic anion transporters in the loop of Henle in the kidney's thick ascending limb, and its diuretic action is mediated by inhibition of both NKCC1 and the renal-specific NKCC2. BTN at low concentrations inhibits NKCCs, without significantly affecting the function of KCCs. A number of studies have employed this drug in an attempt to suppress neonatal seizures on animal models. Some studies (Dzhala et al. 2005, Cleary et al. 2013, Loscher et al. 2013) have suggested that modification of the GABA receptor response by blocking NKCC1 with BTN might be effective. However other data suggest that BTN efficacy is model-specific (Vanhatalo et al. 2009, Kang and Kadam 2014). In contrast, some serious concerns about BTN have been raised. First, BTN functions as a potent loop diuretic with a short half-life in neonates (Pacifici 2012). In humans, NKCC2, another target of BTN, is robustly expressed in the kidney to extract and reabsorb ions from urine. Repeated doses of BTN can nonselectively block NKCC2 as well as NKCC1 (Puskarjov et al. 2014). Second, BTN has poor BBB permeability that results in a less than 1% of BTN penetrating into the brain one hour after an intra-peritoneal injection (Cleary et al. 2013, Puskarjov et al. 2014). Third, a few preclinical studies have also reported that BTN is nonefficacious as an adjunct for antiseizure pharmacotherapy (Mares 2009, Vanhatalo, Hellstrom-Westas, and De Vries 2009, Ben-Ari 2012, Kang et al. 2015). A safety trial of BTN called the NEMO clinical trial (Pressler et al. 2015) was recently terminated because of concern about hearing loss. The same clinical trial also cited BTN inefficacy in improving seizure control as an add-on to phenobarbital for HIE seizures that was associated with the ototoxicity. The putative action of BTN on the NKCC1 expressing inner ear cells has dampened some interest in its antiseizure efficacy studies. The significant role of NKCC1 on inner ear function is well known (Pace et al. 2001). Additionally, the recent evaluation of the BTN prodrug specifically created to bypass the BBB for better brain bioavailability has reported nonefficacy of BTN as an antiseizure agent (Kang and Kadam 2014, Tollner et al. 2014).

ERYTHROPOIETIN

Erythropoietin (Epo) is a hemopoietic growth factor which is widely used in neonatology to stimulate production of red blood cells in preterm infants and has recently emerged as a potential neuroprotective for the brain. The brain has been shown to have a specific receptor for erythropoietin that mediates an adaptive responsive to hypoxia. Clinical trials demonstrated the safety and efficacy of recombinant human Epo in the prevention and treatment of anemia of prematurity (Sun et al. 2005, Iwai et al. 2010). Epo is available clinically, and demonstrates remarkable neuroprotective and neuroregenerative effects in animals (Sun et al. 2005, Iwai et al. 2010). Preclinical data from rodent models of neonatal HIE have demonstrated both short-term and long-term histological and behavioral improvement after treatment with this agent (Gonzalez et al. 2009, Sargin et al. 2010, Xiong et al. 2011). Mikati et al. found Epo to be protective against hippocampal cell loss; it decreased hippocampal apoptosis in rat pups after an acute hypoxic insult, and had the ability to reduce the duration of hypoxic seizures (Mikati MA 2007). Clinical trials of Epo as an add-on medication to moderate hypothermia for infants with asphyxia are being organized (Wu and Gonzalez 2015).

MELATONIN

Melatonin is an indoleamine secreted by the pineal gland. It plays a key role in regulating the circadian rhythm. Melatonin also possesses a broad-spectrum free radical scavenging capacity, antioxidant properties, and anti-inflammatory effects. Seizures can induce markedly increased levels of melatonin in childhood refractory epilepsy and febrile seizures (Ardura et al. 2010, Paprocka et al. 2010). Melatonin has also been reported to be an anticonvulsant (Uberos et al. 2011) and prevents seizure-induced neuronal lesions by limiting NO-induced lipid peroxidation (Skaper et al. 1999). In the recurrent neonatal seizure animal models, pretreatment with melatonin was associated with improved neurobehavioral and cognitive functions. In addition, pretreatment with melatonin showed a significant downregulated expression of ACAT-1, cathepsin-E, and upregulated CaMKII in the hippocampus and the cerebral cortex (Ni et al. 2015). However, there are also reports that melatonin can worsen of seizures (Sheldon 1998). Jain and Besag (2013) reviewed 26 papers reporting an association between melatonin and epilepsy or seizures and some suggested worsening of seizures and others indicated improvement in seizure control with melatonin. All the studies involved relatively small numbers of patients and most were neither blinded nor placebo controlled. Larger randomized studies are needed to evaluate the neuroprotective effects of melatonin, which is used by large numbers of people as an over-the-counter sleep aid.

ANTI-INFLAMMATORY DRUGS

Brain inflammation may be a common substrate contributing to seizures in drug-resistant epilepsies of different etiologies, and recurrent seizures can be a major cause of long-term inflammation (Vezzani et al. 2013). The involvement of inflammation in epilepsy is of great interest because pharmacological interventions targeting inflammation might be of use in treating epilepsy (Diamond et al. 2015). Clinical anti-inflammatory or immunosuppressive treatments can suppress some types of epileptic seizures that are resistant to conventional AEDs (Table 12.4). Pharmacological blockade of specific inflammatory molecules and pathways can significantly reduce seizures in experimental models of seizures and epilepsy (Choi and Koh 2008). From a clinical standpoint (Table 12.4), evidence for a role of inflammation in the pathophysiology of human epilepsy is growing fast (Vezzani and Granata 2005, Vezzani et al. 2013, Diamond et al. 2015). BBB leakage induced by seizures or inflammation allows the entry of compounds with immunogenic or inflammatory potentials, as predicted for example in interferon-induced seizures (Pavlovsky et al. 2005), but it also may facilitate the entry of compounds with therapeutic potential with limited or no access to the CNS. Activation of the ACTH–GC axis in response to antecedent injury or stress, leading to hyperfunction of CRH–neuronal pathways, has been suggested to play a role in the pathogenesis of West syndrome (Baram 1993, 2007). Anti-inflammatory medication could be a new promising treatment for refractory epilepsy (Diamond et al. 2015).

CELL-BASED THERAPIES

Although the use of cell-based therapies for protection against seizure-induced brain injury in neonates is likely to be far into the future, laboratory studies have shown some potential for this approach. Zipancic et al. (2010) transplanted GABAergic precursor cells from the medial ganglionic eminence into the normal neonatal brain and found that they differentiated into functional mature GABAergic interneurons. When grafted into a mouse model of high seizure susceptibility caused by elimination of GABAergic neurons by injection of neurotoxic saporin conjugated to substance P a marked decrease in seizures was reported. Hammad et al. (2014) transplanted GABAergic interneurons from the median eminence of normal mice into the primary visual cortex of mice with the Stargazer mutation that causes them to have absence seizures. Transplantation resulted in a marked decrease in seizures in this model. Cunningham et al. (2014) found that transplantation of hPSC-derived maturing GABAergic interneurons ameliorate seizures and abnormal behavior in mice with epilepsy. These early studies suggest that human cell lines in the future might be prepared to protect or restore areas of the brain damaged by seizures.

Conclusion

Seizures remain a common problem in the neonatal period. Prompt recognition and treatment may help prevent abnormal neurological outcomes. Several pitfalls to attain this goal still exist. Despite the proliferation of the literature on neonatal seizures, there is no consensus regarding the management of neonatal seizures. Treatment of neonatal seizures will always need to focus both on the treatment of the seizures themselves and the treatment of the underlying etiology. Phenobarbital is still the AED of first choice in over 80% of neonatal units worldwide, despite concerns about its adverse effects on the developing brain (Bittigau, Sifringer, and Ikonomidou 2003, Clancy 2006). The efficacy and safety of newer AEDs in neonatal seizure treatment need further evaluation. Other agents such as xenon, erythropoietin, melatonin, and anti-inflammatory agents might be potential therapeutic agents in the future and, especially, may be able to (Clancy 2006) augment the neuroprotection gained by hypothermia after HIE.

REFERENCES

Amess PN, Penrice J, Cady EB et al. (1997) Mild hypothermia after severe transient hypoxia-ischemia reduces the delayed rise in cerebral lactate in the newborn piglet. *Pediatr Res* 41: 803–808. doi: http://dx.doi.org/10.1203/00006450-199706000-00002

Ardura J, Andres J, Garmendia JR, Ardura F (2010) Melatonin in epilepsy and febrile seizures. *J Child Neurol* 25: 888–891. doi: http://dx.doi.org/10.1177/0883073809351315

Aujla PK, Fetell MR, Jensen FE (2009) Talampanel suppresses the acute and chronic effects of seizures in a rodent neonatal seizure model. *Epilepsia* 50: 694–701. doi: http://dx.doi.org/10.1111/j.1528-1167.2008.01947.x

Azzopardi D, Robertson NJ, Kapetanakis A et al. (2013) Anticonvulsant effect of xenon on neonatal asphyxial seizures. *Arch Dis Child Fetal Neonatal Ed* 98: F437–F439. doi: http://dx.doi.org/10.1136/archdischild-2013-303786

Banks P, Franks NP, Dickinson R (2010) Competitive inhibition at the glycine site of the N-methyl-D-aspartate receptor mediates xenon neuroprotection against hypoxia-ischemia. *Anesthesiology* 112: 614–622. doi: http://dx.doi.org/10.1097/ALN.0b013e3181cea398

Baram TZ (1993) Pathophysiology of massive infantile spasms: Perspective on the putative role of the brain adrenal axis. *Ann Neurol* 33: 231–236. doi: http://dx.doi.org/10.1002/ana.410330302

Baram TZ (2007) Go 'West,' young man...The quest for animal models of infantile spasms (West syndrome). *Epilepsy Curr* 7: 165–167. doi: http://dx.doi.org/10.1111/j.1535-7511.2007.00213.x

Barks JD, Liu YQ, Shangguan Y, Silverstein FS (2010) Phenobarbital augments hypothermic neuroprotection. *Pediatr Res* 67: 532–537. http://dx.doi.org/10.1203/PDR.0b013e3181d4ff4d

Bartha AI, Shen J, Katz KH et al. (2007) Neonatal seizures: Multicenter variability in current treatment practices. *Pediatr Neurol* 37: 85–90. doi: http://dx.doi.org/10.1016/j.pediatrneurol.2007.04.003

Ben-Ari Y (2002) Excitatory actions of gaba during development: The nature of the nurture. *Nat Rev Neurosci* 3 (9): 728–739.

Ben-Ari Y, Woodin MA, Sernagor E et al. (2012) Refuting the challenges of the developmental shift of polarity of GABA actions: GABA more exciting than ever! *Front Cell Neurosci* 6, article 35. http://dx.doi.org/10.3389/fncel.2012.00035

Bittigau P, Sifringer M, Ikonomidou C (2003) Antiepileptic drugs and apoptosis in the developing brain. *Ann N Y Acad Sci* 993: 103–114.

Blaesse P, Airaksinen MS, Rivera C, Kaila K (2009) Cation-chloride cotransporters and neuronal function. *Neuron* 61: 820–838. http://dx.doi.org/10.1016/j.neuron.2009.03.003

Boylan GB, Pressler RM (2013) Neonatal seizures: The journey so far. *Semin Fetal Neonatal Med* 18: 173–174. doi: http://dx.doi.org/10.1016/j.siny.2013.05.011

Brassai A, Suvanjeiev RG, Ban EG, Lakatos M (2015) Role of synaptic and nonsynaptic glutamate receptors in ischaemia induced neurotoxicity. *Brain Res Bull* 112: 1–6. doi: http://dx.doi.org/10.1016/j.brainresbull.2014.12.007

Brooks-Kayal AR, Shumate MD, Jin H, Rikhter TY, Kelly ME, Coulter DA (2001) Gamma-Aminobutyric acid(A) receptor subunit expression predicts functional changes in hippocampal dentate granule cells during postnatal development. *J Neurochem* 77: 1266–1278. doi: http://dx.doi.org/10.1046/j.1471-4159.2001.00329.x

Chakkarapani E, Dingley J, Liu X et al. (2010) Xenon enhances hypothermic neuroprotection in asphyxiated newborn pigs. *Ann Neurol* 68: 330–341. doi: http://dx.doi.org/10.1002/ana.22016

Choi J, Koh S (2008) Role of brain inflammation in epileptogenesis. *Yonsei Med J* 49: 1–18. doi: http://dx.doi.org/10.3349/ymj.2008.49.1.1

Clancy RR (2006) Summary proceedings from the neurology group on neonatal seizures. *Pediatrics* 117: S23–S27.

Cleary RT, Sun H, Huynh T et al. (2013) Bumetanide enhances phenobarbital efficacy in a rat model of hypoxic neonatal seizures. *PLoS One* 8: e57148. doi: http://dx.doi.org/10.1371/journal.pone.0057148

Cunningham M, Cho JH, Leung A et al. (2014) hPSC-derived maturing GABAergic interneurons ameliorate seizures and abnormal behavior in epileptic mice. *Cell Stem Cell* 15: 559–573. http://dx.doi.org/10.1016/j.stem.2014.10.006

D'Ambrosio R, Eastman CL, Darvas F et al. (2013) Mild passive focal cooling prevents epileptic seizures after head injury in rats. *Ann Neurol* 73: 199–209. doi: http://dx.doi.org/10.1002/ana.23764

Deisz RA, Lehmann TN, Horn P, Dehnicke C, Nitsch R (2011) Components of neuronal chloride transport in rat and human neocortex. *J Physiol* 589: 1317–1347. doi: http://dx.doi.org/10.1113/jphysiol.2010.201830

Deisz RA, Wierschke S, Schneider UC, Dehnicke C (2014) Effects of VU0240551, a novel KCC2 antagonist, and DIDS on chloride homeostasis of neocortical neurons from rats and humans. *Neuroscience* 277: 831–841. doi: http://dx.doi.org/10.1016/j.neuroscience.2014.07.037

Diamond ML, Ritter AC, Failla MD, Boles JA, Conley YP, Kochanek PM, Wagner AK (2014) IL-1+¦ associations with posttraumatic epilepsy development: A genetics and biomarker cohort study. *Epilepsia* 55: 1109–1119.

Diamond ML, Ritter AC, Failla MD et al. (2015) IL-1beta associations with posttraumatic epilepsy development: A genetics and biomarker cohort study. *Epilepsia* 56: 991–1001. doi: http://dx.doi.org/10.1111/epi.13100

Dzhala VI, Staley KJ (2003) Excitatory actions of endogenously released GABA contribute to initiation of ictal epileptiform activity in the developing hippocampus. *J Neurosci* 23: 1840–1846.

Dzhala VI, Talos DM, Sdrulla DA et al. (2005) NKCC1 transporter facilitates seizures in the developing brain. *Nat Med* 11: 1205–1213. doi: http://dx.doi.org/10.1038/nm1301

Evans D, Levene M (1998) Neonatal seizures. *Arch Dis Child Fetal Neonatal Ed* 78: F70–F75.

Feng HJ, Mathews GC, Kao C, Macdonald RL (2008) Alterations of GABA A-receptor function and allosteric modulation during development of status epilepticus. *J Neurophysiol* 99: 1285–1293. doi: http://dx.doi.org/10.1152/jn.01180.2007

Friedman LK, Koudinov AR (1999) Unilateral GluR2(B) hippocampal knockdown: A novel partial seizure model in the developing rat. *J Neurosci* 19: 9412–9425.

Ghasemi M, Schachter SC (2011) The NMDA receptor complex as a therapeutic target in epilepsy: A review. *Epilepsy Behav* 22: 617–640. doi: http://dx.doi.org/10.1016/j.yebeh.2011.07.024

Gonzalez FF, Abel R, Almli CR, Mu D, Wendland M, Ferriero DM (2009) Erythropoietin sustains cognitive function and brain volume after neonatal stroke. *Dev Neurosci* 31: 403–411. doi: http://dx.doi.org/10.1159/000232558

Gonzalez FF, Ferriero DM (2009) Neuroprotection in the newborn infant. *Clin Perinatol* 36: 859–880, vii. doi: http://dx.doi.org/10.1016/j.clp.2009.07.013

Hammad M, Schmidt SL, Zhang X, Bray R, Frohlich F, Ghashghaei HT (2014) Transplantation of GABAergic Interneurons into the Neonatal Primary Visual Cortex Reduces Absence Seizures in Stargazer Mice. *Cereb Cortex* 25(9): 2970-9. doi: 10.1093/cercor/bhu094

Hasan MR, Kim JH, Kim YJ et al. (2013) Effect of HDAC inhibitors on neuroprotection and neurite outgrowth in primary rat cortical neurons following ischemic insult. *Neurochem Res* 38: 1921–1934. doi: http://dx.doi.org/10.1007/s11064-013-1098-9

187

Helmy MM, Tolner EA, Vanhatalo S, Voipio J, Kaila K (2011) Brain alkalosis causes birth asphyxia seizures, suggesting therapeutic strategy. *Ann Neurol* 69: 493–500. doi: http://dx.doi.org/10.1002/ana.22223

Henson MA, Roberts AC, Perez-Otano I, Philpot BD (2010) Influence of the NR3A subunit on NMDA receptor functions. *Prog Neurobiol* 91: 23–37. http://dx.doi.org/10.1016/j.pneurobio.2010.01.004

Herrero AI, Del Olmo N, Gonzalez-Escalada JR, Solis JM (2002) Two new actions of topiramate: Inhibition of depolarizing GABA(A)-mediated responses and activation of a potassium conductance. *Neuropharmacology* 42: 210–220. doi: http://dx.doi.org/10.1016/S0028-3908(01)00171-X

Holmes GL, Gairsa JL, Chevassus-Au-Louis N, Ben-Ari Y (1998) Consequences of neonatal seizures in the rat: Morphological and behavioral effects. *Ann Neurol* 44: 845–857. doi: http://dx.doi.org/10.1002/ana.410440602

Hrncic D, Rasic-Markovic A, Susic V, Djuric D, Stanojlovic O (2009) Influence of NR2B-selective NMDA antagonist on lindane-induced seizures in rats. *Pharmacology* 84: 234–239. doi: http://dx.doi.org/10.1159/000238055

Iwai M, Stetler RA, Xing J et al. (2010) Enhanced oligodendrogenesis and recovery of neurological function by erythropoietin after neonatal hypoxic/ischemic brain injury. *Stroke* 41: 1032–1037. doi: http://dx.doi.org/10.1161/STROKEAHA.109.570325

Jain S, Besag FM (2013) Does melatonin affect epileptic seizures? *Drug Saf* 36: 207–215. doi: http://dx.doi.org/10.1007/s40264-013-0033-y

Johnston MV (2005) Excitotoxicity in perinatal brain injury. *Brain Pathol* 15: 234–240. doi: http://dx.doi.org/10.1111/j.1750-3639.2005.tb00526.x

Johnston MV, Fatemi A, Wilson MA, Northington F (2011) Treatment advances in neonatal neuroprotection and neurointensive care. *Lancet Neurol* 10: 372–382. http://dx.doi.org/10.1016/S1474-4422(11)70016-3

Johnston MV, Hagberg H (2007) Sex and the pathogenesis of cerebral palsy. *Dev Med Child Neurol* 49: 74–78. doi: http://dx.doi.org/10.1017/S0012162207000199.x

Kahle KT, Deeb TZ, Puskarjov M, Silayeva L, Liang B, Kaila K, Moss SJ (2013) Modulation of neuronal activity by phosphorylation of the K-Cl cotransporter KCC2. *Trends Neurosci* 36: 726–737.

Kahle KT, Staley KJ (2008) The bumetanide-sensitive Na-K-2Cl cotransporter NKCC1 as a potential target of a novel mechanism-based treatment strategy for neonatal seizures. *Neurosurg Focus* 25: E22.

Kaila KS, Norris CM, Graham MM, Ali I, Bainey KR (2014) Long-term survival with revascularization in South Asians admitted with an acute coronary syndrome (from the Alberta Provincial Project for Outcomes Assessment in Coronary Heart Disease Registry). *Am J Cardiol* 114: 395–400. doi: http://dx.doi.org/10.1016/j.amjcard.2014.04.051

Kaila K, Price TJ, Payne JA, Puskarjov M, Voipio J (2014) Cation-chloride cotransporters in neuronal development, plasticity and disease. *Nat Rev Neurosci* 15: 637–654.

Kang S, Kadam S (2014) Pre-Clinical Models of Acquired Neonatal Seizures: Differential Effects of Injury on Function of Chloride Co-Transporters. *Austin J Cerebrovasc Dis Stroke* 1.

Kang SK, Markowitz GJ, Kim ST, Johnston MV, Kadam SD (2015) Age- and sex-dependent susceptibility to phenobarbital-resistant neonatal seizures: Role of chloride co-transporters. *Front Cell Neurosci* 9: 173. doi: http://dx.doi.org/10.3389/fncel.2015.00173

Kendall GS, Mathieson S, Meek J, Rennie JM (2012) Recooling for rebound seizures after rewarming in neonatal encephalopathy. *Pediatrics* 130: e451–e455. doi: http://dx.doi.org/10.1542/peds.2011-3496

Khanna A, Walcott BP, Kahle KT (2013) Limitations of Current GABA Agonists in Neonatal Seizures: Toward GABA Modulation Via the Targeting of Neuronal Cl(-) Transport. *Front Neurol* 4: 78. doi: http://dx.doi.org/10.3389/fneur.2013.00078

Kim JS, Kondratyev A, Tomita Y, Gale K (2007) Neurodevelopmental impact of antiepileptic drugs and seizures in the immature brain. *Epilepsia* 48(Suppl 5): 19–26. doi: http://dx.doi.org/10.1111/j.1528-1167.2007.01285.x

Kimura A, Namekata K, Guo X, Noro T, Harada C, Harada T (2015) Valproic acid prevents NMDA-induced retinal ganglion cell death via stimulation of neuronal TrkB receptor signaling. *Am J Pathol* 185: 756–764. doi: http://dx.doi.org/10.1016/j.ajpath.2014.11.005

Koh S, Tibayan FD, Simpson JN, Jensen FE (2004) NBQX or topiramate treatment after perinatal hypoxia-induced seizures prevents later increases in seizure-induced neuronal injury. *Epilepsia* 45: 569–575. doi: http://dx.doi.org/10.1111/j.0013-9580.2004.69103.x

Liu X, Dingley J, Scull-Brown E, Thoresen M (2015) Adding 5 h delayed xenon to delayed hypothermia treatment improves long-term function in neonatal rats surviving to adulthood. *Pediatr Res* 77: 779–783. doi: http://dx.doi.org/10.1038/pr.2015.49

Loscher W, Puskarjov M, Kaila K (2013) Cation-chloride cotransporters NKCC1 and KCC2 as potential targets for novel antiepileptic and antiepileptogenic treatments. *Neuropharmacology* 69: 62–74. doi: http://dx.doi.org/10.1016/j.neuropharm.2012.05.045

Low E, Boylan GB, Mathieson SR et al. (2012) Cooling and seizure burden in term neonates: An observational study. *Arch Dis Child Fetal Neonatal Ed* 97: F267–F272. doi: http://dx.doi.org/10.1136/archdischild-2011-300716

Lynch NE, Stevenson NJ, Livingstone V, Murphy BP, Rennie JM, Boylan GB (2012) The temporal evolution of electrographic seizure burden in neonatal hypoxic ischemic encephalopathy. *Epilepsia* 53: 549–557. doi: http://dx.doi.org/10.1111/j.1528-1167.2011.03401.x

Mares P (2014) Age and activation determines the anticonvulsant effect of ifenprodil in rats. *Naunyn Schmiedebergs Arch Pharmacol* 387: 753–761. doi: http://dx.doi.org/10.1007/s00210-014-0987-z

Mares P, Folbergrova J, Kubova H (2004) Excitatory aminoacids and epileptic seizures in immature brain. *Physiol Res* 53(Suppl 1): S115–S124.

Mares P (2009) Age-and dose-specific anticonvulsant action of bumetanide in immature rats. *Physiological Research* 58: 927–930.

Mares P, Mikulecka A (2009) Different effects of two N-methyl-D-aspartate receptor antagonists on seizures, spontaneous behavior, and motor performance in immature rats. *Epilepsy Behav* 14: 32–39. doi: http://dx.doi.org/10.1016/j.yebeh.2008.08.013

McDonald JW, Johnston MV (1990) Physiological and pathophysiological roles of excitatory amino acids during central nervous system development. *Brain Res Brain Res Rev* 15: 41–70. doi: http://dx.doi.org/10.1016/0165-0173(90)90011-C

McDonald JW, Silverstein FS, Johnston MV (1987) MK-801 protects the neonatal brain from hypoxic-ischemic damage. *Eur J Pharmacol* 140: 359–361. doi: http://dx.doi.org/10.1016/0014-2999(87)90295-0

Mikati MA, El Hokayem JA, El Sabban ME (2007) Effects of a single dose of erythropoietin on subsequent seizure susceptibility in rats exposed to acute hypoxia at P10. *Epilepsia* 48: 175–181.

Morita Y, Callicott JH, Testa LR et al. (2014) Characteristics of the cation cotransporter NKCC1 in human brain: Alternate transcripts, expression in development, and potential relationships to brain function and schizophrenia. *J Neurosci* 34: 4929–4940. doi: http://dx.doi.org/10.1523/JNEUROSCI.1423-13.2014

Mycrs RE (1972) Two patterns of perinatal brain damage and their conditions of occurrence. *Am J Obstet Gynecol* 112: 246–276.

Ni H, Sun Q, Tian T, Feng X, Sun BL (2015) Prophylactic treatment with melatonin before recurrent neonatal seizures: Effects on long-term neurobehavioral changes and the underlying expression of metabolism-related genes in rat hippocampus and cerebral cortex. *Pharmacol Biochem Behav* 133: 25–30. doi: http://dx.doi.org/10.1016/j.pbb.2015.03.012

Pace AJ, Madden VJ, Henson OW Jr., Koller BH, Henson MM (2001) Ultrastructure of the inner ear of NKCC1-deficient mice. *Hear Res* 156: 17–30. doi: http://dx.doi.org/10.1016/S0378-5955(01)00263-5

Pacifici GM (2012) Clinical pharmacology of the loop diuretics furosemide and bumetanide in neonates and infants. *Paediatr Drugs* 14: 233–246.

Paoletti P, Bellone C, Zhou Q (2013) NMDA receptor subunit diversity: Impact on receptor properties, synaptic plasticity and disease. *Nat Rev Neurosci* 14: 383–400. doi: http://dx.doi.org/10.1038/nrn3504

Paoletti P, Neyton J (2007) NMDA receptor subunits: Function and pharmacology. *Curr Opin Pharmacol* 7: 39–47. doi: http://dx.doi.org/10.1016/j.coph.2006.08.011

Paprocka J, Dec R, Jamroz E, Marszal E (2010) Melatonin and childhood refractory epilepsy–a pilot study. *Med Sci Monit* 16: CR389–CR396.

Pavlovsky L, Seiffert E, Heinemann U, Korn A, Golan H, Friedman A (2005) Persistent BBB disruption may underlie alpha interferon-induced seizures. *J Neurol* 252: 42–46. doi: http://dx.doi.org/10.1007/s00415-005-0596-3

Pressler RM, Boylan GB, Marlow N, et al. (2015) Bumetanide for the treatment of seizures in newborn babies with hypoxic ischaemic encephalopathy (NEMO): An open-label, dose finding, and feasibility phase 1/2 trial. *Lancet Neurol* 14: 469–477. doi: http://dx.doi.org/10.1016/S1474-4422(14)70303-5

Puskarjov M, Kahle KT, Ruusuvuori E, Kaila K (2014) Pharmacotherapeutic targeting of cation-chloride cotransporters in neonatal seizures. *Epilepsia* 55: 806–818. doi: http://dx.doi.org/10.1111/epi.12620

Rakhade SN, Jensen FE (2009) Epileptogenesis in the immature brain: Emerging mechanisms. *Nat Rev Neurol* 5: 380–391. doi: http://dx.doi.org/10.1038/nrneurol.2009.80

Rezvani AH (2006) Involvement of the NMDA system in learning and memory. In: Levin ED, Buccafusco JJ, editors. *Animal Models of Cognitive Impairment*. Boca Raton, FL. doi: http://dx.doi.org/10.1201/9781420004335.ch4

Rice JE III, Vannucci RC, Brierley JB (1981) The influence of immaturity on hypoxic-ischemic brain damage in the rat. *Ann Neurol* 9: 131–141. doi: http://dx.doi.org/10.1002/ana.410090206

Rothman SM (2009) The therapeutic potential of focal cooling for neocortical epilepsy. *Neurotherapeutics* 6: 251–257. doi: http://dx.doi.org/10.1016/j.nurt.2008.12.002

Sanchez RM, Jensen FE (2001) Maturational aspects of epilepsy mechanisms and consequences for the immature brain. *Epilepsia* 42: 577–585. doi: http://dx.doi.org/10.1046/j.1528-1157.2001.12000.x

Sargin D, Friedrichs H, El-Kordi A, Ehrenreich H (2010) Erythropoietin as neuroprotective and neuroregenerative treatment strategy: Comprehensive overview of 12 years of preclinical and clinical research. *Best Pract Res Clin Anaesthesiol* 24: 573–594. doi: http://dx.doi.org/10.1016/j.bpa.2010.10.005

Sarkar S, Barks JD, Bapuraj JR et al. (2012) Does phenobarbital improve the effectiveness of therapeutic hypothermia in infants with hypoxic-ischemic encephalopathy? *J Perinatol* 32: 15–20. doi: http://dx.doi.org/10.1038/jp.2011.41

Scher MS (2003) Neonatal seizures and brain damage. *Pediatr Neurol* 29: 381–390. doi: http://dx.doi.org/10.1016/S0887-8994(03)00399-0

Scher MS, Alvin J, Gaus L, Minnigh B, Painter MJ (2003) Uncoupling of EEG-clinical neonatal seizures after antiepileptic drug use. *Pediatr Neurol* 28: 277–280. doi: http://dx.doi.org/10.1016/S0887-8994(02)00621-5

Scher MS, Painter MJ (1989) Controversies concerning neonatal seizures. *Pediatr Clin North Am* 36: 281–310.

Schubert S, Brandl U, Brodhun M et al. (2005) Neuroprotective effects of topiramate after hypoxia-ischemia in newborn piglets. *Brain Res* 1058: 129–136. doi: http://dx.doi.org/10.1016/j.brainres.2005.07.061

Sheldon SH (1998) Pro-convulsant effects of oral melatonin in neurologically disabled children. *Lancet* 351: 1254. doi: http://dx.doi.org/10.1016/S0140-6736(05)79321-1

Shepherd JD, Huganir RL (2007) The cell biology of synaptic plasticity: AMPA receptor trafficking. *Annu Rev Cell Dev Biol* 23: 613–643. doi: http://dx.doi.org/10.1146/annurev.cellbio.23.090506.123516

Silverman WA, Fertig JW, Berger AP (1958) The influence of the thermal environment upon the survival of newly born premature infants. *Pediatrics* 22: 876–886.

Skaper SD, Floreani M, Ceccon M, Facci L, Giusti P (1999) Excitotoxicity, oxidative stress, and the neuroprotective potential of melatonin. *Ann N Y Acad Sci* 890: 107–118. doi: http://dx.doi.org/10.1111/j.1749-6632.1999.tb07985.x

Smyth MD, Han RH, Yarbrough CK et al. (2015) Temperatures achieved in human and canine neocortex during intraoperative passive or active focal cooling. *Ther Hypothermia Temp Manag* 5: 95–103. http://dx.doi.org/10.1089/ther.2014.0025

Srinivasakumar P, Zempel J, Wallendorf M, Lawrence R, Inder T, Mathur A (2013) Therapeutic hypothermia in neonatal hypoxic ischemic encephalopathy: Electrographic seizures and magnetic resonance imaging evidence of injury. *J Pediatr* 163: 465–470. doi: http://dx.doi.org/10.1016/j.jpeds.2013.01.041

Staley K (2004) Neuroscience. Epileptic neurons go wireless. *Science* 305: 482–483.

Staley KJ (2004) Role of the depolarizing GABA response in epilepsy. *Adv Exp Med Biol* 548: 104–109.

Suda S, Katsura K, Kanamaru T, Saito M, Katayama Y (2013) Valproic acid attenuates ischemia-reperfusion injury in the rat brain through inhibition of oxidative stress and inflammation. *Eur J Pharmacol* 707: 26–31. doi: http://dx.doi.org/10.1016/j.ejphar.2013.03.020

Suda S, Katsura KI, Saito M, Kamiya N, Katayama Y (2014) Valproic acid enhances the effect of bone marrow-derived mononuclear cells in a rat ischemic stroke model. *Brain Res* 1565: 74–81. doi: http://dx.doi.org/10.1016/j.brainres.2014.04.011

Sun Y, Calvert JW, Zhang JH (2005) Neonatal hypoxia/ischemia is associated with decreased inflammatory mediators after erythropoietin administration. *Stroke* 36: 1672–1678. doi: http://dx.doi.org/10.1161/01.STR.0000173406.04891.8c

Talos DM, Fishman RE, Park H et al. (2006a) Developmental regulation of alpha-amino-3-hydroxy-5-methyl-4-isoxazole-propionic acid receptor subunit expression in forebrain and relationship to regional susceptibility to hypoxic/ischemic injury. I. Rodent cerebral white matter and cortex. *J Comp Neurol* 497: 42–60. doi: http://dx.doi.org/10.1002/cne.20972

Talos DM, Follett PL, Folkerth RD et al. (2006b) Developmental regulation of alpha-amino-3-hydroxy-5-methyl-4-isoxazole-propionic acid receptor subunit expression in forebrain and relationship to regional susceptibility to hypoxic/ischemic injury. II. Human cerebral white matter and cortex. *J Comp Neurol* 497: 61–77. doi: http://dx.doi.org/10.1002/cne.20978

Thibeault-Eybalin MP, Lortie A, Carmant L (2009) Neonatal seizures: Do they damage the brain? *Pediatr Neurol* 40: 175–180. http://dx.doi.org/10.1016/j.pediatrneurol.2008.10.026

Thoresen M, Satas S, Puka-Sundvall M et al. (1997) Post-hypoxic hypothermia reduces cerebrocortical release of NO and excitotoxins. *Neuroreport* 8: 3359–3362. doi: http://dx.doi.org/10.1097/00001756-199710200-00033

Tollner K, Brandt C, Topfer M, Brunhofer G, Erker T, Gabriel M et al. (2014) A novel prodrug-based strategy to increase effects of bumetanide in epilepsy. *Ann Neurol* 75(4): 550–62. doi: 10.1002/ana.24124.

Uberos J, Augustin-Morales MC, Molina Carballo A et al. (2011) Normalization of the sleep-wake pattern and melatonin and 6-sulphatoxy-melatonin levels after a therapeutic trial with melatonin in children with severe epilepsy. *J Pineal Res* 50: 192–196.

Vanhatalo S, Hellstrom-Westas L, De Vries LS (2009) Bumetanide for neonatal seizures: Based on evidence or enthusiasm? *Epilepsia* 50: 1292–1293.

Vezzani A (2005) Inflammation and epilepsy. *Epilepsy Curr* 5: 1–6.

Vezzani A, Aronica E, Mazarati A, Pittman QJ (2013) Epilepsy and brain inflammation. *Exp Neurol* 244: 11–21. doi: http://dx.doi.org/10.1016/j.expneurol.2011.09.033

Vezzani A, Granata T (2005) Brain Inflammation in Epilepsy: Experimental and Clinical Evidence. *Epilepsia* 46: 1724–1743.

Weiner SP, Painter MJ, Geva D, Guthrie RD, Scher MS (1991) Neonatal seizures: electroclinical dissociation. *Pediatr Neurol* 7: 363–368.

Williams K (1993) Ifenprodil discriminates subtypes of the N-methyl-D-aspartate receptor: Selectivity and mechanisms at recombinant heteromeric receptors. *Mol Pharmacol* 44: 851–859.

Wu YW, Gonzalez FF (2015) Erythropoietin: a novel therapy for hypoxic-ischaemic encephalopathy? *Dev Med Child Neurol* 57(Suppl 3): 34–39. doi: http://dx.doi.org/10.1111/dmcn.12730

Wyllie DJ, Livesey MR, Hardingham GE (2013) Influence of GluN2 subunit identity on NMDA receptor function. *Neuropharmacology* 74: 4–17. doi: http://dx.doi.org/10.1016/j.neuropharm.2013.01.016

Xiong T, Qu Y, Mu D, Ferriero D (2011) Erythropoietin for neonatal brain injury: Opportunity and challenge. *Int J Dev Neurosci* 29: 583–591. doi: http://dx.doi.org/10.1016/j.ijdevneu.2010.12.007

Yager JY, Armstrong EA, Miyashita H, Wirrell EC (2002) Prolonged neonatal seizures exacerbate hypoxic-ischemic brain damage: Correlation with cerebral energy metabolism and excitatory amino acid release. *Dev Neurosci* 24: 367–381. doi: http://dx.doi.org/10.1159/000069049

Zavanella C, Subramanian S (1978) Review: Surgery for transposition of the great arteries in the first year of life. *Ann Surg* 187: 143–150. doi: http://dx.doi.org/10.1097/00000658-197802000-00008

Zipancic I, Calcagnotto ME, Piquer-Gil M, Mello LE, Alvarez-Dolado M (2010) Transplant of GABAergic precursors restores hippocampal inhibitory function in a mouse model of seizure susceptibility. *Cell Transplant* 19: 549–564.

INDEX

Note: Locators followed by '*f*' and '*t*' refer to figures and tables, respectively

International Review of Child Neurology Series

Published for the International Child Neurology Association by Mac Keith Press www.mackeith.co.uk

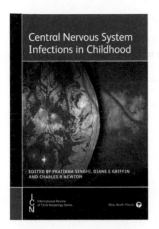

Central Nervous System Infections in Childhood
Pratibha Singhi, Diane E. Griffin and Charles R. Newton (Editors)

2014 ▪ 390pp ▪ hardback ▪ 978-1-909962-44-6
£95.00 / €128.30 / $159.95

This title has been developed with the International Child Neurology Association to provide information on common central nervous system (CNS) infections. It covers almost all CNS infections commonly seen in children across the world, in both developed and resource poor countries. It provides a concise, state of the art overview of viral, bacterial, tubercular, fungal, parasitic and many other infections of the CNS. The book is intended to be of practical use to residents, physicians, paediatricians and paediatric neurologists across the globe.

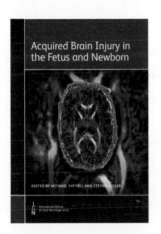

Acquired Brain Injury in the Fetus and Newborn
Michael Shevell and Steven Miller (Editors)

2012 ▪ 330pp ▪ hardback ▪ 978-1-907655-02-9
£125.00 / €168.80 / $200.95

Given the tremendous advances in the understanding of acquired neonatal brain injury, this book provides a timely review for the practising neurologist, neonatologist and paediatrician. The editors take a pragmatic approach, focusing on specific populations encountered regularly by the clinician. They offer a 'bench to bedside' approach to acquired brain injury in the preterm and term newborn infant. The contributors, all internationally recognized neurologists and scientists, provide readers with a state-of-the art review in their area of expertise.

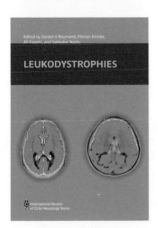

Leukodystrophies
Gerald V. Raymond, Florian Eichler, Ali Fatemi and Sakkubai Naidu (Editors)

2011 ▪ 240pp ▪ hardback ▪ 978-1-907655-09-8
£80.00 / €108.00 / $125.00

This book is the only up-to-date, comprehensive text on leukodystrophies. Its purpose is to summarize for the reader all aspects of the inherited disorders of myelin in children and adults. After a comprehensive overview of myelin and the role of oligodendrocytes, astrocytes and microglia in white matter disease, chapters are then devoted to individual disorders, covering their biochemical and molecular basis, genetics, pathophysiology, clinical features, diagnosis, treatment, and screening. The final chapters address therapeutic approaches in leukodystrophies and present a clinical approach to diagnosing leukoencephalopathies in children and adults.

Recent titles from Mac Keith Press www.mackeith.co.uk

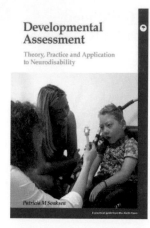

Developmental Assessment: Theory, Practice and Application to Neurodisability
Patricia M. Sonksen

A practical guide from Mac Keith Press
2016 ▪ 384pp ▪ softback ▪ 978-1-909962-56-9
£39.95 / €56.50

This handbook presents a new approach to assessing development in preschool children that can be applied across the developmental spectrum. The reader is taught how to confirm whether development is typical and if it is not, is signposted to the likely nature and severity of impairments with a plan of action. The author uses numerous case vignettes from her 40 years' experience to bring to life her approach with clear summary key points and helpful illustrations.

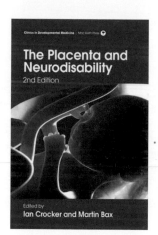

The Placenta and Neurodisability, 2nd Edition
Ian Crocker and Martin Bax (Editors)

Clinics in Developmental Medicine
2015 ▪ 176pp ▪ hardback ▪ 978-1-909962-53-8
£50.00 / €67.50 / $80.00

This comprehensive and authoritative book discusses the critical role of the utero-placenta in neurodisability, both at term and preterm. It examines aspects of fetal compromise and possible cerebro-protective interventions, recent evidence on fetal growth and mental illness, as well as cerebro-therapeutics. Throughout the book, information from the basic sciences is placed within the clinical context.

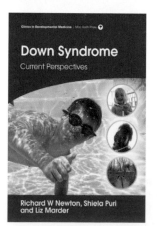

Down Syndrome: Current Perspectives
Richard W Newton, Shiela Puri and Liz Marder (Editors)

Clinics in Developmental Medicine
2015 ▪ 320pp ▪ hardback ▪ 978-1-909962-47-7
£95.00 / €128.30 / $150.00

Down syndrome remains the most common recognisable form of intellectual disability. The challenge for doctors today is how to capture the rapidly expanding body of scientific knowledge and devise models of care to meet the needs of individuals and their families. *Down Syndrome: Current Perspectives* provides doctors and other health professionals with the information they need to address the challenges that can present in the management of Down syndrome.